Models of Oculomotor Behavior and Control

Editor

B. L. Zuber, Ph.D.
Professor of Bioengineering
Bioengineering Program
University of Illinois
Chicago Circle Campus
Chicago, Illinois

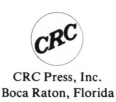

CRC Press, Inc.
Boca Raton, Florida

Library of Congress Cataloging in Publication Data
Main entry under title:

Models of oculomotor behavior and control.

    Includes bibliographies and index.
    1.   Eye—Movements—Regulation.   I.   Zuber, Bert L.
[DNLM: 1. Eye movements.   2.   Oculomotor muscles.
3.   Oculomotor nerve.   4.   Model, Neurological. WW 400
M689]
QP477.5.M63   599.01'823   80-39734
ISBN 0-8493-5679-2

    Direct all inquiries to CRC Press, Inc., 2000 N.W. 24th Street, Boca Raton, Florida 33431.

© 1981 by CRC Press, Inc.

International Standard Book Number 0-8493-5679-2

Library of Congress Card Number 80-39734
Printed in the United States

FOREWORD

Presenting as it does the most recent models of ocular motility, described by some of the field's most active investigators, this book contains important reading for all of us: students, teachers, professionals alike, whose business, in one way or another, is understanding something about eye movements. But there is a larger message here instructive even to more general readers.

In contrast to many more recent aspects of neurobiology, applications of the methods of scientific inquiry to oculomotor behavior and control extend back nearly two centuries. Well over a hundred years ago Helmholtz devoted a substantial chapter in the 3rd volume of his monumental *Handbuch der Physiologischen Optik* to this subject. It is still well worth rereading in the context of Westheimer's discussion of Donder's, Listing's and Hering's Laws in the current volume.

As Westheimer makes clear, Helmholtz's incessant antagonist, the physiologist Ewald Hering, made important contributions to the subject in the latter half of the last century. His law of equal innervation to yoked muscles of the two eyes was described in *Die Lehre vom Binokularen Sehen* in 1868; the law of identical visual directions of the foveas of the two eyes appeared in his 'chapter' on *Der Raumsinn und die Bewegungen des Auges* written for L. Hermann's *Handbuch der Physiologie* in 1879. It enlarges considerably our perspective of the subject by introducing problems about space localization with moving eyes and of binocular coordination, problems still *au courant.*

Shortly thereafter, the 'oculist' E. E. Maddox introduced his model of vergence movements. It became the point of departure for the great body of investigations which are brought up to date by Rashbass' cogently reasoned analysis and by Semmlow's discussion of the near triad, in this volume.

At the turn of the century the physiologist Sherrington added one more principle of oculomotor behavior and control: the dogma that when eyes move, antagonistic extra-ocular muscles are reciprocally innervated. We still know little or nothing of the organization detail of these innervation patterns. But the chapters by Westheimer, Raphan and Cohen, and especially by Keller, in a sense the entire book, testify to their intricacy and beauty.

Scientific photography introduced methods for measuring the position of the human eye objectively and noninvasively. This attracted experimental psychologists to the subject. They brought to it a different emphasis as well as different kinds of experimental questions. Analysis began of eye movements in more complicated — and more natural — viewing conditions.

The different varieties of conjugate movements were quickly identified and it was soon fairly obvious that depending upon the task (tracking a moving target, say, or reading) the relative dominance of smooth pursuit or saccadic movements changed. In the first quarter of the present century many details of these phenomena were made explicit. A good summary can be found in Woodworth's classic textbook of experimental psychology. The early hopes that by defining eye movement differences between efficient and poor readers, the reading problems of school children would become manageable if not eliminated, have yet to be fulfilled. But they did lead to the establishment of a fruitful field in experimental cognitive psychology which is slowly elucidating the reading process as Zuber and Wetzel, on the one hand, and Rayner and Inhoff, on the other, emphasize in these pages.

During this period the neural pathways devoted to the control of eye movements were being specified by tools sharpened in the clinical analysis of patients with abnormal eye movements and by the classical neuroanatomical and physiological methods of lesions, electrical stimulation and gross electrode recording with common laboratory mammals, mainly cat and monkey. Studying patients is an especially valuable approach which only recently has begun to suggest how its potential can be fully exploited. Some feeling for the excitement in this very rapidly expanding method to understand eye movement control is found in the chapters by Dell' Osso and Daroff as well as the one by Zee in this Volume. On the other hand, what one could learn from the traditional mammalian anatomical and physiological laboratories had obvious limitations.

The explosion of technology during and immediately following the second war had remarkable consequences which expanded the study of eye movements far beyond such constraints.

Physical system control theory was an important part of this technology and psychologists such as the late Paul M. Fitts quickly saw innovative ways to apply it to the study of man-machine systems. Inevitably it found a niche in efforts to understand oculomotor behavior and control. One major theme of this volume is concerned with precisely the significance of that place. Most of the models one meets here derive directly in this tradition; bioengineers such as Robinson, Keller, Semmlow, Stark, Young, and Zuber are distinguished members of a discipline concerned with the application of the theory of physical systems to biology. This is by no means the only way to model eye movement control but the numerous examples of such work found in this volume show how heuristic this way of modeling can sometimes prove.

This variety of model building was greatly facilitated by a closely related second war development: the digital computer. Differential equations without formal solution now became easy to manage. Computers are not only revolutionizing the experiments one does (as for example, in the experiments outlined in the Rayner-Inhoff chapter), but also the theoretical structure into which experimental results are ordered. With the exponential growth in computer capacity and the paradoxical reduction both in its size and price, even those insensitive to trends can see that the immediate future will witness accelerated expansion of this kind of model structuring. All of this is to the good. These pages help us anticipate the power of understanding we may well look for in the next decade from this approach. If a skeptical reader were to identify a possible caveat, perhaps it is in the difficulties facility with computers can put in the way of model builders anxious to make the sharpest possible cut with Occam's razor. Putting the full power of modern computers to work as a slave of one's own brain is both a technical skill and an art, but once it is mastered the processes of developing, simulating, even testing a complicated theoretical model is not all that much more difficult than doing the same with a very simple one. Thus, the borderlines between elegant mathematics used in description as distinct from analysis, between breadth and depth, between fitting curves and finding general principles of organization, in a word between the second and the first rate, have become — superficially at least — fuzzier, more difficult to see. But they are still there; they will always be there.

However this may be, no one can read this book intelligently and not be impressed with the potential strength of analysis made available by the application of modern computers and the theory of control of physical systems to oculomotor behavior. Indeed, there are those who argue that this approach to human neurobiology is all we need, that the traditional approach (i.e., anatomical and neurophysiological experiments on laboratory animals) is both obsolete and redundant.

Since these arguments are timely, I will return to them shortly, but consider first the current status of precisely these anatomical and neurophysiological studies of oculomotor control. Here too technological advances — in electronics and in operant conditioning, among other things — have liberated research from traditional constraints. When last I wrote a summary of this literature a decade or so ago, it seemed possible, perhaps even likely, that a major thrust forward, even a breakthrough, was eminent.

Techniques had then been developed for recording inside — or very near to — neurones in the brain of alert behaving (i.e., unanesthetized) primates trained (with the help of these very same computers) to hold their eyes fixed or to move them in specified ways. Moreover, the historical background of which I have just written, specified in great detail both the characteristic of the few and highly stereotyped varieties of eye movements that occur, and the precise neuroanatomy of the pathways most relevant to their execution. So one optimistically looked forward to a monumental neurobiological discovery, nothing less than the unveiling of the unequivocally documented circuit diagram of the primate (if not the human) oculomotor control network.

That no such diagram is among the models within the following pages does not contradict a decade of enormously productive research. Hints of the current excitement can be gleaned in the chapters by Robinson, by Keller, and by Raphan and Cohen. Much of what is emerging, as is true of the best of normative science, are results which crisply exclude various ways ocular motor control might well have been wired, but clearly is not.

What is obvious from reading this book is the enormous dependence advancement in modeling eye movements has upon results from laboratory animal research and vice versa. A striking example of the mutual benefits accruing from the exchanges between the results of laboratory physiology, model building and the clinical examination, is to be found in the pathophysiology of the interaction of optokinetic and vestibular data. Although Colleweijn approaches it as a physiologist who studies afoveate rabbits and Zee as clinical neurologist, their respective chapters show how strongly they (along with Raphan and Cohen, who work on foveate monkeys) rely on these exchanges. One has the impression that as a result perhaps here, at least, a general pattern of organization may soon emerge.

One cannot help but ponder after reading Zee and Dell'Osso and Daroff what enormous clinical benefits are to reaped in the understanding, diagnosis and treatment of human disease by the definitive circuit diagram of the oculomotor control system. Is it reasonable to suppose then that a discovery with such clear benefits for the relief of human suffering can be derived exclusively from computer simulation and models of physical systems alone without any recourse whatsoever to the fundamental results of primate neurobiological research? This book teaches us that it is not.

Robinson, for example, makes the explicit point that current models of even the dynamics of eye mechanics suffer from lack of good physiological data. The same point is implicit in the much more complicated control of refixation saccadic movements illustrated in Figure 17 in Young's chapter on the sampled data model. Even a definitive choice among the models of the *Naheinstellungsreaktion* discussed by Semmlow beg for neurophysiological resolution from experiments on laboratory primates.

Keller's chapter, indeed, deals only with these kinds of experiments and their impact for model builders is plain enough to every reader. He has, for instance, very neatly (and for me personally painfully) excluded in this way any model requiring the final common path for different kinds of eye movements to a given position in the orbit to be distinct. Or witness the process by which Raphan and Cohen derive an organizational scheme of the slow phase of nystagmus by relating variables in their model to unit activity in the vestibular nucleus.

Voluntary nystagmus as viewed by Stark, Hoyt, Ciuffreda, Kenyon, and Hsu is a paradigm for the control modeling of bioengineering in its "purest" form, i.e., without any but the most superficial references to animal neurophysiology. Yet even here at the heart of the ability of the model to treat these movements as saccadic, on the one hand and, on the other, to be consistent with the sampled data behavior of the saccades of normal refixation Young describes, is the *ad hoc* hypothesis that nystagmus command "signals" bypass the "supranuclear" sampled data mechanisms, whatever they are. The *ad hoc* hypothesis is, of course, a familiar tool of the trade for model builders, as well as the rest of us. But it is of value only when it is also capable of experimental testing; the most straightforward ways of doing it in this particular case all seem to this reader, at least, to involve laboratory animals.

Why is it then that after ten years, the circuit diagram of the oculomotor network is not to be found in this book devoted to models of eye movement control? What do we still need to know to realize the definitive model? Each neurophysiologist who studies these phenomena, each model builder, indeed each reader, will answer this question for himself. For what it is worth my own view is that it may well be liberation from the frustration implicit in the surprising result that wherever one looks in regions of the primate nervous system driven by a visual stimulus, the visual field has an oculocentric (i.e., retinotopic) map. But when we move our eyes, the sweep of the image of the world around us across the retina is unperceived while the world which is perceived is seen as stationary. This familiar fact means to me, that at the very heart of the circuit which controls oculomotor behavior will be found a region in the primate nervous system in which visual stimuli excite cells which in their ensemble produce an egocentric, rather than a retinotopic, map of the visual world. (As Young emphasizes saccades are egocentrically — spatiotopically — organized. Implicit in Rashbass' analysis is the concept that the disparities in the egocentric maps of the visual field excited by each of the two eyes drive fusional eye movements.) Where in the primate central nervous system this region is and how it functions remains to be worked out. But I have little doubt that the answer to such questions will be sorted out some day, in some way: perhaps by studying vergence eye movements with the ^{14}C-2-deoxyglucose audioradiographic technique, perhaps by using the enzyme horseradish peroxidase to examine the synaptic imputs Westheimer discusses with regard to the cell illustrated in his Figure 3, perhaps by techniques of the neurobiological laboratory not yet developed.

I do not pretend that these speculations are at all prescient of a major neurobiological discovery. The point in recalling them here is only that however the question raised at the beginning of the preceding paragraph is to be dealt with, the answer (to the extent it is a reasonable and a viable answer) will have one thing in common with the fantasy I have supplied as an example: In one way or another it will lend itself to examination and experimental testing by neurophysiological research on laboratory primates.

However powerful the application of the theory of physical systems control to biology is, however much computers extend the range and the usefulness of our models, it detracts not one iota from the value and importance of this impressive volume on modeling to say that one puts it down convinced that these techniques alone without assistance from ongoing results of laboratory animal research will never define the definitive circuit diagram of the human oculomotor control system. Given the tradition of almost two centuries of the study of eye movements and the strong influence system theory and computers have already had in bringing understanding to the levels of which we read here, levels, I submit, as high as those of the neurobiology of any human activity, if this kind of understanding cannot be achieved in this way in the study of oculomotor behavior and control, it will not be so achieved for any other human activity either. That is the larger message of this book.

Mathew Alpern

Ann Arbor, Michigan
July 24, 1980

INTRODUCTION

The oculomotor system is perhaps the most extensively studied of all physiological control systems. The comprehensive nature of our knowledge of this system is, I hope, reflected in this Volume, where the reader will find detailed descriptions of single cell behavior as well as treatment of the intricacies of the input-output behavior of the overall system. This Volume is intended to be comprehensive both in coverage and in approach to the system. While modeling is a major emphasis in these pages, models of a system are meaningful only within the context of our overall knowledge of a system's behavior, both descriptive and quantitative. Each author was encouraged to place his contribution in historical perspective so as to make the book as useful as possible to the wide variety of scientists having an equally wide variety of interests in and approaches to the oculomotor system. Additional historical perspective is provided by the inclusion of many chapters written by investigators with longstanding and well-established records of contributions to the field.

I am indebted to my colleagues, who responded so graciously to invitations to be a part of this work. I only hope that the sum of their collected efforts will serve to justify their commitments of time and toil. Finally, to Aaron and Gregory my appreciation for their patience and understanding.

B. L. Zuber, Ph.D.
Chicago, 1980

THE EDITOR

B. L. Zuber, Ph.D., is Professor of Bioengineering in the Bioengineering Program at the University of Illinois, Chicago Circle Campus. He received the B.A. in Liberal Arts and the B.S. in Chemical Engineering from the University of Pennsylvannia in 1960 and 1961, respectively. At M.I.T. he was awarded the M.S. in Biochemical Engineering in 1963, and the Ph.D. in Bioengineering in 1965.

Dr. Zuber has held appointments at Presbyterian-St. Luke's Hospital in Chicago, at the Medical Center Campus of the University of Illinois in Chicago and at Bell Laboratories in Murray Hill, New Jersey. He has consulted extensively throughout the country in the field of Bioengineering. In addition to his current appointment at the University of Illinois, he is a Lecturer in the Department of Orthopedics, Loyola University Stritch School of Medicine, Maywood, Illinois, and is a Biomedical Engineer at the Hines Veterans Administration Hospital, Hines, Illinois.

Dr. Zuber is a member of the American Physiological Society, the Institute of Electrical and Electronics Engineers, the Association for Research in Vision and Ophthalmology, the International Brain Research Organization and the Biomedical Engineering Society.

CONTRIBUTORS

Kenneth Ciuffreda, O.D., Ph.D.
Department of Physiological Optics and
  Engineering Science
University of California
Berkeley, California

Bernard Cohen, M.D.
Morris B. Bender Professor of
  Neurology
Mount Sinai School of Medicine
New York, New York

Han Collewijn, M.D., Ph.D.
Professor of Physiology
Erasmus University
Rotterdam, Netherlands

Louis F. Dell'Osso, Ph.D.
Director, Ocular Motor
  Neurophysiology Lab
Veterans Administration Medical
  Center
Professor of Neurology and Biomedical
  Engineering
Case Western Reserve University
Cleveland, Ohio

Robert B. Daroff, M.D.
Neurology Service, Cleveland Veterans
  Administration Medical Center
Department of Neurology
Case Western Reserve University
  School of Medicine
Cleveland, Ohio

William Hoyt, M.D.
Professor, Department of Neurology,
  Neurosurgery, and Ophthalmology
University of California
San Francisco, California

Frederick Hsu, B.M.E.
Department of Physiological Optics and
  Engineering Science
University of California
Berkeley, California

Werner Inhoff
Department of Psychology
University of Massachusetts
Amherst, Massachusetts

Edward L. Keller, Ph.D.
Professor, Electrical Engineering and
  Computer Sciences
University of California
Berkeley, California

Robert Kenyon, Ph.D.
Department of Physiological Optics and
  Engineering Science
University of California
Berkeley, California

Theodore Raphan, Ph.D.
Assistant Professor Department of
  Neurology
Mount Sinai School of Medicine
New York, New York

Keith Rayner, Ph.D.
Professor of Psychology
University of Massachusetts
Amherst, Massachusetts

Cyril Rashbass, M.A., M.D.
Professor, Department of
  Neurophysiology
University of Groningen
Groningen, The Netherlands

David A. Robinson, Ph.D.
Professor, Departments of
  Opthalmology and Biomedical
  Engineering
The Johns Hopkins University School
  of Medicine
Baltimore, Maryland

John L. Semmlow, Ph.D.
Associate Professor of Electrical
  Engineering
Rutgers University
Associate Professor of Surgery
Rutgers Medical School
Piscataway, New Jersey

Lawrence Stark, M.D.
Professor of Physiological Optics and
  Engineering Science
University of California
Berkeley, California
and Department of Neurology
University of California
San Francisco, California

Gerald Westheimer, Ph.D.
Professor of Physiology
University of California
Berkeley, California

Paul A. Wetzel, M.S.
Department of Aeronautics and
  Astronautics
Massachusetts Institute of Technology
Cambridge, Massachusetts

Laurence R. Young, Sc.D.
Professor of Aeronautics and
  Astronautics
Massachusetts Institute of Technology
Cambridge, Massachusetts

David S. Zee, M.D.
Associate Professor of Ophthalmology
  and Neurology
The Johns Hopkins School of Medicine
Baltimore, Maryland

B. L. Zuber, Ph.D.
Professor of Bioengineering
Bioengineering Program
University of Illinois
Chicago Circle Campus
Chicago, Illinois

TABLE OF CONTENTS

Chapter 1

OCULOMOTOR NEURON BEHAVIOR

Edward L. Keller

TABLE OF CONTENTS

I. INTRODUCTION

The extremely high velocity displacement and remarkable precision manifest in eye movements have long interested neurophysiologists in their neuromuscular control mechanisms. Early studies involving the recording of oculomotor neurons* with microelectrodes were carried out in anesthetized or brain-transected animals by inducing vestibular nystagmus.[1-3] These studies shed some light on the organization of this level of the oculomotor system. However, with developments in the technique for recording single neurons in alert behaving animals,[4] it has recently become possible to study these mechanisms in detail at the neuronal level during natural eye movements. The initial successful applications of this technique to the oculomotor system were made in studies concerning the behavior of oculomotor neurons. Extensive literature on this subject in a variety of species has appeared in the short time since the original reports on the functional behavior of oculomotor neurons in primates[5-7] were published. The present review will summarize this literature, as well as placing it into the context of a broader understanding of the oculomotor system, by including pertinent information on oculomotor neurons supplied through anatomical or electrophysiological techniques.

The use of systems and modeling techniques to analyze and present the alert animal data, and even to aid in the design of crucial experiments, has been the additional major factor contributing to the rapid advance in understanding the operation of the final common path of the oculomotor system. These techniques will be reviewed in the text where they contribute to clarity of the exposition.

II. CELLULAR ORGANIZATION OF OCULOMOTOR NEURONAL POOLS

A. Anatomy

Oculomotor neurons reside in three nuclear complexes located along the caudal to rostal axis of the brain stem. The most caudally located, the abducens nuclei, consists of two distinct, off-midline cellular groups. Each nucleus sends fibers to the ipsilateral lateral rectus muscle (LR). Proceeding rostrally, the next cellular groups, the trochlear nuclei, are also paired structures located off the midline. Fibers from each nucleus project dorsally, decussate in the anterior medullary velum, and innervate the contralateral superior oblique muscle (SO). The oculomotor nucleus, situated at the level of the superior colliculus, is a more complex structure of paired cellular columns which fuse together on the midline. Fibers from this nucleus innervate the remaining extraocular muscles, the medial (MR) and inferior rectus (IR) and inferior oblique (IO) (all ipsilateral) and the superior rectus (SR) (contralateral). The main somatic portion of this nuclear complex forms a structure somewhat similar to an inverted V. Masses of smaller cells form a dorsal cap which extends into a midline position between the two paired somatic columns at certain levels of the nucleus. These cells send preanglionic autonomic fibers to the orbit.

Within the somatic motor columns, the exact location of specific cellular groups innervating each of the remaining four extraocular muscles (EOM) has been the subject of considerable controversy. Warwick[8] has reviewed the earlier literature on this sub-

---

* The term "oculomotor neuron" will be used to denote motoneurons innervating any of the extraocular muscles. When specific reference is intended to neurons located in the third-nerve nucleus, the term oculomotor nucleus neuron will be used. Neurons innervating the retractor bulbi muscles will not be considered in this chapter.

ject. His own research utilizing the retrograde degeneration technique following extirpation of individual EOM, has established what is generally considered the most reliable map of the representation of each of the muscles in the oculomotor complex in primates.[9] Cells sending fibers to each muscle are arranged in dorsal to ventral or lateral to medial strips or columns. According to his scheme, the most ventrally situated group of cells innervates the MR, while the cells projecting to the IR are grouped most dorsally. Cells for the IO are interposed between the former and latter groups. Superior rectus motoneurons are found in a medially located cellular column on the contralateral side. This exact representation of muscles has received confirmation from microelectrode recordings in monkeys.[6]

The dorsalventral arrangement of individual muscle motoneurons has also been observed in a degeneration study in the cat.[10] However, these authors noted a rearrangement of the muscle representation in that the MR column was situated most dorsally, while the IR representation was most ventral. The authors also comment on the very low percentage of cells marked by positive retrograde changes even in the kitten, so that the boundaries of their cellular groups are rather imprecise. A more recent study in the cat utilizing the retrograde transport of horseradish peroxidase (HRP), which had been injected into individual muscles in the orbit,[11] supports this apparent species difference with respect to the MR and IR representations between cat and monkey. A slight rearrangement of the location of the cells for the IO from the previous cat study was noted particularly at rostral levels of the nucleus. At this level, the cells for IO assumed a more medial location instead of their interposed location between the MR and IR cellular groups.

The situation in primates has not been reconfirmed with the more sensitive HRP and autoradiographic techniques. However, these techniques have been put to good use in the cat in disclosing several additional anatomic features of the organization of the oculomotor neuron pools. Warwick claimed that almost all cells in each of the oculomotor nuclei showed signs of degenerative change, leading to the conclusion that the abducens and trochlear nuclei and somatic columns portion of the oculomotor nuclei were substantially pools of only lower motor neurons.[8] More recently, it has been shown that both the abducens and the oculomotor nuclei in cat contain significant numbers of oculomotor interneurons.[12-15] Even the trochlear nuclei apparently contain significant numbers of nonmotoneuronal neurons.[16]

Morphologically oculomotor neurons appear as both large (40 to 60 μm) multipolar and small to medium (15 to 40 μm) circular or pyriform-shaped cells.[15,17] Interneurons overlap this range in size (25 to 50 μm) and are not clearly distinct in appearance from motoneurons even at the ultrastructural level.[15] Spencer and Sterling estimate that approximately 25% of the cells in the abducens nucleus are interneurons.[15]

B. Electrophysiology

Electrophysiological techniques have demonstrated a number of interesting features concerning the structural details of oculomotor neurons.[18-23] As expected on the basis of the wide distribution in somata size, these neurons show a broad range of conduction velocities from 2 to 120 m/sec.[20] Their postspike membrane-potential trajectories suggest special evolution to permit high-discharge frequencies and, indeed, intracellular current injections can drive these specialized motoneurons to fire at 400 spikes/sec.[20,22] Antidromic stimulations suggest a total absence of any recurrent inhibitory feedback which may also play a role in allowing high-discharge frequencies. The total lack of electrophysiologically demonstrated axon collaterals in oculomotor neurons supports similar earlier anatomical observations on these motoneurons.[24] Interestingly, intracellular single-cell injections of HRP have now demonstrated the presence of axon collaterals in all oculomotor neurons in the IR, SR, and MR pools, but their absence in IO, SO, and LR groups.[16] These collaterals terminate within their parent nuclei, but always on interneurons and not other motoneurons.

Also, in contrast to spinal motoneurons, oculomotor neurons do not show orthodromically activated synaptic potentials following electrical stimulation of their motor nerves.[19-21] Although Sasaki[18] claimed to have observed very rarely such a response in motoneurons innervating the IO, the overwhelming weight of the evidence argues against his observation.

One study has found circumstantial electrophysiological evidence that electronic coupling exists between cat oculomotor neurons.[25] However, other studies have failed to find electrophysiological[19,20] or morphological[15] support for this arrangement. The presence of such coupling would tend to synchronize the discharge of the entire pool of motoneurons, an obvious functional disadvantage in the very rapid EOM during attempted steady fixation. Therefore, in the absence of more convincing evidence, one should probably consider oculomotor neurons to be functionally separate subunits.

C. Mechanical Studies

The mechanical properties of individual oculomotor units is of great interest to the present review, since much of the discussion in subsequent sections on primates will focus on the activity patterns of the motoneurons innervating these mechanical entitites. In the studies to be reviewed, it was not technically possible to determine the mechanical properties of the isolated unit under study. The mechanical properties of individual oculomotor units have been examined in cat.[26,27] Maximum tetanic tension of different units varied from 50 to 400 mg (one order of magnitude). The extent of this range in EOM closely resembles that in skeletal muscles like the soleus, which are composed of more uniform muscle fiber type.[28] In comparison, the gastrocnemius, a muscle with heterogeneous fiber types like the EOM, has a distribution of individual motor unit tensions that range over 2½ orders of magnitude.[29] The smaller size of the EOM is indicated by the fact that the absolute values of units tensions are 3 to 40 gm in soleus and 0.5 to 120 gm in the gastrocnemius. As shown in Figure 1, unit tensions in the EOM are more uniformly distributed than in either soleus or gastrocnemius and have a mean tension of 173 mg. One should also be able to calculate a similar value of mean unit tension by dividing the total muscle tetanic tension by the number of motor units in the muscle. When this is done for the LR from published data, total muscle tension = 100 g,[30] and the number of motor units = 1400.[31] Therefore, the mean unit tension = 72 mg, a figure much lower than the expected value of 173 mg. This must indicate that the unit physiological studies[26,27] tended to sample a population biased toward the larger units. Nevertheless, it is clear that the range of unit tensions in EOM are more narrowly distributed than in skeletal muscles like the gastrocnemius. It is important to note that Figure 1 also shows that the two highest tension groups of EOM units (300 to 350 and 350 to 400-mg) with only about 11% of the total number of units can generate 23% of the maximum muscle tension. This disproportionate share of the total tension generated by large units should be kept in mind when the mechanical properties of EOM, based on average motoneuron discharge rates, are discussed.

In terms of the dynamic properties of individual motor units, these same studies have measured a number of parameters for cat EOM, including twitch-contraction time and fusion frequency.[26,27] A more important variable for the purpose of this chapter is the time constant of the rise in isometric force in response to step increases in stimulation frequency to fusion rates. This value can be extracted from figures given for LR motor units.[27] The estimated time constant seems to vary only from about 15 to 25 msec from "fast" to "slow" units, suggesting rather uniform mechanical properties of the population of motor units. Unfortunately, length-tension diagrams and

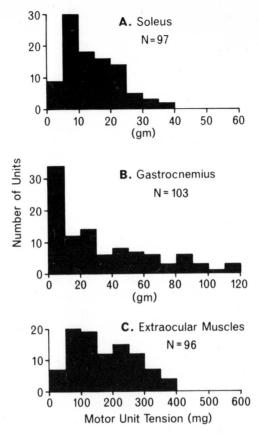

FIGURE 1. A comparison of the distribution of
single-motor unit tetanic tensions in several types of
cat muscle. (A) Soleus muscle, data from Mc-
Phedran, et al.[28] (B) Gastrocnemius muscle, data
from Wuerker, et al.[29] (C) Combined data from lateral rectus[27] and the inferior oblique.[26]

force-velocity measurements were not made, and thus, estimates of the range of actual
mechanical time constants are not available. The very important finding was reported,
that although fusion frequency varied from 50 to 350 pps, maximum tetanic tension
continued to increase in the low-fusion frequency units even at stimulation rates up to
200 pps.[26] This observation will be important when the natural firing rates of motoneurons is discussed later.

III. MOTONEURON DISCHARGE CHARACTERISTICS DURING FIXATION

The remainder of this review will be concerned with the description of the firing
patterns of oculomotor neurons during natural eye movements, mostly in primates,
but also comparisons to cats and man will be made when such data is available.

A. Rate-Position Relationship

During steady fixation each oculomotor neuron discharges at a constant rate in monkey,[5-7,32-35] cat,[36] and man.[37] An example for monkey is shown in Figure 2A. The
standard deviation of the interspike interval variability is typically only 6% of the

mean (range: 3.7 to 17.2%) in monkey[32] and a similar value has now been reported for cat.[36] When an animal repeatedly refixates a steady target, the unit's firing rate returns to a mean rate with a variability of only 5%.[32]

In describing the relationship between eye fixation position and unit discharge rate, the terms on-and-off-directions will be used to designate eye movements in, or away from, the direction of action of the muscle innervated by the unit. When unit discharge rate is measured at a series of fixation angles at successively greater positions in the on-direction, a rather fixed, approximately linear relationship results as shown in Figure 2B. The data points for each individual motoneuron may be fit with a linear regression line of slope, k, and threshold, θ_T. Within a pool of oculomotor neurons there is a broad distribution of these parameters. Slope values, k, vary from 1.1 to 14.5 spikes sec^{-1}/deg in monkey[6] and from 2.4 to 9.1 in cat.[36]

The largest thresholds, θ_T, (unit d, Figure 2B) are about 20 to 25 deg[5,32] so that gaze deviations beyond this angle are mediated by increased firing rates rather than recruitment. Some units continue to discharge even at extreme gaze deviations into the off-direction, and thus, have no thresholds (unit a, Fig. 2B). Hypothetical values of θ_T can be calculated for these units by extrapolation of the linear rate-position line to its intercept on the horizontal axis. Values of θ_T are thus found to be distributed between -60 and $+25$ deg, but with 79% having thresholds in the off half-field as shown in Figure 2C. Antidromically identified cat motoneurons show a much narrower distribution of thresholds, reflecting its more limited oculomotor range.[36]

The data of Collins[37] obtained from multiunit EMG recordings indicates a similar mechanism at work in human extraocular muscle, namely, successive recruitment of additional motor units and increased discharge frequency from previously recruited units as the eye moves to a series of fixation positions further into the on-direction. In fact, if the recruitment of new units were distributed uniformly over the oculomotor range and each recruited unit increased its discharge rate linearly for increasing values of fixation angle, then a square law relationship between total integrated muscle activity and eye position would be expected, which is the relationship found by Collins over the whole range ($\pm$ 50 deg) of human ocular motility.[37]

The animal single-unit data suggests, however, that the majority of units are already recruited at the primary position and that beyond about 20 to 25 deg into the on-field unit frequency increase must provide all the additional muscle activity. Thus, one would expect to find a significant decrease in the rate of increase of the slope of the relationship between total integrated muscle activity and eye position for on-direction fixations eccentric to the primary position. The increasing slope in this relationship found by Collins even at 40 and 50 deg fixation angles may have resulted from an artifact known to influence multiple-unit EMG recordings. The extracellular potential of higher threshold, single motor units will be larger than that recorded from lower threshold units[38] due to their increased size (more muscle fibers). This would result in an apparent increase in integrated EMG activity. It should also be noted that the relationship shown by Collins, while definitely described by a power law over the whole range of fixation positions ($\pm$ 50 deg), could be equally well fit by a linear relationship from $+20$ to $+50$ degs, i.e., the far on-field.

While supporting the basic concept of discharge frequency being proportional to fixation position in each motoneuron, Eckmiller in the monkey[39] and Collins in man[37] have published data that suggest that hysteresis exists in the rate-position relationships of oculomotor neurons. When separate regression lines are plotted through discharge rates for the same set of fixation positions reached by opposite direction saccades, a slight separation of data points results. Thus, at a given position, the firing rates tend to be higher when the position was reached with the motoneuron acting as the agonist, than when it was reached with the motoneuron acting as an antagonist. The description of this effect in monkey[39] is based on an extremely small sample and shows a difference of only about 10% or less of the mean firing rate. Since variations of 6% in unit discharge rate are common even for a single fixation interval, it is not clear if the hypothesized hysteresis is significant. The data of Collins[37] on the other hand, show differences of 100% or more between the levels of integrated EMG for the muscle acting as agonist and then as antagonist at the same position, but only at large eccentricies (>20 deg). It is again difficult to judge the significance of this finding since the number of measurements is not stated and the values from only one muscle of a patient with strabismus are plotted.[37] Resolution of this question is of considerable interest since ocular muscles show a mechanical hysteresis (at constant innervation) with the muscle developing more tension at a given position when extended to that position, than when shortened to the position. Collins[37] has suggested that hysteresis in the innervational input would act to compensate for this mechanical hysteresis since the net effects would tend to cancel each other.

B. Comparison to Spinal Motoneurons

In comparison to spinal motoneurons, oculomotor neurons possess several distinctive features. The maximum steady rates reached during fixation are much higher (250 to 300 for a typical oculomotor neuron) in comparison to the 20 to 30 reached during static contractions of fast spinal muscles.[38,40] This is to be expected on the basis of the higher fusion frequency of EOM. The same shared mechanism of increased unit recruitment and increased discharge frequency seems to be present in spinal muscle motor-unit pools, but on the whole, frequency increases seem to play a lesser role.[38,40] Perhaps this observation is related to the smaller absolute range of effective frequencies due to the lower fusion rates in spinal muscles.

IV. DISCHARGE CHARACTERISTICS DURING PURSUIT MOVEMENTS

A. Rate-Velocity Relationship

During smooth pursuit movements, the instantaneous discharge rate shows an additional increment or decrement at a given position if the eye is not fixating at the position, but moving in the on- or off-direction, respectively.[6] An example of these different rates for different directions of the movement is shown in Figure 2D. The discharge rate at time epoch 1 is quite different from that at epoch 2, although the eye has the same position at both times, due to the opposite directions of movement through this position. If one plots instantaneous discharge rates as the eye passes through a fixed point at different velocities, one obtains a rather linear relationship[6] (Figure 2E). The values of the slope, r, of the rate-velocity relationship were distributed from 0.25 to 5.0 spikes sec^{-1}/deg sec^{-1} in the monkey.[34]

B. Development of the Descriptive Equation

From the results of the static and the tracking measurements, each motoneuron's instantaneous firing rate can be related to eye position and velocity by a first-order differential equation:[6]

$$IR = k(\theta - \theta_T) + r\frac{d\theta}{dt} \tag{1}$$

where IR is motoneuron discharge rate, θ is eye position, $d\theta/dt$ is eye velocity and k, r and θ_T are as previously defined. The mean ratio r/k found by averaging over many

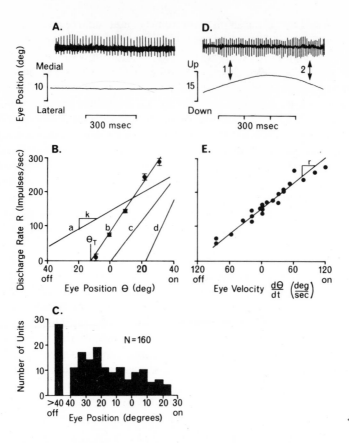

FIGURE 2.   The behavior of oculomotor neurons in alert monkey during fixation and pursuit eye movements. (A) A typical neuron (upper
trace) fires steadily during fixation. (B) Discharge rate plotted against eye
position during steady fixations on a series of target lamps from four
cells showing extremes of threshold, θ_T, and slope, k. Typical means and
standard deviations of rate are shown for cell b. (C) Distribution of firing
threshold (in terms of eye position) for a large number of oculomotor
neurons.[5-7,32] (D) Discharge behavior during a continuous pursuit movement. The eye has the same position at times 1 and 2, but the relationship
between rate and eye velocity causes firing to be higher at 2 when eye
velocity is in the on-direction. (E) Discharge rate of one typical cell plotted against velocity (through one position). (A, B, D, and E from Robinson, D. A. and Keller, E. L., *Bibliotheca Opthalmologia,* 82, 7, 1972.
With permission.)

motoneurons is an estimate of the neural output to the orbital mechanics consisting
of the eyeball, extraocular muscles, and passive orbital tissues. As previously noted, k
ranged over values with a ratio of 13:1 and r varied by over 15:1 in the monkey, but
values of the ratio r/k ranged only over 4:1 with a mean value of about 200 msec.[6]

Although more exact descriptions of the orbital mechanics (the active state tension
to eye position relationship requires at least fourth-order differential equations and
the inclusion of some nonlinear elements (see Robinson this volume), for lower velocity
movements, the system may be approximated by a linear, first-order equation:

$$F = K\theta + R \frac{d\theta}{dt} \qquad (2)$$

$$T_m = R/K \qquad (3)$$

where F is net active state muscle force and θ and $d\theta/dt$ are the same as above. K is an elastic and R a viscous coefficient whose ratio R/K is the time constant (T_m) of the orbital mechanics. If the assumption is made that motoneuron discharge rate is converted directly into active state tension, then the neural time constant r/k should be equal to the mechanical time constant R/K. The mechanical time constant has been measured in the monkey from the application of force steps to the globe and is reported to be about 95 msec.[32] This 2:1 discrepancy in time constants can be partially explained as an artifact of the method of simple averaging over the sample of individual motoneuron time constants (r/k). The data given in Section I indicate a variability of generated tension among ocular motor units over a ratio of 4:1. This indicates that the larger (higher tension) motor units need to be weighed more heavily in the calculation of the overall neural time constant. The data of Lennerstrand[26] indicate that there exists a tendency for the larger units to also be the more rapidly contracting (shorter time constant). If the time constant data from our previous study[41] are weighed according to the scheme 4× for units with time constants <100, 3× for time constants 100 to 150, 2× for time constants 150 to 200, and 1× for time constants >200 msec, the value of overall motoneuronal time constant is 137 msec, which is much closer to the measured mechanical time constant.

V. DISCHARGE CHARACTERISTICS DURING VESTIBULARLY ACTIVATED SLOW PHASE MOVEMENTS

A. Sinusoidal Analysis

The vestibular pathways influencing oculomotor neurons have been intensively studied,[42] and therefore, it is of interest to determine if the behavior of these motoneurons differs under vestibularly generated eye movements from that just described for visually guided movements. In their detailed study in the monkey, Skavenski and Robinson[43] report that there was no qualitative difference in motoneuron behavior during the slow phase of vestibular nystagmus and during pursuit movements. Approximately the same value for r is obtained by measuring discharge rate for various eye velocities through a given position during pursuit movements and during slow-phase vestibularly driven eye movements. This was further confirmed by rotating the animal sinusoidally and measuring the phase angle between motoneuron discharge rate and eye position. The measured phase shifts conformed generally to those phase angles, $\varnothing$ predicted from Equation 1, namely:

$$\phi = \tan^{-1} 2 \Pi f \left(\frac{r}{k}\right) \qquad (4)$$

where f is the frequency of head rotation and r and k are the values determined from visually guided eye movements as previously explained.

However, there were slight quantitative differences in the values obtained for r during vestibular as opposed to pursuit movements in a number of abducens neurons. The authors interpreted this to be indicative of local variations in synaptic density of the supranuclear fibers relaying input from the two sources of eye-velocity commands to the oculomotor neurons.

In this same study[43] the authors determined the frequency response of abducens unit discharge for sinusoidal rotation of the head over the frequency range from 0.3 to 1.5

Hz. The phase-angle relationship for eye position with respect to unit discharge rate was closely fit by a first order lag:

$$\phi (f) = \tan^{-1} 2 \Pi f T \qquad\qquad (5)$$

where f is frequency of head rotation and T is the lag time constant. The value of T was varied for each unit to provide the best fit of the curve $\varnothing$ (f) to the measured values of $\varnothing$ as shown in Figure 3. A mean value of T = 160 msec was determined from 10 units.

B. Comparison in Monkey and Cat

In a subsequent study of the same relationship in decerebrate cat, Shinoda and Yoshida[44] plotted the frequency response of a number of abducens units. The mean values they obtained are also shown in Figure 3. Although the two studies covered rather separate ranges of frequency, the lack of correspondence in the data at a frequency of around 0.25 Hz. suggested a much slower nature for the cat orbital mechanics (a larger value of T_m in Equation 3). It should be noted that in this latter study the eye movement measurements were made in different animals than the abducens unit measurements. This complication, and the uncertainty of the decerebrate animal's state, casts considerable doubt on the validity of this conclusion. In a more recent study in alert, intact cat on antidromically identified motoneurons, a datum set more similar to that of the monkey was obtained (Figure 3).[36] From this study a mean motoneuronal time constant of about 200 msec can be estimated for the cat orbit. Direct measurement of the cat orbital mechanics based on eye movement measurements obtained by sinusoidal stimulation of the oculomotor nerve suggested a time constant of 64 msec.[45] However, it should be noted that electrical stimulation of the motor nerve probably favors the larger axons (larger tension motor units), which tend to innervate faster muscle fibers, over the natural recruitment order which is the opposite. Thus, stimulation studies tend to underestimate the muscle functional time constant.

VI. DISCHARGE CHARACTERISTICS DURING VERGENCE MOVEMENTS

A. Activity Patterns in Medial and Lateral Rectus Motoneurons

A number of basic relationships concerning the organization of vergence eye movements at the level of the final common paths have been clarified by recording from motoneurons in alert primates trained to make vergence movements.[41,46] It was found that all abducens and oculomotor nucleus neurons (medial rectus subdivision) followed the behavior predicted by Equation 1 obtained during version movements. Thus, during a convergence movement as shown on the left in Figure 4, medial rectus units increase their discharge rates and lateral rectus units (not shown) decrease their rates. Moreover, the change in discharge rate in the steady state is exactly that which would have occurred if this eye had made a version movement between the same initial and final gaze positions. During divergence movements, as shown on the right in Figure 4, the opposite patterns in the MR and LR (not shown) appear. In this sense, divergence movements result from active increases in the LR and not just from passive relaxation of the MR.

Quantitative calculations based on analysis of the discharge rate before and after separate vergence and version movements between the same two points indicated that the value of k in Equation 1 was the same for the two classes of movement. Often the vergence movements were roughly exponential in trajectory (after an initial period of

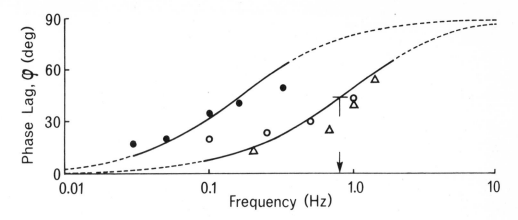

FIGURE 3. The phase lag, ∅, of eye position with respect to discharge rate of oculomotor neurons during sinusoidal rotations of the head. Filled circles show the average data points for neurons in decerebrate cat from Shinoda and Yoshida,[44] open circles the average data points for neurons in the alert, intact cat from Goldberg,[36] and triangles the average data points for neurons in alert monkey from Skavenski and Robinson.[43] The curves, representing Equation 5, are adjusted along the frequency axis to give the best fit by eye to the data points from the decerebrate animals (solid curve on the left) and to the points from the intact animals (solid curve on the right). The dashed portions show the extensions (Equation 5) of the two curves. The vertical arrow indicates the value of frequency where the phase lag first increases to 45 deg. The value of the time constant, T, in Equation 5 may be determined from the reciprocal of this frequency.

acceleration), while the motoneuronal command was a step change in discharge rate as shown in Figure 4. Values of r in Equation 1 during vergence movements could be calculated from:

$$r = \frac{\Delta IR}{V_o} \qquad (6)$$

where ΔIR is the change in firing rate and V_o is the value of vergence velocity measured just after the period of initial acceleration. There was no statistical difference between the set of values for r obtained in this manner and for similar measurements of r for the same units obtained during pursuit movements.[46] The similarity in values of these estimates for k and r during version and vergence movements led to the suggestion that the supranuclear control signals for these two classes of eye movement must be combined at some central site and not at the level of the motoneuron.[46] Recently, direct measurements of the discharge pattern of identified interneurons (IN) in the abducens nucleus in cat[47] or the axons of these neurons in the MLF in monkey (Keller, unpublished observations) have been made. While each of these neurons closely resembles motoneurons during pursuit and fixation, none change rate during vergence movements. Since these IN form the major supranuclear input to MR motoneurons for version movements, it appears that the earlier suggestion of the supranuclear combination of vergence and version control signals is not correct. Instead, these two classes of control signal must be integrated at the motoneuron. The fact that *each* individual motoneuron receives almost exactly the same effective synaptic input (as shown by the similar values of both r and k) from these supranuclear inputs so distinctly different in origin (one from higher level accommodative centers and the other from brain stem IN of the abducens nucleus) suggests a remarkably specific developmental process for oculomotor neurons.

B. Refinement of the Descriptive Equation

The unique property that vergence movements result from a step change in motor-

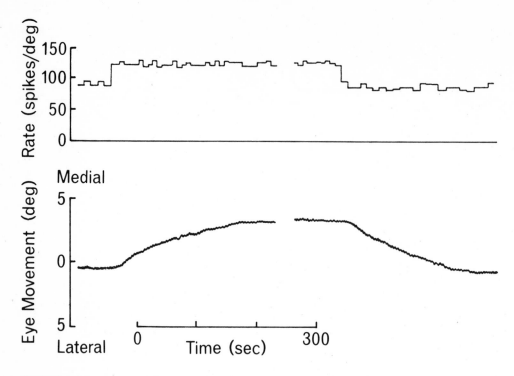

FIGURE 4.   Instantaneous discharge rate (upper curves) of a medial rectus motoneuron during a convergence movement (lower-left trace) and a divergence movement (lower-right trace). (From Keller, E. L., *Vision Res.,* 13, 1565, 1973. With permission.)

unit firing rate offers an opportunity to estimate the higher-order terms in the relationship between motoneuron discharge rate and eye movements.[46] When Equation 1 is rewritten to include the effect of eye acceleration, Equation 7 results:

$$IR = k(\theta - \theta_T) + r\, d\theta/dt + md^2\theta/dt^2 \qquad (7)$$

As shown in Figure 4, the eye accelerates from 0 to 30°/sec in about 20 msec at the beginning of a typical accommodate vergence movement. During this brief interval, the change in firing rate is determined almost exclusively by acceleration. This method suggests that a typical value of m is 0.012 spikes sec^{-1}/deg sec^{-2}. Factoring the second-order Equation 7 after inserting the appropriate values of k, r, and m for each unit led to an estimate of 16.2 and 179 msec for the average value of the two time constants.[46] By the reasoning already discussed, these two time constants should also be the neural reflexion of mechanical dynamics of the orbit. Thus, during more rapidly changing eye velocities when accelerations become more important, an alteration of Equation 2 to incorporate these two time constants would be appropriate.[48,49] (See also, Robinson, this volume.)

VII. DISCHARGE CHARACTERISTICS DURING SACCADES

A. Peak Discharge Rates and Discharge Profiles

Figure 5 shows in schematic form the activity patterns that are typical for all monkey oculomotor neurons during two saccades in the on-direction and one saccade in the off-direction (far right).[5-7,34] Saccades in the on-direction are created by high-fre-

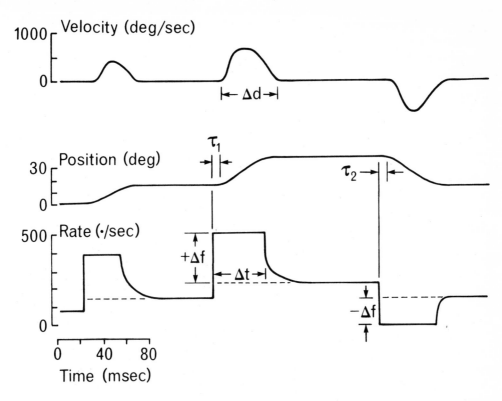

FIGURE 5. Discharge rate of a typical oculomotor neuron (lower trace) during two saccades in the on-direction (on the left and center) and during one saccade in the off-direction (right). Eye position and velocity shown by middle and upper traces, respectively. Other symbols discussed in the text.

quency bursts of motoneuron discharge ($+\Delta f$) on top of the step change in fixation rates associated with the change in eye position so that the net time course of neural activity is approximately a pulse-step. During saccades in the off-direction, most motoneurons are completely inhibited ($-\Delta f$) and then resume discharge at a lower rate associated with the new fixation position. This profile is, in effect, a negative pulse-step. The onset of the pulse leads the initiation of the saccadic movement (τ_1 and τ_2) by about 5 to 8 msec. All investigators of saccade-related discharge in monkey agree on these qualitative points, but a number of discrepancies have appeared in the various reports with respect to the quantitative measurement of the discharge parameters.

A typical velocity for a large (>20 deg) monkey saccade is 800 deg/sec,[50] while a typical value for r is 0.6 spikes sec^{-1}/deg sec^{-1}. Thus the term, r dθ/dt, in Equation 1 would predict a burst rate of 480 spikes/sec, which is, in fact, a typical value for the saccadic burst rate. Neurons recorded in the oculomotor nucleus burst with frequencies distributed between 200 to 600 spikes/sec,[6,7] while abducens neurons show a bimodal distribution with one group distributed over a frequency range similar to oculomotor nucleus neurons, and another group from 600 to 850 spikes/sec.[5,34] Fuchs and Luschei[5] suggested that this latter group of neurons were interneurons (IN) and not motoneurons. This hypothesis has been supported by the subsequent demonstration of the existence of IN in the abducens nucleus.[12,13]

B. Relationship of Burst Rate and Duration to Saccade Size

Robinson[6] reported that burst frequency was related to saccade size in most motoneurons. This relationship is predicted by Equation 1 because smaller saccades have lower velocities[50] (far left saccade in Figure 5) which results in a smaller r $d\theta/dt$ term. Other authors have not supported this finding,[5,7,35] although Schiller[7] found that burst rate was correlated with saccadic velocity. Since it is well established that larger saccades reach higher peak velocities, it is difficult to see how he did not find a positive correlation between saccade size and burst frequency.

Each of the three laboratories report that burst duration (Δt in Figure 5) is just about equal to saccade duration (Δd in Figure 5).[5-7] Since larger saccades have longer durations,[50] burst duration is observed to increase with saccade size.

Henn and Cohen[35] have reported that burst duration was not well correlated with saccade size in their sample of oculomotor neurons, but it should be noted that they collected data on saccades in all directions, not just in the on — and off — directions for each unit as done by previous authors. Although it has not been well publicized, the tight correlation between saccade size and duration for horizontal movements[50] breaks down during oblique movements.[35,51,52] For example, a large, slightly off-vertical oblique saccade will normally have a small horizontal component of long duration (as compared to a pure horizontal saccade of the same size). In a random mixture of oblique saccades, the correlation between vertical and horizontal component size and movement duration would be lost, as would the correlation between burst duration and component size. Nevertheless, burst duration would still be equal in duration to component duration.

C. Tonic and Phasic Motoneurons

Henn and Cohen[35] also divide their sample of motoneurons into four classes based on the relative size of the saccade burst (pulse) to the step (change in fixation rates). Their two intermediary classes correspond to the continuum of motoneuron types reported by others.[5-7] Their two extreme classes, the pure tonic (with no saccadic burst over or undershoot) and the pure phasic (which only discharge in bursts during saccades), have not been observed by others.[5-7,32] Since their monkeys were not trained, their data probably does not contain fixations beyond the 25 deg eccentricities required to bring some motoneurons over tonic (fixation) firing threshold (unit d in Figure 2B). Thus, their phasic class probably represents the high threshold (large θ_T) continuum of motor units seen by others. It appears from their published data that their pure tonic class shows small saccadic overshoots (particularly inhibitory pulses during off-saccades), but if absolutely tonic units exist, they may be supranuclear neurons similar to those reported to exist in the reticular formation surrounding the motoneuron pools.[53,54] The discrepancy here is a small point, but the use of the terms pure phasic and tonic leads to confusion in the literature, particularly in the clinical area where the incorrect concept of separate motor pools and muscle fibers for fast (saccadic) eye movements is just beginning to be corrected.

D. Burst Lead Times

The final parameter of interest is saccadic lead time (τ_1 and τ_2 in Figure 5), which represents the time interval from the onset of the saccadic burst or inhibition to the initiation of the eye movement. There is general agreement that the change in unit activity in all units precedes the onset of the saccade, and hence, saccades are created by a synchronous pulse of motoneuron activity.[5,6,41] Units are not recruited during the movement. A typical mean value for τ_1 is 5.5 msec (range = 4 to 10 msec) and the value of τ_2 is found to the same[6] or slightly longer.[32,41] Thus, antagonist inhibition does not significantly precede agonist excitation in the monkey.

The activity patterns of motoneurons during saccades in the plane perpendicular to a unit's on-off-direction have not been carefully studied. The information that does exist is contradictory. Robinson[6] reported that no charges in unit discharge rate occurred during such orthogonal movements, but Westheimer and Blair[55] claimed that rate changes occurred in all units during saccades in any direction. Fuchs and Luschei also reported small and variable bursts in trochlear nerve fibers[33] during both medial and lateral horizontal movements. In any case, the small transients that appear in motoneurons during movements in the plane perpendicular to their on-off direction are clearly distinct from the large bursts and pulses of inhibition that occur for movements in the latter plane, and may reflect the inability to resolve small, on-axis components in the electrooculogram movement registration system.[55]

E. Comparison to Data from Cat and Man

In general, the saccadic data from other species is similar to that reported for monkey. Collins[37] reports that in man both the smaller orbital and larger globally located muscle fibers burst during on-direction saccades, the latter to a greater extent than the former. His EMG data indicate, however, that the burst duration in motor units is only about one half the saccadic movement duration. The reason for this apparent difference from the monkey, where the burst is nearly equal to saccade duration, is not clear. The human EMG data of Sinderman, et al.,[56] supposedly from single motor units, shows burst durations about equal to saccade durations. This point is of some concern since saccades are such rapid movements that exact specification of the controller burst profile is required in order to specify the appropriate orbital mechanical model during saccades.

The human EMG data[37,56] support the contention of Robinson[6] that motoneuron burst rates increase during larger (higher velocity) saccades.

Recordings in the abducens nucleus indicate that cat saccades are also created by a pulse-step motoneuronal control signal.[36,57] Burst duration is found to be about equal[36] or slightly longer[57] than saccade duration. Just as in the monkey, the results showing the relationship of burst rate to saccade size are contradictory. In an early study in nonintact cat, burst frequencies were shown to increase very little or not at all with saccade size.[57] It should be noted that all the rapid eye movements generated in this study were fast-phase movements of vestibular nystagmus in decerebrate cat. This preparation appears to be peculiar in that eye velocity did not increase with fast-phase movement size.[57] Thus, higher burst frequencies (which code higher movement velocities) should not be expected. On the other hand, when motor unit activity during spontaneous saccades in the alert, intact cat were studied,[36] a clear correlation between burst frequency and saccade size (and velocity) were obtained.

Reinhart and Zuber[57] reported that the average value of τ_1 in the cat was 31.7 msec, an unexpectedly large value based on the monkey studies. Goldberg[36] recording from antidromically identified motoneurons in the cat in my laboratory found an average value of burst lead to be 10 msec, a value much closer to the value in monkey.

VIII. EVIDENCE AGAINST A STRETCH REFLEX IN OCULOMOTOR NEURONS

No other single area of oculomotor neuron physiology has been the subject of a wider and more confused literature. It is beyond the scope of the present paper to review this background here, but the interested reader can find much of the material discussed in a previous paper.[32] In that report, experimental evidence obtained in the fully alert, intact monkey is presented that shows unequivocally that there is no stretch reflex in the extraocular muscles of the monkey. These data were obtained on a variety of unit types (high and low threshold) during both fixation and saccades. Since the monkey has been shown to have extraocular muscle spindles,[58] it seems likely that other primates, including man, also lack an ocular stretch reflex. These findings do not dispute the existence of orbital (including muscle) proprioceptive receptors, but in contrast to other spinal muscles, these afferent inputs seem to project more centrally without sending collaterals to motoneurons. It appears that extraocular muscle proprioceptive input goes to the cerebellum[59,60] along with the mass of similar input from other muscles, but its functional utilization here is, at present, unknown.

Because the extraocular muscles are unique in having no antigravity function and deal, throughout life, with the same mechanical load, the basic function of the stretch reflex is inapplicable for them. Thus, from a functional standpoint, it should not be surprising to find the stretch reflex absent in these muscles. In the broader integrative sense of motor physiology, the extraocular muscles may not be so unique and the answer to the function of extraocular muscle proprioception may be found when the higher function of proprioception in other limb muscles is found.

IX. CONCLUSIONS

The overall conclusion gained from the sum total of oculomotor neuron recording experiments in a variety of species is indeed very simple. Motoneurons fire in a rather machine-like way at rates which directly reflect the tension desired in their innervated muscle without regard to the type of movement being generated. No type of eye movement (or fixation) is the exclusive product of a certain subset of motoneurons. By allowing for a continuum in variation of parameters, the discharge of all motoneurons may be simply described during fixation or slow constant-velocity movements by Equation 1. A small hysteresis may effect the value of k, but more evidence is required on this point. During accelerations, Equation 7 will give a more accurate description of firing rate. If sufficient latitude is given to weighting of the individual units on the basis of their relative tensions (and assuming that larger units are also more rapidly contracting[26]), then a very accurate prediction of the dominant orbital mechanical time constant (Equation 3) is produced by averaging the individual motoneuron time constants.

The identification of higher-order features in a model of orbital mechanics during saccadic eye movements can only be approximated from the data described herein, because of the highly nonlinear behavior of rapidly shortening and lengthening muscle. Nevertheless, Equation 1 or 7 predicts a high-frequency burst in agonist and a complete inhibition of discharge in antagonist motoneurons, a fact readily agreed upon by all investigators. Questions concerning the exact profile of the burst (exact duration, how flat the intraburst frequency remains, and the instantaneous frequency relation to instantaneous eye velocity) require further study for reconcilation of differences among investigators and species.

In terms of further system analysis, oculomotor neurons offer the distinct advantage over other motoneurons in that they form an open-loop projection to their muscles. The total lack of recurrent collaterals and proprioceptive feedback to oculomotor neurons requires that the stereotyped discharge patterns observed during each type of eye movement be generated by synaptic input from various supranuclear centers. The study of the source and organization of these higher central nervous system inputs to the oculomotor neurons is now proceeding on the firm foundation supplied by the knowledge of final common path behavior as described in this chapter.

REFERENCES

1. Schaefer, K.- P., Die Erregungsmuster einzelner Neurone des Abducens-Kerns beim Kaninchen, *Pflügers Arch.*, 284, 31, 1965.
2. Precht, W., Grippo, J., and Richter, A., Effect of horizontal angular acceleration on neurons in the abducens nucleus, *Brain Res.*, 5, 527, 1967.
3. Horcholle, G. and Tyo-Dumont, S., Activites unitaires des neurones vestibulaires et oculomoteurs au cours du nystagmus, *Exp. Brain Res.*, 5, 16, 1968.
4. Evarts, E. V., A technique for recording activity of subcortical neurons in moving animals, *Electroencephalogr. Clin. Neurophysiol.*, 24, 83, 1968.
5. Fuchs, A. F. and Luschei, E. S., Firing patterns of abducens neurons of alert monkeys in relationship to horizontal eye movement, *J. Neurophysiol.*, 33, 382, 1970.
6. Robinson, D. A., Oculomotor unit behavior in the monkey, *J. Neurophysiol.*, 33, 393, 1970.
7. Schiller, P. H., The discharge characteristics of single units in the oculomotor and abducens nuclei of the unanesthetized monkey, *Exptl. Brain Res.*, 10, 347, 1970.
8. Warwick, R., Oculomotor organization, in *The Oculomotor System,* Bender, M., Ed., Harper & Row, New York, 1964, chap. 7.
9. Warwick, R., Representation of the extraocular muscles in the oculomotor nuclei of the monkey, *J. Comp. Neurol.*, 98, 449, 1953.
10. Tarlov, E. and Tarlov, S. R., The representation of extraocular muscles in the oculomotor nuclei: experimental studies in the cat, *Brain Res.*, 34, 37, 1971.
11. Gacek, R. R., Localization of neurons supplying the extraocular muscles in the kitten using horseradish peroxidase, *Exp. Neurol.*, 44, 381, 1974.
12. Graybiel, A. M. and Hartwieg, E. A., Some afferent connections of the oculomotor complex in the cat: an experimental study with tracer techniques, *Brain Res.*, 81, 543, 1974.
13. Baker, R. and Highstein, S., Physiological identification of interneurones in the abducens nucleus, *Brain Res.*, 91, 292, 1975.
14. Maciewicz, R. J., Kaneko, C. R. S., Highstein, S., and Baker, R., Morphophysiological identification of interneurones in the oculomotor nucleus that project to the abducens nucleus in the cat, *Brain Res.*, 96, 60, 1975.
15. Spencer, R. F. and Sterling, P., An electron microscope study of motoneurones and interneurones in cat abducens nucleus identified by retrograde intraaxonal transport of horseradish peroxidase, *J. Comp. Neurol.*, 176, 65, 1977.
16. Baker, R., personal communication, 1979.
17. Tredici, G., Pizzini, G., and Milanesi, S., The ultrastructure of the nucleus of the oculomotor nerve (somatic efferent portion) of the cat, *Anat. Embryol.*, 149, 323, 1976.
18. Sasaki, K., Electrophysiological studies on oculomotor neurons of the cat, *Jpn. J. Physiol.*, 13, 287, 1963.
19. Baker, R. G., Mano, N., and Shimazu, H., Intracellular recording of antidromic responses from abducens motoneurons in the cat, *Brain Res.*, 15, 127, 1969.
20. Baker, R. and Precht, W., Electrophysiological properties of trochlear motoneurons as revealed by IVth nerve stimulation, *Exp. Brain Res.*, 14, 127, 1972.
21. Goldberg, S. J., Hull, C. D., and Buchwald, N. A., Afferent projections in the abducens nerve: an intracellular study, *Brain Res.*, 68, 205, 1974.
22. Remmel, R. S. and Marrocco, R. T., Impulse generation properties of abducens motoneurons, *Vision Res.*, 15, 1039, 1975.
23. Grantyn, R. and Grantyn, A., Morphological and electrophysiological properties of cat abducens motoneurons, *Exp. Brain Res.*, 31, 249, 1978.
24. Cajal, S. R. y., *Histologie dul Systeme Nerveux de l'Homme et des Vertebres,* Maloine, Paris, 1911.
25. Gogan, P., Gueritaud, J. P., Horcholle-Bossavit, G., and Tyc-Dumont, S., Electrotonic coupling between motoneurones in the abducens nucleus of the cat, *Exptl. Brain Res.*, 21, 139, 1974.
26. Lennerstrand, G., Electrical activity and isometric tension in motor units of the cat's inferior oblique muscle, *Acta Physiol. Scand.*, 91, 458, 1974.
27. Goldberg, S. J., Lennerstrand, G., and Hull, C. D., Motor unit responses in the lateral rectus muscle of the cat: intracellular current injection of abducens nucleus neurons, *Acta Physiol. Scand.*, 96, 58, 1976.
28. McPhedran, A. M., Wuerker, R. B., and Henneman, E., Properties of motor units in a homogeneous red muscle (soleus) of the cat, *J. Neurophysiol.*, 28, 71, 1965.
29. Wuerker, R. B., McPhedran, A. M., and Henneman, E., Properties of motor units in a heterogeneous pale muscle (m. gastrocnemius) of the cat, *J. Neurophysiol.*, 28, 85, 1965.
30. Barmack, N. H., Bell, C. C., and Rence, B. G., Tension and rate of tension development during isometric responses of extraocular muscle, *J. Neurophysiol.*, 34, 1072, 1971.

31. Steinacker, A. and Bach-y-Rita, P., The fiber spectrum of the cat VI nerve to the lateral rectus and retractor bulbi muscles, *Experientia,* 24, 1254, 1968.

32. Keller, E. L. and Robinson, D. A., Absence of a stretch reflex in extraocular muscles of the monkey, *J. Neurophysiol.,* 34, 908, 1971.

33. Fuchs, A. F. and Luschei, E. S., The activity of single trochlear nerve fibers during eye movements in the alert monkey, *Exp. Brain Res.,* 13, 78, 1971.

34. Robinson, D. A. and Keller, E. L., The behavior of eye movement motoneurons in the alert monkey, in *Cerebral Control of Eye Movements and Motion Perception,* Dichgans, J. and Bizzi, E., Eds., S. Karger, Basel, 1972, 7.

35. Henn, V. and Cohen, B., Quantitative analysis of activity in eye muscle motoneurons during saccadic eye movement and positions of fixation, *J. Neurophysiol.,* 36, 115, 1973.

36. Goldberg, J., Activity of abducens nucleus in the alert cat, Ph.D. Diss., University of California, Berkeley, 1980.

37. Collins, C. C., The human oculomotor control system, in *Basic Mechanisms of Ocular Motility and Their Clinical Implications,* Lennerstrand, G. and Bach-y-Rita, P., Eds., Pergamon Press, Oxford, 1975, 145.

38. Clamann, H. P., Activity of single motor units during isometric tension, *Neurol.,* 20, 254, 1970.

39. Eckmiller, R., Hysteresis in the static characteristics of eye position coded neurons in the alert monkey, *Pflügers Arch.,* 350, 249, 1974.

40. Milner-Brown, H. S., Stein, R. B., and Yemm, R., Changes in firing rate of human motor units during linearly changing voluntary contractions, *J. Physiol. (London),* 230, 371, 1973.

41. Keller, E. L. and Robinson, D. A., Abducens unit behavior in the monkey during vergence movements, *Vision Res.,* 12, 369, 1972.

42. Precht, W., Neuronal operations in the vestibular system, in *Studies in Brain Function,* Vol. 2 Springer-Verlag, Basel, Berlin, 1978, chap. 5.

43. Skavenski, A. A. and Robinson, D. A., Role of abducens neurons in vestibuloocular reflex, *J. Neurophysiol.,* 36, 724, 1973.

44. Shinoda, Y. and Yoshida, K., Dynamic characteristics of responses to horizontal head angular acceleration in the vestibuloocular pathway in the cat, *J. Neurophysiol.,* 37, 653, 1974.

45. Zuber, B. L., Eye movement dynamics in the cat: the final motor pathway, *Exp. Neurol.,* 20, 255, 1968.

46. Keller, F. L., Accommodative vergence in the alert monkey: motor unit analysis, *Vision Res.,* 13, 1565, 1973.

47. Delgado-Garcia, J., Baker, R., and Highstein, S. M., The activity of internuclear neurons identified within the abducens nucleus of the alert cat, in *Control of Gaze by Brain Stem Neurons,* Baker, R. and Berthoz, A., Eds., Elsevier, Amsterdam, 1977, 291.

48. Van Gisbergen, J. A. M. and Robinson, D. A., Generation of micro and macrosaccades by burst neurons in the monkey, in *Control of Gaze by Brain Stem Neurons,* Baker, R. and Berthoz, A., Eds., Elsevier, Amsterdam, 1977, 301.

49. Zee, D. S. and Robinson, D. A., An hypothetical explanation of saccadic oscillations, *Annu. Neurol.,* 5, 405, 1979.

50. Fuchs, A. F., Saccadic and smooth pursuit eye movements in the monkey, *J. Physiol. (London),* 191, 609, 1967.

51. Keller, E. L., Oculomotor specificity within subdivisions of the reticular formation, in *The Reticular Formation Revisited: Specifying Function for a Non-Specific System,* Hobson, J. A. and Brazier, M. A. B., Eds., Raven Press, New York, 1980, 227.

52. King, W. M., personal communication, 1979.

53. Luschei, E. S. and Fuchs, A. F., Activity of brain stem neurons during eye movements of alert monkeys, *J. Neurophysiol.,* 35, 445, 1972.

54. Keller, E. L., Participation of medial pontine reticular formation in eye movement generation in monkey, *J. Neurophysiol.,* 37, 316, 1974.

55. Westheimer, G. and Blair, S. M., Concerning the supranuclear organization of eye movements, in *Cerebral Control of Eye Movements and Motion Perception,* Dichgans, J. and Bizzi, E., Eds., S. Karger, Basel, 1972, 28.

56. Sindermann, F., Geiselmann, B., and Fischler, M., Single motor unit activity in extraocular muscles in man during fixation and saccades, *Electroencephalogr. Clin. Neurophysiol.,* 45, 64, 1978.

57. Reinhart, R. J. and Zuber, B. L., Abducens nerve signals controlling saccadic eye movements in the cat, *Brain Res.,* 34, 331, 1971.

58. Green, T. and Jampel, R., Muscle spindles in the extraocular muscles of the macaque, *J. Comp. Neurol.,* 126, 547, 1966.

59. Fuchs, A. F. and Kornhuber, H. H., Extraocular muscle afferents to the cerebellum of the cat, *J. Physiol. (London),* 200, 713, 1969.

60. **Baker, R., Precht, W., and Llinas, R.,** Mossy and climbing fiber projections of extraocular muscle afferents to the cerebellum, *Brain Res.,* 38, 440, 1972.

Chapter 2

MODELS OF THE MECHANICS OF EYE MOVEMENTS

David A. Robinson

TABLE OF CONTENTS

I. INTRODUCTION

In this volume, E. L. Keller has already described the relationship between the observed input to the oculomotor plant (the motoneurons, muscles, and passive tissues of the eye and orbit) — taken here to be the discharge rate, R_m, of a representative motoneuron — and the output which is eye position, E. This relationship may be summarized by the equation,

$$R_m = R_0 + kE(t + \tau) + r\dot{E}(t + \tau) + m\ddot{E}(t + \tau) \qquad (1)$$

R_0 is the discharge rate when the eye is in the primary position (E equal to zero) and is typically 100 spikes/sec. The coefficient k reflects the elasticity of orbital tissues, most of which is in the length-tension relationship of the muscles, and is 4.0 (spikes/sec)/(deg) for the average motoneuron. The viscosity of the tissues is reflected in r which is typically 0.95 (spikes/sec)/(deg/sec). The acceleration term m reflects higher-order phenomena (not necessarily inertia) and has a typical value of 0.054 (spikes/sec)/(deg/sec²). The eye follows the motor command by a delay τ which is about 8 msec.

As a result of this empirical description, one can regard the plant as a black box, define the input signal to be the modulation R_m less R_0, or ΔR_m, and, by taking the Laplace transform of Equation 1, arrive at the transfer function:

$$\frac{E}{\Delta R_m} = \frac{\frac{1}{k} e^{-s\tau}}{(sTe_1 + 1)(sTe_2 + 1)} \qquad (2)$$

The time constant Te_1 is approximately equal to r/k and has a value of about 0.2 sec. Te_2 is approximately m/r and is about 0.016 sec. This equation, at least for the monkey, allows one to deduce what motoneurons are doing for any kind of eye movement or to know what sort of eye movement would be produced by the activity of neurons in the central nervous system.

For many purposes, Equation 2 is unnecessarily complicated since τ and Te_2 are small and only become important when the details of saccadic waveforms are considered. The simpler equation,

$$\frac{E}{\Delta R_m} = \frac{\frac{1}{k}}{(sTe_1 + 1)} \qquad (3)$$

is adequate for many purposes. This is the case, for example, for clinical considerations. Many eye movement abnormalities resulting from changes in orbital mechanics or altered input signals due to brainstem or cerebellar lesions can be readily explained through the use of Equation 3.[1,2]

One might wonder, in light of these observations, why one should bother to make a model of the mechanics of eye movements. The neurophysiologist only needs a black box description which spans the bridge between neural signals and eye movements, and Equation 3 or 2 is adequate for all but very special purposes. Clinically, Equation 3 is adequate for examining the effects of central lesions and peripheral lesions as well (such as a muscle palsy), as long as one can deduce what the lesion has done to the viscosity (r) and elasticity (k) at various eye positions. The major interest in abnormalities of peripheral mechanics is in the diagnosis and management of strabismus, but this problem requires a model of the *statics* of eye mechanics in three dimensions;[3] the models considered here are one-dimensional, *dynamic* models.

One suspects that the basic reason one tries to model the dynamics of eye mechanics is simply that the problem is there. It seems, on the surface, easy to analyze, and modeling is fun. However, I offer one caveat: I hope to show that current models suffer from an indeterminacy that is caused by a lack of good physiological data. Progress cannot be made until those data are available. However, those data are also difficult to obtain as witnessed by the lack of any significant advances in a quantitative description of eye muscle behavior in recent years. One might be more tempted to exert the effort to do the required difficult experiments if a significant benefit would result, but refining these models with better data will not, in my opinion, result in any basic advance in oculomotor physiology or be of any use in the clinic. Of course, one never knows.

One interesting point does arise from trying to make a model of eye mechanics: it illustrates how shockingly ignorant we are of how muscles behave. Most research in muscle physiology is, naturally enough, devoted to discovering the electrochemical means by which muscles are able to generate force and shorten. Little attention has been paid to an accurate description of how muscles, *in situ,* rotate joints in real-life situations, probably because of the complicated ways in which muscles, fascia, and tendons are arranged around most joints. The eye, however, presents a rather simple situation. In each plane of action there are two, parallel-fibered muscles, one "joint", and, because the muscle tendons wrap around the globe, each muscle has a constant moment arm. Also, the only load on these muscles is that of the eye itself, which is constant. Thus, in the eye, it is reasonable to attempt to describe mathematically how naturally-innervated muscles make real, every-day movements. However, when one attempts this, one suddenly discovers that very little is known about this situation and the muscle models based on length-tension and force-velocity relationships derived from isotonic and isometric experiments on artificially activated muscles are just too simplistic. Consequently, the modeling described in this chapter tries to point out in rather specific ways many of the things which remain unknown about the way in which muscles behave in the body.

II. TOPOLOGY OF THE MODEL

Figure 1 shows the basic arrangement of the elements which are thought to be important in plant mechanics. The muscles are shown unwrapped from the globe as though they were translating it, but that is only for convenience and all variables refer to angular movements. Changes in actual muscle lengths in mm can be found by multiplying the angle of eye rotation, E, from the primary position, converted to radians, by the globe radius which is about 12.4 mm. The conversion factor is 0.216 mm/deg. Forces in g can be converted to moments by multiplying by the globe radius. However, it is more intuitive to measure all length changes in equivalent eye rotation in deg and moments by the equivalent force in g at the globe's surface.

In Figure 1, J is the moment of inertia of the eyeball which is acted upon by three forces: the tendon force of the two muscles which will play the role of agonist (F_1) and antagonist (F_2), and the force of the nonmuscular passive tissues, P. Each muscle's force is composed of the force of its passive tissues, F_p, and its neurally controlled, developed force F_d. The limp leash elements, LL, represent the fact that muscles can only pull and not push. Muscle length, L, is conceptually divided into two parts: L_s, the length of the series-elastic element, and L_c, the length of the contractile element.

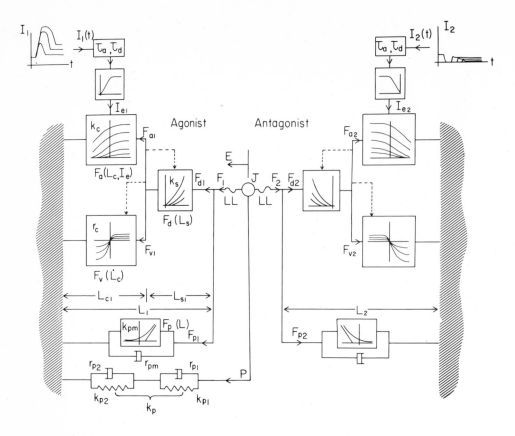

FIGURE 1.   The basic organization of the mechanical elements of the orbit. The agonist and antagonist variables are denoted by subscripts 1 and 2, respectively. The series-elastic element is denoted by $F_d(L_s)$ and the force-velocity relationship by $F_v(\dot{L}_c)$. Dashed lines indicate both elements are parametrically modulated by F_a. The length-tension-innervation curves are denoted by $F_a(L_c, I_e)$. Wave-forms for the innervations I_1 and I_2 are shown for saccades of different sizes. Time constants τ_a and τ_d represent activation and deactivation time constants. The stiffnesses k and viscosities r with various subscripts indicate mean or local slopes of functions often used in linear approximations. See text for further description.

(For those unfamiliar with this phenomenological description of muscle behavior, one could consult any physiology textbook or a brief review by Lännergren[4] aimed at oculomotor physiologists.) The series-elastic element acts like a stiff, nonlinear, undamped spring. The contractile element is conceptually divided into two parts. One is described by the force-velocity relationship which acts like a viscosity in that it produces a force, F_v, that is related to its velocity $\dot{L}_c$. The other generates a force called active-state tension, F_a. The dependence of F_a on L_c is called the length-tension relationship. In the steady state, F_d equals F_a, since F_v is zero. The most important variable that determines F_a is innervation, I, which is related to R_m, but must include other things such as the number of motoneurons active and the sizes of various types of muscle fibers. There are also activation and deactivation dynamics which are interposed between I and F_a. One must, of course, know the time courses of I_1 (t) and I_2 (t) associated with various types of eye movements.

III. MODEL ELEMENTS

As one might suppose, we have very poor descriptions, in some cases no description at all, of the elements in Figure 1. This means that it is quite literally necessary to just guess how some of these elements behave. This estimation is usually done by tweaking constants until the model makes realistic eye movements. This would be a correct procedure if the input, output, and all constants but one were known but, in fact, the input is not known exactly; and there are many constants, function, and relationships in current models which are approximated or guessed. It is not difficult to adjust all these unknowns to obtain a reasonable model output. However, the usefulness of the model is in a sensitivity analysis in which one probes, which assumptions have a strong effect on model behavior and what degree of indeterminacy exists between such elements. This job still remains to be done and the following discussion does not provide answers, but simply points out the problems.

A. Inertia of the Globe

If the eyeball were a rigid sphere of density 1.0, its moment of inertia, J, would be 6.12×10^{-5} g/(deg/sec^2). The eye is not rigid and, during a saccade, most of the vitreous is momentarily left behind. However, if one added the inertia of the optic-nerve head, Tenon's capsule, and the distal ends of the muscles, the above value could still be roughly correct. Fortunately, the value of J is so small that estimating its value is not very critical. J must be artificially raised by a factor of almost a thousand before it significantly affects eye movements.[5] For a typical peak acceleration of 50,000 deg/sec^2 the inertial force is only 3 g, which is small compared to other forces (e.g., F_a, which is about 100 g at such times).

Thomas and collaborators[6-8] used an accelerometer mounted on a contact lens. By vibrating the eye sinusoidally, they found a resonance at about 60 Hz with a damping coefficient of 0.51. Various models of the plant[9-11] contain a pair of complex poles (in the Laplace transform) at a similar frequency and damping ratio. The main source of this resonance is probably the moment of inertia, J, and the stiffness of the series-elastic element, k_s. The latter is estimated at 5 g/deg for the stiffness, $2 k_s$, of a pair of muscles (see below) so that the resonant frequency $\sqrt{2k_s/J}/2\pi$, using the above value of J, would be 45 Hz. The agreement with the observed value is close enough, considering the roughness of the approximations, to make it likely that these spring-mass elements cause the resonance.

However, it must be stressed that the effect of this resonance on eye movements is negligible because of the large amount of damping contained in all other elements of the plant. The behavior of models is insensitive to J and this element could probably even be ignored.

B. Passive Orbital Tissues

The passive tissues include all nonmuscular suspensory tissues such as Tenon's capsule, the optic nerve, the fat pad, and the conjunctiva. Together, they form some sort of viscoelasticity. The force-displacement curve of the net elasticity has been measured[12] and has the form,

$$P = 0.48 E + 1.56 \times 10^{-4} E^3 \qquad (4)$$

Out to about 20 deg, the cubic term may be neglected. The linear slope k_p may vary considerably among individuals. The value 0.48 g/deg came from eyes in which the total stiffness, measured by pulling on an intact, covered eye while the opposite eye fixated, was around 1.5 g/deg. However, Collins[13] finds that 1.0 g/deg is more representative of the population so that a value for k_p of 0.32, determined by scaling all springs down together, may be more correct for the average eye.

When the human eye, with horizontal recti detached, is displaced and suddenly released, it returns rapidly by about 61% of the way with a time constant of about 0.02 sec, and then creeps the rest of the way with a time constant of about 1 sec.[14] This behavior indicates that at least two viscoelastic elements are needed as shown in Figure 1. From the above values, one can deduce the following: k_{p1}, 0.79; k_{p2}, 1.22; r_{p1}, 0.0158; r_{p2}, 1.22. (Note that k_p is the stiffness of k_{p1} and k_{p2} in series.)

If the model is to be used to look at events during and just after a saccade, the elements (k_{p2}, r_{p2}) with a one-second time constant can be ignored. Taking into account the elasticity in the muscles, k_{p2} would cause the eye to creep, after a saccade, by a total of 17% of the saccade size. However, the rate of creep is very slow, only 3.4% after 0.2 sec (the usual intersaccadic interval) which can be neglected. Presumably, some adjustment of innervation is needed to prevent this post-saccadic creep. Such a change has not been noticed in the discharge rate of motoneurons, but it has probably been overlooked because it is so small. However, such a phenomenon could account for reports of hysteresis in R_m (see below).

C. Passive Muscle Tissues

The force-displacement curve of passive human eye muscles has been measured.[3,12] It is shown in Figure 3 as the curve marked F_p and in the box $F_p(L)$ in Figure 1. For computational purposes, the curve may be described by the hyperbola,

$$F_p = \frac{k}{2}(\Delta \ell - 6.4) + \sqrt{\frac{k^2}{4}(\Delta \ell - 6.4)^2 + a^2} \qquad (5)$$

where k is the slope of the asymptote for lengthening muscle and a determines the curvature of the hyperbola. In order to extrapolate from one muscle to another of different length, it is best to express length changes $\Delta \ell$ not in mm, but as a percent of the muscle's length in the primary position. For the lateral rectus, for example, which has a fleshy portion 49.11 mm long, the conversion factors are 2.04%/mm or 0.44%/deg. The variable $\Delta \ell$ in Equation 5 and Figure 3 is expressed in % in which case k has the value 1.8 g/% and a the value 6.24 g. In terms of equivalent eye rotation, the ascending asymptote has a slope of k (denoted by k_{pm} in Figure 1) of 0.79 g/deg and it intercepts the abscissa at ±14.5 deg. The slope of the line at the primary position is 0.13 g/deg.

Collins studied this element in the cat[14] and found that 71% of the stiffness of the element was undamped. All the components in his model of this element were very nonlinear and depended on the applied force. In view of these complications the viscosity of this element, r_{pm}, has simply been neglected in plant models.[11,15] However, Collins and colleagues have implanted a strain gauge in series with a human extraocular muscle during the course of strabismus surgery[15] and found that during a saccade the tension in the antagonist tendon did not fall to zero. It rose initially, probably because the muscle's force-velocity element had not yet been totally deactivated, but the force continued to be maintained at around 12 to 20 g throughout the duration of the saccade, during which time, of course, the contractile element should be unable to exert any force because the muscle is electrically silent. This force is probably due, then, to r_{pm} indicating that this element is far from negligible. At the moment, there is considerable uncertainty about the viscosity of passive muscle and how it depends on velocity, direction, and length. There seems little doubt that the value chosen for this viscosity will have a considerable effect on a model's behavior and our lack of any certain knowledge of its properties is certainly a source of indeterminacy in any model.

D. The Series-Elastic Element

When a tetanized muscle is suddenly released, it shortens almost instantaneously by about 5% of its normal operating length. Using the lateral rectus as an example (which converts at 0.44%/deg) this amounts to 11.3 deg of eye rotation. It is estimated that the tetanic tension of a human eye muscle is about 100 g (see below). Thus, the mean series-elastic stiffness, k_s, would be about 100 g/11.3 deg or 8.8 g/deg. However, this element shown as $F_d(L_s)$ in Figure 1 is very nonlinear. The results of Wilkie,[16] for example, can be fit by,

$$F_d = c\, L_s^2 \tag{6}$$

where c is a constant. The slope of Equation 6 is twice the mean slope when the muscle is bearing a lot of tension, so that 17.6 g/deg is a better estimate of k_s in a working situation.

Collins measured the stiffness k_s in a human eye muscle and found 2.5 g/deg.[15] The discrepancy between calculated and measured values (almost 10:1) can easily be accounted for if one realizes that the normally innervated eye muscle is far from tetanized. In the primary position, the force is only 12 g,[3] almost 1/10 the tetanic value. Scaling 17.6 down by 12/100 yields 2.12 g/deg, which is quite close to the measured value. However, this scaling only applies if one assumes that the series-elastic element is not in the tendon, but in the muscle fiber. If k_s were in the tendon, its value would be independent of the number of fibers active, while if it were in the sarcomere, it should be roughly proportional to developed force (neglecting the variations in size and types of muscle fibers). The fact that scaling k_s by muscle force works so well indicates that most of the series-elastic element resides inside the sarcomere and not in the tendon. Collins' study[14] shows rather clearly that the stiffness of $F_d(L_s)$ varies directly with F_a and more evidence to this effect will appear below.

If one accepts this hypothesis (and it is generally accepted by muscle physiologists that at least a large portion, if not all, of k_s is in the sarcomere) then the series-elastic element becomes a beast of hitherto unsuspected complexity because L_s is no longer just a function of F_d, but is also a function of F_a as indicated by the dashed lines in Figure 1. The notion of using a linear, time-invariant spring to model this element becomes rather questionable. It is claimed that k_s, which is the stiffest spring in the plant, is so stiff that nonlinearities or other variations are not important. However, using the value 2 g/deg, a change in muscle force of only 20 g can stretch this element by 10 deg. That is hardly negligible. Now, if the stiffness of this element can drop to zero in an antagonist when the innervation (or F_a) is zero, or can rise by a factor of 10 in an agonist, maximally excited, the approximation by a fixed spring approaches the absurd. Unless proven otherwise, this element forms a very large source of indeterminacy in any model and such a model would simulate saccades correctly in spite of, not because of, the state of our knowledge about the behavior.

The fact that $F_d(L_s)$ is modulated by F_a raises some fascinating and unexplored avenues in muscle mechanics. F_a can change in three ways: (1) by recruitment of new fibers, (2) a change in muscle length, or (3) a change in discharge rate. If the elastance were, say, in the actin filaments, k_s would vary in condition 1, but not 2 or 3, where F_a varies with the number and rate of active bridges formed. If k_s were in the bridges (which seems likely, just looking to see which is the weakest structure morphologically), then it would vary in all three situations. Collins[14] has shown that k_s does vary when the frequency of stimulation was altered while keeping recruitment and L constant, which is good evidence that the series-elastic element not only resides in the sarcomere, but in the actin-myosin bridges. There is an interesting consequence of this:

in the steady state, the series-elastic element will always be stretched by the same length regardless of muscle force.

This result can be seen from Equation 6. If the elasticity is mainly in the bridges, then the coefficient c should not be a constant, but should be directly proportional to F_a. If this substitution is made, F_a and F_d, which are equal in the steady state, cancel out which means that L_s is a constant. Put another way, individual bridges are either made or broken in an all-or-none fashion. When made, they therefore exert their maximum tension and are maximally extended in the steady state. The muscle's force is varied only by changing the rate at which the bridges are remade or the number of bridges active. However, since the bridges are all in parallel, the series-elastic element, which is the combined elasticity of all the bridges, is also maximally extended regardless of the number of bridges active.

It is not surprising that modelers of the oculomotor system have not included the parametric modulation of $F_d(L_s)$ by F_a in their models since muscle physiologists themselves have apparently neither described or investigated the phenomenon, but the experimental results described above make it quite certain that the stiffness of the series-elastic element is not independent of F_a. The effect on model performance of allowing $F_d(L_s)$ to be nonlinear and parametrically modulated by F_a has not been investigated, but there is little doubt that the effects would not be negligible.

E. The Force-Velocity Relationship

The way in which the force of the contractile element, F_d, depends on its rate of change of length, $\dot{L}_c$, has been described by Hill[17] by the hyperbola,

$$v = \frac{b(F_0 - F_d)}{F_d + a} \tag{7}$$

where a and b are constants, F_0 is the maximum tetanic value of F_a, and v is the velocity of shortening, $-\dot{L}_c$. This curve is the right-hand curve in the upper half of Figure 2A. The following treatment is that of Cook, Stark and Clark.[11,18] The force F_v lost to the muscle's viscous-like element is found by,

$$F_v = F_d - F_0 = -\frac{(a + F_0)}{b + v}\, v = \frac{(a + F_0)}{b - \dot{L}_c}\, \dot{L}_c \tag{8}$$

This relationship is the most negative curve in the lower half of Figure 2B. An important, but still unresolved question, is what happens in a normal, nontetanized muscle where F_0 is replaced by F_a which can change through recruitment, changes in length, and changes in motoneuron discharge rate. Abbott and Wilkie[19] changed F_0 (or F_a) by changing muscle length and found that the force-velocity curve for each value of F_0 tended to cross the v axis at a constant intercept v_{max} which is off-scale in Figure 2A.

It should be remarked that the finding of a constant v_{max} is not generally accepted. Carlson[20] felt that v_{max} decreased with F_0 and the curves measured by Bahler et al.,[21] for example, show the same result. However, the region of disagreement is in a region that is difficult to reach experimentally, since even a totally unloaded muscle will usually not shorten at more than about $\frac{2}{3}\, v_{max}$. Since muscles do not operate in this region and Equation 7 is a good approximation in the region in which they do operate, one might as well adopt the hypothesis that v_{max} is fixed.

In that case, v_{max} may be found from Equation 7 by setting F_d to zero:

$$v_{max} = \frac{b}{a}\, F_a \tag{9}$$

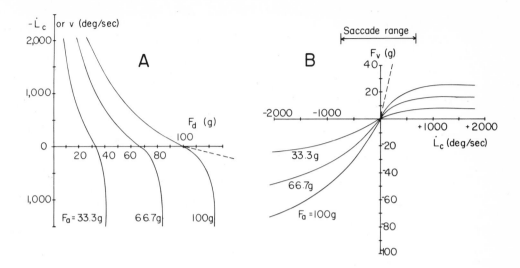

FIGURE 2. The force-velocity relationship. (A) The upper-half shows the conventional plot of velocity of shortening v (or $-\dot{L}_c$) plotted against developed force F_d, as shown in Equation 7. The right-hand curve assumes that a tetanized, isometric human eye muscle exerts about 100 g. The other two curves pertain to a partially innervated muscle in which active-state tension F_a is varied to ⅔ and ⅓ of maximum. If extended upward, all curves would cross the ordinate at v_{max} which, according to Close and Luff[22] would be near 5689 deg/sec. When partially innervated muscle is forcibly extended, the muscle slips (curves in lower half). These curves have been roughly extrapolated from data by Joyce and Rack;[23] (B) The same curves as in A, but with F_v (the force $F_d - F_a$) plotted against $\dot{L}_c$ to emphasize that this element is a nonlinear viscosity. The lower curves are described by Equation 8. The saccadic range is ±700 deg/sec which is the peak velocity for most large, human saccades. The muscles are never asked to work outside this range. The dashed lines indicate data from Katz[33] in tetanized muscle who failed to observe slipping.

where F_0 is now replaced by F_a. If v_{max} is to be constant as F_a changes, either a or b must also change and experimental curves could be matched if one assumed that the value of a was 1.25 F_a.[19] Note that with this assumption, v_{max} has the value 4 b. Equation 8 becomes,

$$ F_v = \left(\frac{1.25\ F_a}{b - \dot{L}_c} \right) \dot{L}_c \tag{10} $$

Curves of this equation for several values of F_a are shown in Figure 2B. Collins,[14] in cat eye muscle, showed that $F_v(\dot{L}_c)$ changed with F_a when the latter was altered by changing only the frequency of stimulation and, in human eye muscle he observed the same effect when F_a was altered naturally by both firing rate and recruitment.[15] Consequently, we may assume that Equation 10 applies no matter how F_a is caused to change, and this parametric modulation is shown by a dashed line in Figure 1.

A fairly good estimate can be made for the value of b. Human saccades can easily reach 700 deg/sec and the agonist is far from unloaded at such times. Thus, v_{max} should be well in excess of 2000 deg/sec so that b (which equals 0.25 v_{max}) must be larger than 500. It is difficult to extrapolate from experiments on other muscles since v_{max} depends critically on temperature and the composition of muscle fiber types, so that even correcting for muscle length (by expressing v_{max} in percent change of muscle length/sec), many different values of v_{max} may be found in the literature.

However, Close and Luff[22] examined the force-velocity relationship of rat extraocular muscle at 35°C. The value of v_{max}, assuming a sarcomere length of 2.2 μm, at L_0

was 28.1 $L_0's/sec$ (L_0 is the length at which maximal F_a occurs). If this were the value appropriate for the human lateral rectus of 49.11 mm length, this value would convert to 1380 mm/sec or 6377 deg/sec. The medial rectus is shorter (38.51 mm) so its v_{max} would be 5001 deg/sec. Perhaps the average of 5689 deg/sec would be more appropriate if, as usual, one assumes that the two antagonist muscles are identical. Lacking any better evidence directly dealing with cat, monkey, or human eye muscles, this value for v_{max} must be accepted until something better comes along.

Although our muscles spend almost as much time lengthening, while activated, as shortening, little attention has been paid to their behavior in this situation. Joyce and Rack[23] showed that in a condition resembling normal innervation, muscles slip. At a certain force above F_a, the muscle acts as though the bridges were forcibly broken, lessening the time during which they can bear tension, and allowing the muscle to extend at higher and higher velocities as F_d increases beyond F_a. These curves for various F_a, shown in the lower half of Figure 2A and the upper half of Figure 2B, have not been fit by an equation or used in any model of the oculomotor plant.

F. Length-Tension Curves

The curves which relate total muscle force, F, to changes in muscle length $\Delta\ell$ (expressed as a percentage of the muscle's length in the primary position) have been measured[12] and can be fit by the hyperbolae,[3]

$$F = \frac{k}{2}(\Delta\ell + e) + \sqrt{\frac{k^2}{4}(\Delta\ell + e)^2 + a^2} \qquad (11)$$

This equation is similar to Equation 5 and the values of k and a are the same (1.8 g/% and 6.24 g, respectively). The variable e is a dummy variable that slides the curve in the direction of shorter muscle lengths and, thus, simulates an increased innervation as shown by the thin lines in Figure 3. The force F_a is total force less passive force,

$$F_a = F - F_p \qquad (12)$$

By substituting Equations 11 and 5 in 12, one can generate the family of length-tension curves (active-state tension) for various levels of innervation shown by the thick lines in Figure 3 and in the box marked F_a (L_c, I_e) in Figure 1. The relationship between I and e will be described shortly.

Experimentally, force was plotted against changes in muscle length $\Delta\ell$ and that is the variable used in the above equations, but F_a should be plotted against changes in L_c which must be done by subtracting out changes in L_s. If one approximated the series-elastic element by a fixed, linear spring of stiffness k_s, then each point on the curves in Equation 12 (thin lines, Figure 3) should be displaced to the left by the amount F/k_s. Or, one could use the nonlinear fixed spring described by Equation 6. However, if most of L_s is in the bridges then, in the steady state, L_s is a constant which is about 5% of the primary-position, muscle length and is equivalent to 11.3 deg. Thus, in my opinion, the curves of Equation 12 should all be shifted to the left *en bloc* by 5% (in the dimensions of $\Delta\ell$ and e) or 11.3 deg, and this is what has been done in Figure 3 to obtain the heavy lines.

The slope of the curves $F_a(L_c,I_e)$ approaches zero as L_c becomes large in either direction. The maximum slope, for large I_e in the range of L_c just less than the primary position length, is 0.79 g/deg. The slope at the primary position for large I_e approaches 0.66 g/deg but for normal, primary-position innervation the slope is 0.42 g/deg. Consequently, the model eye described by these equations has a total stiffness of 1.58 g/

deg: the passive muscle tissues contributing 0.13 for each of two muscles, the contractile components contributing 0.42 each, while k_p contributes 0.48. It has already been remarked[13] that subsequent studies show 1.0 g/deg more representative of the average total stiffness and the curves $F_a(L_c,I_e)$ should perhaps be scaled down accordingly.

It will be noted that recruitment of parallel, identical muscle fibers should not result in a set of $F_a(L_c,I_e)$ curves which map into each other by sliding along the L_c axis. It has been argued by some, who feel that a stretch reflex is obligatory for every muscle in the body,[24] that only such a reflex could produce such curves despite the fact that this reflex cannot be discovered in eye muscles by the great majority of researchers (see especially Reference 25). However, when one sees the great variety of lengths of muscle fibers in an eye muscle and considers that they contribute force over a wide spread of ranges centered about different lengths at which peak force is developed, it is not difficult to see how the observed behavior of $F_a(L_c,I_e)$ can come about by the order of recruitment of various muscle fiber types. More empirically, parallelism between length-tension curves for different levels of innervation has been observed in eye muscles in which any hypothetical stretch reflex could play no role.[5,14]

G. The Time Course of Innervation

It is, of course, necessary to know the input wave-form if one is going to use a correct model output to argue that the model is correct. The bandwidth of most natural input signals which cause, say pursuit or vergence movements, is so low that a model's response tells one nothing about many of the elements which only affect behavior in the high-frequency region and saccades are the only type of eye movement that contain such high-frequency signal components. Yet, until recently, only the crudest characteristics of the input wave-form for saccades was known. Individual motoneurons begin bursting at high discharge rates (e.g., 400 spikes/sec) about 8 msec before the eye is seen to move, continue to fire at a high rate during the saccade and, roughly 8 msec before the end, abruptly drop their rate back to a constant postsaccadic rate. (The 8 msec dead-time can be ignored for the purposes of this chapter.) Thus, the rate $R_m(t)$, has been approximated as a rectangular pulse with a flat top and vertical leading and trailing edges followed by a step, and this waveform has been accepted as sufficiently realistic to be useful.[5,11,18]

However, a rectangular pulse and step is certainly a rather crude approximation of the actual wave-form of $R_m(t)$. Variations in saccade size are effected by changes in peak firing rate,[26,27] as well as the duration of the high-frequency burst. Examples of averaged wave-forms of $R_m(t)$ for saccades of various sizes for one motoneuron are shown in Figure 4. The intrasaccadic rate is not constant; the rate falls off slowly and then more rapidly toward the end of a saccade.[27] There is also a spread of about ±4 msec in the time by which R_m leads saccade onset for a given neuron from saccade to saccade and among different neurons for a single saccade. This suggests that averaging across time for a single neuron, as in Figure 4, is equivalent to averaging over the population for a single saccade. In that case, the net innervation, I, which accounts for both the discharge rate modulation and recruitment, rises from the pre- to the per-saccadic rate smoothly over about 8 msec. Thus, the wave-form I(t) does not have an abrupt rise. A similar 8 msec spread at saccade offset is largely masked by the fact that the net innervation falls to the post-saccadic rate, rather slowly, toward the end of a saccade. The end result is that the approximation of an abrupt jump-up and jump-down in innervation is quite incorrect and imposes an unrealistic situation on any model.

A problem which remains unresolved is the fact that experiments in which an eye muscle or its nerve is artificially stimulated indicate that such muscles do not develop

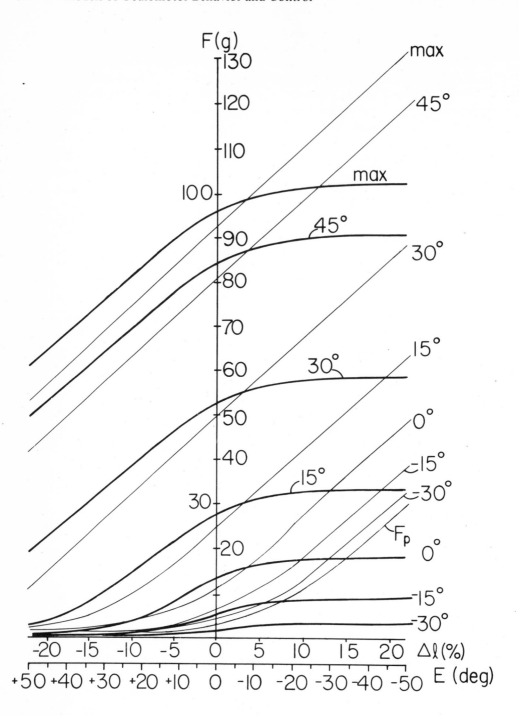

FIGURE 3.   The length-tension-innveration curves of a human, lateral-rectus, eye muscle. The force F_a in g (ordinate) is plotted as a function of muscle length Δl, expressed as a percentage of primary-position length, or its equivalent in degrees of eye rotation E. Thin lines represent total muscle force F when innervation is varied by attempts to look straight ahead (0°) and 15, 30, and 45° left and right. The curve for −45° is omitted for clarity. The curve F_p represents a totally passive muscle. The curve max is an estimate of behavior when the muscle is maximally innervated. The thick lines were obtained by subtracting F_p from each thin line to obtain active state tension F_a and then shifting the result to the left by 5% or 11.3° to correct for the length of the series elastic element. The thick lines then represent the curves $F_a(L_c, l_e)$.

SPIKES SEC⁻¹

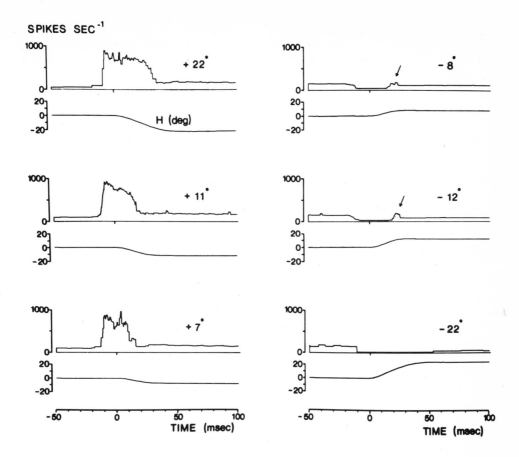

FIGURE 4. The time course of $R_m(t)$ for saccades of various sizes and directions. These records came from unpublished observations by J. A. M. van Gisbergen, S. Geelen, and the author. The instantaneous discharge rate $R_m(t)$ of an abducens motoneuron (upper traces) and eye position (lower traces) were averaged over about 10 saccades, all of the same size and direction, made by a trained monkey. The motoneuron burst at typically 800 spikes/sec when its muscle is an agonist (saccade sizes $+22°$, $+11°$, $+7°$) and is totally inhibited for saccades in the other direction ($-8°$, $-12°$, $-22°$). Arrows point to a brief excitatory pulse in the antagonist at the end of a saccade which probably acts to dynamically brake the eye. The origin of the time base is the beginning of the saccade.

additional tension, F_a, for stimulus frequencies above 200 Hz. One may then ask what is the point of motoneurons bursting at 400 Hz? The answer currently accepted is that while F_a may not increase, the rate of change, dF_a/dt, in an isometric muscle, continues to increase as stimulus rate increases.[28] In any case, there is obviously a saturation phenomenon and above a certain level, I(t) no longer causes an increase in the curve $F_a(L_c)$. This is shown by a nonlinearity in Figure 1 which relates an effective innervation, I_e, to the net neural innervation I. I_e may be measured in terms of the force which it creates. Since F_a depends on length as well as innervation, one can define innervation I_e as that force which a muscle can produce at a given length, in this case, the length in the primary position where $\Delta\ell$ is zero. Thus, from Equation 11,

$$I_e = \frac{k}{2} e + \sqrt{\frac{k^2}{4} e^2 + a^2} - F_p(0) \qquad (13)$$

where $F_p(0)$ is the passive force from Equation 5 evaluated when $\Delta\ell$ is zero (about 1.3 g).

Equation 13 forms a link between e, which is a dummy variable representing inner-vation, and I_e which is, at least, a more intuitive way of expressing innervation at the level of the muscle. If one wished to run a numerical simulation, I_e would be first determined for each muscle at any instant of time and e may be found from the inverse of Equation 13:

$$e = \frac{(I_e + F_p(0))^2 - a^2}{k(I_e + F_p(0))}$$

(14)

After this, one may then use Equations 11 and 12 to find F_a.

The most important part of the nonlinearity between I and I_e is the level of satura-tion. How much force can an eye muscle exert? Collins attempted to determine this by measuring the isometric muscle force in the agonist during attempted 45 deg sac-cades.[15] He found that the maximum value of I_e was about 92 g. Because of the length-tension curve, the maximum value of total force F drops to 55 when the muscle is shortened by 45 deg and rises to 130 g when the muscle is lengthened by 45 deg (Figure 3, uppermost curve).

It is also known that active-state tension lags behind when I changes rapidly. This can be simulated (Figure 1) by allowing I_e to lag I by an activation process $[1/(s\tau_a + 1)]$ when I is increasing and a deactivation process $[1/(s\tau_d + 1)]$ when I is decreasing. The processes are probably related to the diffusion and resequestering of C_a^{++} ions in the excitation-contraction process. Unfortunately, essentially nothing is known about τ_a and τ_d. It is generally thought that τ_a is smaller than τ_d on the basis of the rise and fall of isometric force during stimulation by stimulus trains of sudden onset and offset, but muscle physiologists have not, I believe, measured these values in muscles operat-ing in a situation resembling the in vivo condition.

The wave-form of $I_e(t)$ also depends on initial eye position and saccade direction because the model is clearly nonlinear [primarily because of $F_a(L_c,I_e)$]. Therefore, the presumed amplitude and duration of the burst, even assuming a rectangular pulse and step, should differ depending on the location of the initial and final eye position. Some information is available on this subject from human emg studies,[15] but no models have been tested to probe the nonlinearity of the elasticities, the effects of which become important as the eye moves further away from the primary position.

At one time, it was thought that the eye was actively checked at the end of a saccade by a pulse of activity in the lengthening muscle. When it was discovered that the inertia of the eyeball was negligible,[5] the notion of active checking or braking was abandoned. Too quickly, as it now turns out. When $R_m(t)$ is averaged over many saccades made by a trained monkey, there emerges a small, but distinguishable increase in $R_m(t)$ just at the end of a saccade in antagonist motoneurons (arrows, Figure 4). The pulse occurs in most, but not all motoneurons. A corresponding inhibition of the agonist is not seen. The pulse is so small that it is not noticeable in individual recordings of spike trains even when one is looking for it. A similar observation has been reported in single-unit, emg recordings in human eye muscles.[29] The effect of this pulse is not to make a second, small saccade in the opposite direction — which does occur in certain situations,[30] is called dynamic overshoot, and is generated neurally[27] — but simply to brake the on-going saccade and bring the eye to rest more quickly. This rather recent finding has not yet been incorporated in models of eye mechanics.

In summary, there are a large number of uncertainties about the shape of the driving wave-form during saccades and how the innervation is transformed into active-state tension. Since the behavior of any model will be directly affected by all the phenomena discussed in this section, it is important to resolve these uncertainties, since one can hardly be certain that the parameters of the model are correctly chosen if one is still unsure about the shape of the input signal.

H. Hysteresis

There is a curious problem that has so far been ignored by all modelers: when most biological tissues, in this case muscle and fascia, are extended to a given length, they exert more force than when shortened to that length. One might suppose then that, in the monkey, R_m which generates muscle force, would be different when the eye came to a given position from one or another direction. One study has reported such an hysteresis in the amount of up to 15%.[31] Oddly, many other studies of ocular motoneurons in the monkey have failed to observe this phenomenon (e.g., Reference 32). Yet, mechanical and innervational hysteresis of large amounts (e.g., 50% in force and ±12 deg in eye position) have been reported in studies of human eye muscles.[13,15] There is something very wrong here. In the face of such contradictory evidence, it is no wonder that modelers have simply ignored hysteresis. However, the possibility that hysteresis may somehow play a role in plant mechanics is very real and, if that is the case, the models proposed so far could be ghastly caricatures of the real situation. It is a pity that this threat has not yet induced anyone to get to the bottom of this puzzle through physiological experiments.

IV. PUBLISHED MODELS

There currently exists two fairly complete models of the oculomotor plant.* One is by Cook and Stark,[18] first published in 1967. In 1974, it was modified by Clark and Stark[11] and will be referred to as the Cook-Clark-Stark model. The other model was presented by Collins in 1975.[15] I shall not include comments on my own early model in 1964,[5] since it was very elementary and was only designed to emphasize two points not realized at the time: the major impedance to movements of the eye is viscous, not inertial, and to move such a load rapidly, one needs a pulse-step input of innervation. In many other regards, my model was too simple and could not benefit from the physiological findings which have appeared since.[3,12]

A. Inertia of the Globe

The Cook-Clark-Stark model used 4.3×10^{-5} g/(deg/sec²) for the inertia J. Collins ignored J. As mentioned, J is almost negligible but nevertheless, a sensitivity analysis should be done to see if J really can be left out without causing some small but noticeable effect.

B. Passive Orbital Tissues

Both models used a single viscoelasticity and ignored the slow creep element (r_{p2}, k_{p2}). Both ignored the nonlinearity, which is reasonable for a start, and rounded k_p off to 0.5 g/deg. The main discrepancies are in the viscosity. The Cook-Clark-Stark model used data from experiments on the cat eye and used a 30 msec time constant. This would make r_{p1} equal to 0.015 g/(deg/sec) but 0.018 was actually used. Collins chose a time constant of 120 msec so that r_{p1} was 0.06 g/(deg/sec). The former figure would seem more appropriate since, if one is ignoring creep, the short time constant of the human quick-release response is only 20 msec.

C. Passive Muscle Tissues

Despite the ease in modern digital simulation of incorporating nonlinearities, both models approximated $F_p(L)$ by straight-line segments. Collins let F_p be zero for L less than 25 deg and rise linearly with L at a rate of 1.2 g/deg. The latter figure is based

---

* See Addendum.

on the assumption that the series-elastic element was in series with $F_p(L)$. Collins assumed that the former had the value of 2.5 g/deg which, in series with the latter, would give the correct net stiffness of 0.79 g/deg. It is very likely that, as already discussed, the series-elastic element is in the sarcomere and in parallel with $F_p(L)$. The intercept of 25 deg is rather large and, from Equation 5 and Figure 3, $F_p(L)$ is by no means zero for E less than $+25$ deg. The slope of $F_p(L)$ for a pair of muscles at the primary position is 0.26 g/deg which is not negligible. The effect of Collins' approximation on the saccadic behavior of the model is unknown.

The Cook-Clark-Stark model over-estimates k_{pm}. This model assumes that the slope of the rising asymptote is 1.0 g/deg (rather than 0.79 g/deg). This is not the problem: the asymptote is assumed to cut the abscissa at 0 deg. When two antagonist muscles are put together, the net result is a constant slope of 1.0 g/deg for all eye positions. Thus, this model has a slope of $F_p(L)$ for two muscles in the primary position of 1.0 g/deg rather than the actual value of 0.26 g/deg. Again, the consequences of this approximation are not known. The approximations in both models seem quite unnecessary, since $F_p(L)$ is known and the compromise caused by using straight-line approximations with incorrect intercepts having not been evaluated. One would assume that using the measured values of $F_p(L)$ would have been appropriate unless it were clear that it made no difference and one is reluctant to assume, when, at 15 deg eccentric gaze, one model predicts that F_p will be zero and the other predicts it will be 15 g (the correct value is in between), that these assumptions do not make a difference.

An even worse problem concerns viscosity. The Cook-Clark-Stark model assumes that the viscosity r_{pm} is zero. The evidence from implanted strain gauges found by Collins shows that the deactivated antagonist, during a saccade, still exerts a large resistance to lengthening so r_{pm} is clearly not zero. Collins put this viscosity into the force-velocity relationship of muscle and assigned it a value of 0.12 g/(deg/sec) (see below). The disagreement here is obvious. The Cook-Clark-Stark model badly underestimates r_{pm} and their model's behavior (concerning antagonist per-saccadic force) is quite incompatible with Collins' strain gauge data. Collins retains a passive muscle viscosity but assigns it to the wrong muscle element.

D. The Series-Elastic Element

Both models used a fixed, linear spring. Collins used a stiffness of 2.5 g/deg; the Cook-Clark-Stark model used 1.8 g/deg. Neither model investigated the notion of parametric modulation of this spring. It is difficult to guess what would be the effects in these models of letting $F_d(L_s)$ be both nonlinear and modulated by F_a. It is hard to imagine that the effects would not be significant. This is a case where the results of experimental muscle physiology are badly needed, since it would be less than useful to second-guess the outcome of experiments not yet done.

E. The Force-Velocity Relationship

The Cook-Clark-Stark model estimates v_{max} to be 3600 deg/sec (or b in Equation 10 to be 900 deg/sec). This value could be an underestimate in view of the values found in rat eye muscle, at 35°C, equivalent to 5689 deg/sec (see above). This value pertains primarily to fast-twitch fibers,[22] but it is they which probably generate most of the saccadic force. If this value of v_{max} does pertain to human eye muscle, the Cook-Clark-Stark model underestimates it by 37%. Perhaps some of the viscosity in this model should be taken out of this element and put in r_{pm}.

This model used a description of lengthening muscle reported by Katz[33] who failed to observe the slipping phenomenon and reported a large increase in viscosity of forcibly-lengthened, tetanized muscle indicated by dashed lines in Figure 2. However, using this incorrect description in this model made little difference because when F_{a2}

drops to a value close to zero (2 g was assumed in this model), the force F_{v2}, which is still directly proportional to F_a, becomes so small as to be negligible (less than 3.3 g for a 500 deg/sec saccade). However, during the time of deactivation there will be a transient viscous drag, and that could be in error if the correct description for lengthening muscle is not used.

Collins tried to estimate the force-velocity relationship in human eye muscles by observing the recovery of force after a quick lengthening. This method is not very accurate compared to the classical isotonic method and one should note that the results pertain to lengthening muscle although they were applied, in the model, to muscle that was either lengthening or shortening. This is certainly incorrect. The results were fit by

$$F_v = \frac{0.12 + 0.0052\, F_a\, (1 - e^{-t/0.02})}{1 + \dfrac{|\dot{L}_c|}{200}}\; \dot{L}_c \qquad (15)$$

This equation has been modified from that first put forward by Collins[15] by personal communication with him. The major change is in the denominator: the variable $\dot{L}_s$ is replaced by $\dot{L}_c$ because F_v can only, by definition, depend on the latter. The absolute value sign prevents the denominator from becoming zero when $\dot{L}_c$ is -200 deg/sec. The original intent was to let F_a in the numerator reflect only changes in innervation I, but that would neglect the fact that F_a also changes with $\dot{L}_c$, so I suggest the simpler and broader interpretation of using F_a rather than I here.

The exponential term $(1 - e^{-t/0.02})$ is meant to reflect a 20 msec lag between F_a and its effect on F_v (time, t, starts after each abrupt change in F_a). Little is known about τ_a and τ_d and Collins evidently felt that his data were best approximated if both time constants equalled 20 msec. Unfortunately, little evidence was provided to support this choice.

If the lag element is ignored (or built into the relationship between I and F_a), Equation 15 can be rewritten,

$$F_v = \frac{24 + 1.04\, F_a}{200 + |\dot{L}_c|}\; \dot{L}_c \qquad (16)$$

This form is quite similar to Equation 10 for shortening muscle ($\dot{L}_c$ negative) except for the constant term in the numerator. The equation reflects the main nonlinearity of Hill's equation: as v increases, the slope d F_v/dv decreases. In fact, it assigns to b in Equation 10 the value 200 which makes v_{max} equal to 800 deg/sec. This is obviously much too slow since muscles can shorten at this or higher speeds during saccades. A minimum estimate for v_{max} is 2000 deg/sec. Thus, Collins' model is much too heavily damped.

The constant term of 24 g in the numerator of Equation 16 must reflect a viscosity in the passive muscle tissues since its presence is still felt when F_a is zero. When $\dot{L}_c$ is small, it has the value, r_{pm}, of 24/200 or 0.12 g/(deg/sec). This viscosity is not small. In Equation 16, if F_{a2} is zero (the antagonist) and eye velocity is 500 deg/sec, F_{v2} is 17 g. As mentioned, the Cook-Clark-Stark model ignored r_{pm}. Collins appears to have done the same but would seem to have, in fact, hidden it in the force-velocity relationship. It is this constant term that allows his model to simulate the fact, discovered by an implant strain gauge, that the force of a lengthening, inactivated, antagonist muscle remains in the vicinity of 12 to 20 g during a saccade.

F. Length-Tension Curves

The Cook-Clark-Stark model assumes that F_a does not depend on L_c so the heavy curves, Figure 3, would be replaced by a family of horizontal lines. It is easy to see why this approximation was made in 1967[18] (I did the same in 1964),[5] but it is not clear why it was retained in 1974[11] after the length-tension curves had been measured. In the primary position, 53% of the total stiffness of an eye is due to the length-tension curves $F_a(L_c, I_e)$.

When one assumes that F_a does not depend on L_c, difficulties arise. If, for example, the eye is at $+30$ deg and makes a saccade back to zero, the antagonist muscle has a stiffness dF_a/dL_c of about 0.79 g/deg just before the saccade and this stiffness drops to zero when the muscle is deactivated. There is no corresponding rise in agonist stiffness, since it is operating in a region where dF_a/dL_c is nearly zero. It is hard to believe that the sudden loss of 50% of the total orbital stiffness will not influence the time course of the saccade. Another problem is that, in Equation 10, F_v depends on F_a which in turn depends on L_c. However, if F_a is not allowed to vary with L_c, an important source of modulation of $F_v(L_c)$ is removed. During a 30 deg saccade from the primary position, the per-saccadic decrease of F_a in the agonist is about 30% just due to shortening. The fact that the Cook-Clark-Stark model was so successful in generating normal saccadic wave-forms with an incorrect set of curves $F_a(L_c, I_e)$ indicates how little correct output behavior tells one about the uniqueness of the model's elements.

Collins used a slope dF_a/dL_c of 1.2 g/deg so that when put in series with k_s with a value of 2.5 g/deg, the net result would yield the observed value of 0.79 g/deg. I have already suggested that this adjustment could be incorrect if the series-elastic element always has a fixed steady-state extension. Collins approximated the curves in the box $F_a(L_c, I_e)$ in Figure 1 by two straight line segments:

$$F_a = I_e \qquad\qquad , E > 25 \text{ deg}$$

$$F_a = I_e + 1.2\,(E - 25) \quad , E \leq 25 \text{ deg} \qquad\qquad (17)$$

Unfortunately, this equation allows F_a to become negative if E is less than $(25 - 0.833\ I_e)$ which is a situation that can easily occur (for example, in an antagonist, where I_e is zero, it occurs for any E smaller than 25 deg, such as the primary position). The limp leash (LL, Figure 1) does not allow the muscle to push on the globe, but does allow the length-tension element to push on the force-velocity relationship which is, of course, quite unphysiological. The fact that the antagonist can help lengthen itself in this way allows the viscosity of the force-velocity relationship and/or r_{pm} to be overestimated since their effect, at least during lengthening, would be partially overcome by the pushing action of F_a. It would appear that in both models the attempt to simplify by linearization has created more problems than simplifications.

G. The Time Course of Innervation

Neither model has recognized the saturation between I and I_e, one effect of which is to allow dI_e/dt to continue to increase as dI/dt increases even though I_e itself goes into saturation. How important this phenomenon might be is unknown.

Collins used emg recordings to construct the time course of $I(t)$ for saccades of different sizes, directions, and starting positions. He recreated these wave-forms electronically to drive his model. This is certainly a realistic way to simulate the input. He evidently assumed that I_e did not saturate until I itself did, which is unlikely. Collins permitted an activation and deactivation lag to affect $F_v(\dot{L}_c)$, but not to affect $F_a(L_c, I_e)$ itself, which is not correct the use of F_a in Equation 15 is my own, not Collins'). The emg wave-forms measured by Collins show a rather long, exponential tail following the pulse for some saccades. This does not agree with the behavior of $R_m(t)$ seen in monkeys (Figure 4) and one wonders if the discrepancy is a species difference or could be methodological.

The Cook-Clark-Stark model assumes that $I(t)$ is a rectangular pulse and a step. The sharp leading and trailing edges would cause unwanted transients in the output wave-forms. To avoid these, τ_a and τ_d were introduced. There is very little physiological data on the time course of the activation and deactivation processes and the values of 4 and 8 msec, respectively, probably represent those that gave satisfactory output wave-forms. Probably τ_a and τ_d also help to simulate the slower rise and fall of $I(t)$ in a population of cells that one does not see in a single cell [$R_m(t)$]. This model also assumes that I_e rises to 100 g for saccades of all sizes. This is certainly not correct for I,[15,26,27] and for small saccades where I is below saturation, the peak value of I_e would also change with saccade size. Since the model does not allow F_a to depend on L_c, the assumed pulse height would be quite incorrect for saccades starting from different initial positions. Although it is known that the antagonist muscle is totally deactivated during a saccade, these authors, for some reason, allowed F_a to remain at 2 g during this time.

A final remark is necessary concerning Collins' model. Its performance has never been accurately tested against human saccadic wave-forms. The one example given of the model's output shows a saccade with a peak velocity which is much too small for its size; probably because of the large viscosity of the force-velocity relationships.

V. DISCUSSION

The main conclusion to be drawn from the above considerations would seem to be that more physiological data are needed. Muscle is still a poorly understood motor. Its behavior has not been described in a variety of situations. Specifically, the activation and deactivation time courses are not understood, even qualitatively, let alone quantitatively. The dependence of the force-velocity relationship on the active state, especially during transients, has not been studied. This relationship has not been quantitated in eye muscles in states of partial innervation. The idea that the series-elastic element is parametrically modulated by the active state is unexplored. Hysteresis remains unexamined.

I have not even mentioned the problem of muscle fiber types but, since they are recruited in some order related to type, the mechanical characteristics of that part of muscle which is active depends on innervation level, and by how much and in what way we simply do not know. A number of uncertainties about the driving wave-form itself have been mentioned. The comments on the published models are made only to underline in a specific way, the things we do not know about how muscle behaves.

I would suggest that models of the plant have gone about as far as they can go at the moment. They have served their original purpose — a major function of models — of illustrating how much the available data can explain. They reveal, in a very precise way, what we do and do not know about how muscles work, and this is especially revealed in the problem of eye movements where so much is known, that what is not known becomes glaringly obvious.

At the moment, further theoretical analysis can serve only one function: it is possible to determine whether a model's performance is compatible with the various assumptions that it is necessary to make by trying other assumptions or varying the currently assumed parameters. The main purpose of this exercise is to eliminate proposals in the model which are incompatible with actual behavior and help to focus on those parameters which are most deserving of further physiological investigation. So far, little of this has been done. However, I believe that we are now at the point where we need more facts about how muscles behave, rather than more modelling.

ADDENDUM

This article was written in the spring of 1979. Since then, another model has been put forth by Bahill, Latimer, and Troost.[34] It would be most inappropriate not to cite this contribution and comment upon it. This model is a modification of the Cook-Clark-Stark model: the missing length-tension curve was added. The other major change was to approximate the force-velocity relationship by a straight line the slope of which is independent of F_a; thus removing a feature which was claimed to be a major step toward realism in the Cook-Clark-Stark model. Slipping of the lengthening antagonist was recognized but since that muscle is essentially passive at that time, the viscosity used should really be assigned to r_{pm} (Figure 1) rather than the force-velocity relationship. The series-elastic element continues to be modeled by a fixed, linear spring. The length-tension curves unfortunately fail to distinguish between passive and developed muscle force so that the former is treated as though it were part of F_a. Like the Cook-Clark-Stark model, it is designed to model only saccades starting from the primary position. Without further modificaton, the model misbehaves (such as muscles pushing) if the saccade starts elsewhere. The model uses an agonist pulse which is very large and brief (e.g., 275 g for 30 msec for a 20 deg saccade). It is doubtful that the muscles are capable of such large forces. The duration of a 20 deg saccade is 70 msec and many studies in monkey indicate that pulse and saccade duration should be equal. This model lends further support to the need for more knowledge on muscle behavior. It takes yet another arrangement of model elements, approximated in new ways, driven by an unrealistic input signal and, because there are so many parameters to adjust, can make an excellent match of saccadic waveforms. It is now even more clear, looking at the three models together, that a variety of arrangements and parameter choices can all produce realistic saccades and the correct one can only be determined by experimental data.

REFERENCES

1. **Zee, D. S. and Robinson, D. A.**, Clinical applications of oculomotor models, in *Topics in Neuro-ophthalamology*, Thompson, H. S., Ed., Williams & Wilkins, Baltimore, 1979.
2. **Robinson, D. A.**, The functional behavior of the peripheral oculomotor apparatus: a review, in *Disorders of Ocular Motility*, Kommerell, G., Ed., Bergmann Verlag, München, 1978, 43.
3. **Robinson, D. A.**, A quantitative analysis of extraocular muscle cooperation and squint, *Invest. Ophthalmol.*, 14, 801, 1975.
4. **Lännergren, J.**, Structure and function of twitch and slow fibres in amphibian skeletal muscle, in *Basic Mechanisms of Ocular Motility and their Clinical Implications*, Lennerstrand, G., and Bach-y-Rita, P., Eds., Pergamon Press, Oxford, 1975, 63.
5. **Robinson, D. A.**, The mechanics of human saccadic eye movement, *J. Physiol. (London)*, 174, 245, 1964.
6. **Stone, S. L., Thomas, J. G., and Zakian, V.**, The passive rotatory characteristics of the dog's eye and its attachments, *J. Physiol.*, 181, 337, 1965.
7. **Thomas, J. G.**, The torque-angle transfer function of the human eye, *Kybernetik*, 3, 254, 1967.
8. **Thomas, J. G.**, The dynamics of small saccadic eye movements, *J. Physiol. (London)*, 200, 109, 1969.
9. **Robinson, D. A.**, The oculomotor control system: a review, *Proc. IEEE*, 56, 1032, 1968.
10. **Childress, D. S. and Jones, R. W.**, Mechanics of horizontal movement of the human eye, *J. Physiol. (London)*, 188, 273, 1967.

11. Clark, M. R. and Stark, L., Control of human eye movements. I. Modelling of extraocular muscles; II. A model for the extraocular plant mechanism; III. Dynamic characteristics of the eye tracking mechanism, *Math. Biosci.*, 20, 191, 1974.

12. Robinson, D. A., O'Meara, D. M., Scott, A. B., and Collins, C. C., Mechanical components of human eye movements, *J. Appl. Physiol.*, 26, 548, 1969.

13. Collins, C. C., unpublished observations.

14. Collins, C. C., Orbital mechanics, in *The Control of Eye Movements*, Bach-y-Rita, P. and Collins, C. C., Eds., Academic Press, New York, 1971, 283.

15. Collins, C. C., The human oculomotor control system, in *Basic Mechanisms of Ocular Motility and their Clinical Implications*, Lennerstrand, G. and Bach-y-Rita, P., Eds., Pergamon Press, Oxford, 1975, 145.

16. Wilkie, D. R., The mechanical properties of muscle, *Br. Med. Bull.*, 12, 177, 1956.

17. Hill, A. V., The heat of shortening and the dynamic constants of muscle, *Proc. R. Soc., Ser. B*, 126, 136, 1938.

18. Cook, G. and Stark, L., Derivation of a model for the human eye-positioning mechanisms, *Bull. Math. Biophys.*, 29, 153, 1967.

19. Abbott, B. C. and Wilkie, D. R., The relation between velocity of shortening and the tension length curve of skeletal muscle, *J. Physiol. (London)*, 120, 214, 1953.

20. Carlson, F. D., Kinematic studies of mechanical properties of muscle, in *Tissue Elasticity*, Remington, J. W., Ed., American Physiology Society, Washington, D.C., 1957, 55.

21. Bahler, A. S., Fales, F. T., and Zierler, K. L., The dynamic properties of mammalian skeletal muscle, *J. Gen. Physiol.*, 51, 369, 1968.

22. Close, R. I. and Luff, A. R., Dynamic properties of inferior rectus muscle of the rat, *J. Physiol. (London)*, 236, 259, 1974.

23. Joyce, G. C. and Rack, P. M. H., Isotonic lengthening and shortening movements of cat soleus muscle, *J. Physiol. (London)*, 204, 475, 1969.

24. Granit, R., The probable role of muscle spindles and tendon organs in eye movement control, in *The Control of Eye Movements*, Bach-y-Rita, P. and Collins, C. C., Eds., Academic Press, New York, 1971, 3.

25. Keller, E. L. and Robinson, D. A., Absence of a stretch reflex in extraocular muscles of the monkey, *J. Neurophysiol.*, 34, 908, 1971.

26. Keller, E. L., Participation of the medial pontine reticular formation in eye movement generation in monkey, *J. Neurophysiol.*, 37, 316, 1974.

27. Gisbergen, J. A. M. van and Robinson, D. A., Generation of micro- and macrosaccades by burst neurons in the monkey, in *Control of Gaze by Brain Stem Neurons*, Baker, R. and Berthoz, A., Eds., Elsevier, Amsterdam, 1977, 301.

28. Lennerstrand, G., Motor units in eye muscles, in *Basic Mechanisms of Ocular Motility and their Clinical Implications*, Lennerstrand, G. and Bach-y-Rita, P., Eds., Pergamon Press, Oxford, 1975, 119.

29. Sindermann, F., Geiselmann, B., and Fischler, M., Single motor unit activity in extraocular muscles in man during fixation and saccades, *Electroencephalogr. and Clin. Neurophysiol.*, 45, 64, 1978.

30. Bahill, A. T., Clark, M. R., and Stark, L., Dynamic overshoot in saccadic eye movements is caused by neurological control signal reversals, *Exp. Neurol.*, 48, 107, 1975.

31. Eckmiller, R., Hysteresis in the static characteristics of eye position coded neurons in the alert monkey, *Pflügers Arch.*, 350, 249, 1974.

32. Keller, E. L. and Robinson, D. A., Abducens unit behavior in the monkey during vergence movements, *Vision Res.*, 12, 369, 1972.

33. Katz, B., The relation between force and speed in muscular contraction, *J. Physiol. (London)*, 96, 45, 1939.

Chapter 3

THE SAMPLED DATA MODEL AND FOVEAL DEAD ZONE FOR SACCADES

Laurence R. Young

TABLE OF CONTENTS

I. INTRODUCTION

A sampled data model for the generation and control of saccadic eye movements was introduced in 1962 to provide a simple mathematical description of one dominant feature of the system — the psychological refractory period. The most direct evidence for this psychological refractory period, and the strongest support for a discrete approximation to saccadic control, came from the staircase-like saccadic temporal behavior in response to a sudden target displacement during open loop tracking. This elementary approximation served also to predict the predominant, although not exclusive, eye movement patterns observed in several other tracking situations. These included responses to target position steps, pulses of varying durations, saccadic corrections to position errors involved in pursuit tracking such as ramp and step-ramp stimuli, and the relative increase in gain of the eye movement frequency response at about 2.0 to 2.5 Hz attributable to sampling aliasing. The general behavior of eye tracking instabilities for both positive and negative feedback was approximately described by the sampled model.

The major features of the original sampled data model for saccadic tracking were few and rather simple. Retinal error would not normally be corrected unless it lay outside of an effective "dead zone" of approximately ±0.3 degrees. The size of this error was sampled periodically and processed to generate a step-like eye movement one reaction time later. New information concerning retinal error, which occurred between samples, had to wait until the next sampling time before being processed. The system worked in conjunction with pursuit eye movements, which were at that time envisioned as responsible for making smooth eye movements to minimize retinal slip velocity. The earliest sampled data model also included a sampled version of pursuit tracking.[40,45] Since that time, due in large part to the suggestion of the continuous nature of pursuit tracking by Robinson,[29] and the further evidence provided by Brodskey and Stark,[6] the discrete model for pursuit tracking has been abandoned and a continuous version substituted.[44] Furthermore, our entire conception of the goals of pursuit tracking have changed. Instead of minimizing retinal slip velocity in a closed loop fashion, we now conceive of the pursuit system in terms of open loop ocular velocity control to match the eye speed to the perceived angular velocity of the target of interest with respect to the head.[39,42,43]

The first sampled data model was simple enough to be treated analytically, and analysis formed the basis for its predictions both in the frequency domain and in response to simple deterministic targets. The limitations of the simplified models were stated explicitly at the time, including the functional position of the sampler, the constancy of sampling rate, the relationship between pursuit and saccadic samples, and the nature of the dead zone; these were largely ignored by many early users of the model. Since the early 1960s, a wealth of new experimental data has been generated in the area of oculomotor control and a generation of investigators has tested the specific predictions of the original and succeeding sampled data models. Neurophysiological evidence has been forthcoming concerning both the control of the individual saccade and the "latching mechanism" responsible for the usual intersaccadic intervals. A number of the detailed experiments on saccadic tracking, especially concerning the distribution of latencies to primary and secondary saccades and the generation of corrective saccades to double pulse experiments, has clarified the nature of the control mechanism and necessitated some amplification of the sampled data concept. The purpose of this Chapter is to put in perspective some of the more critical experimental developments of the intervening period and point out the modifications of the original sampled data model that have been necessary to account for them. It must once again be pointed out that the purpose of this level of modeling is to be functionally accurate, rather than to present physiologically based descriptions. To the extent that this or similar models lead to searches for the physiological correlates, as has been the case for the sampled data model, they may be considered as successful.

In his discussion of the range of successful predictions of the sampled data model for saccades, Fuchs[12] summarized many of the limitations of the fixed sampling rate, instantaneous sample model. He concluded that continued exploitation and further enhancement of the model, beyond the Young, Forster, and van Houtte version, would be less productive than to merely consider the system as discontinuous and to concentrate on the underlying neurophysiological bases for the discontinuity. In the intervening period, substantial new information has been produced. The pulse-step nature of reciprocal innervation signals at the oculomotor nuclei has been demonstrated. A growing number of brain stem units associated with the planning and execution of saccades have been categorized — including pausers, bursters, long-lead bursters, and others. The interface between the brain stem "machinery" and the generation of saccadic commands from supranuclear areas, especially the collicular, thalamic, and cortical influences, raises new and, as yet, unresolved issues concerning the visual frame of reference, as well as the timing issues in generating saccades. (See the Workshop Syntheses in Baker and Berthoz (1977) for summaries of this area.[2]) The approach of synthesizing the eye movement control mechanism out of the individual neuron categories is to be encouraged and may eventually lead to a model which explains, rather than describes. Meanwhile, although equivalent network descriptions for the intersaccadic interval have been proposed (e.g., Robinson[30]), no general model has replaced the sampled data formulation. Our early attempts to localize the site of the sampling operation[46] were not very successful and the neurophysiological correlate of the "sampling" can still not be inferred from the model.

The basic notion of sampling in the saccadic eye tracking system continues to survive and to be included in various more extensive models. Morasso et al.[25] incorporate the sampler and saccade generator into their eye-head coordination model. Selhorst et al.[31] and Hsu et al.[17] provide evidence that certain oculomotor pathologies are well described by maladjusted gains in the sampled data feedback model. Zuber and Djordjevich[48] used asymmetrical fusional vergence stimuli to support the idea of a dead zone (0.2°) and sampling interval (191 ms). The shortcomings of the model are largely those which were pointed out when it was introduced. The presence of different classes of response to identical stimuli requires a stochastic sampling description — and the exact distribution and synchronization rules have yet to be determined. The evidence supports parallel processing of saccades in some cases, but this requires extensive modifications of the model as discussed below. The neurophysiological implementation of the sampling cannot be inferred from the model. Finally, neither the sampled data model, nor others known to us, predict the distribution of open loop saccadic gains — made evident by overshoot and undershoot, as well as by the external visual feedback required to initiate and sustain oculomotor oscillations.

II. EVIDENCE FOR THE SAMPLING HYPOTHESIS

A. Step and Pulse Responses

The eye tracking response to a step position displacement of a small fixation target generally consists of a time delay from 150 to over 500 ms, followed by a saccade in the direction of the target. Undershoot is common for target amplitudes exceeding 10 degrees, and the primary saccade is frequently followed by a secondary or corrective saccade some 150 to 250 ms later. This characteristic is describable in terms of a system containing a pure dead time or transport delay. However, when the initial target step is followed by a return to its initial position, as described first by Westheimer,[36] the

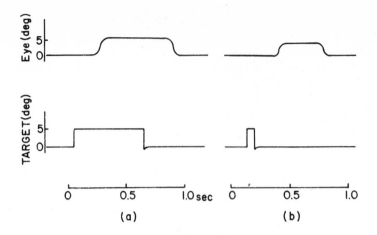

FIGURE 1.   Pulse responses. Top traces, horizontal target angle. Bottom traces, horizontal eye position.

typical eye movement pattern is as shown in Figure 1. The eye deviates to the displaced target position and remains there for a minimum time, normally not less than 200 ms and sometimes as long as 400 ms, before returning to its initial position. Notice that, for brief pulses on the order of 100 ms or so, this frequently means that the target has returned to its initial position, with zero retinal error, before the eye ever initiated the first saccade. In fact, the eye movement pattern which may result from this stimulus is not always the same, and may at times be a shortened return latency, a decreased amplitude saccade, or a complete absence of response. A system responding such as that in Figure 1b cannot be a linear continuous system with only time delays to account for the interval between stimulus and response, since the response to a pulse is not the superposition of the response to two equal and opposite steps, delayed with respect to one another by the pulse width. The discrete nature of the response suggests that saccadic corrections to retinal error are processed, perhaps over a finite time interval, to produce a sudden correction, rather than a continuous update. Finally, the fact that the eye movement system may launch a saccadic movement to a displaced position, even though the target had already been returned to the initial position, suggests that these discrete movements, once calculated, may not be cancelled after a certain period. All of these conclusions are consistent with a sampled data system, which either receives or sends out signals at discrete time intervals.

B. Open Loop Tracking

Perhaps the most persuasive simple experiment supporting the sampled data hypothesis is that associated with open loop tracking of displaced targets. The normal eye movement control system loop is closed through the simple geometrical relationship between changes in eye position and changes in corresponding retinal position of the image. This feedback loop can be opened in a number of ways in order to study the forward loop characteristics directly. Eye position can be prevented from movement, even though the efferent motor commands are delivered, either by restraining the eye or by paralyzing the extraocular muscles. A particularly useful form of this experiment is one in which the restrained eye is presented the visual target and the unrestrained eye is blinded to the target. In this manner, the movements of the unrestrained eye faithfully record the commanded versional movements, but do not affect the retinal error signal imposed upon the seeing restrained eye. The use of after-images as tracking targets provides an easier method of investigating the open loop tracking situation.

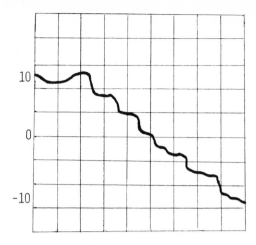

FIGURE 2. Experimental step responses under variable feedback, K = 0.0.

Since an after-image is fixed with respect to the retina, any attempts to fixate it, if the image is not already in the center of the macula, will result in open loop eye movement tracking, since the resulting movements do not reduce retinal error. Similarly, attempts to track any other object fixed to the eye, such as the shadows of the vascular tree will lead to open loop tracking. Open loop tracking conditions have also been produced conveniently, although less precisely, by adding an artificial external-feedback loop which measures eye position and moves the target by an angle just equal to the eye deviation. This may be accomplished through electronic measurement of eye position and control of target position or by optical means through the use of mirrors connected to the eye. If the target stabilization is not perfect, image fading will not occur.

Regardless of the means used to generate open loop tracking, the results for tracking of targets displaced more than a few degrees from the center of the fovea appear the same. The first attempt to fixate a perifoveal target initiates a staircase of approximately equal amplitude saccades, generally decreasing slightly in magnitude with time. These saccades march the eye, often to the periphery of its range, with a series of jumps separated by an intersaccadic interval of approximately 200 ms. Since the retinal error remains constant but the output changes only at discrete times, this open loop step response is clear evidence for discontinuous control. Notice that treatment of this response as the step output of a sampled data system does not imply anything about the site of the sampler, whether it be at the processing of sensory information, the calculation of the responses, or the motor end. As seen in the typical example of Figure 2, the steps continue, frequently slightly abated, until reaching either the end of the eye movement range or the range of the measurement instrument used to open the loop.

Open loop tracking situations may also give rise to smooth eye movements in an attempt to pursue the apparent velocity of the retinally fixed target. These pursuit movements appear to be superimposed upon the saccadic tracking and not to interfere with it.

C. Variable Feedback Oscillation

The technique of measuring eye position and feeding it back as immediate changes

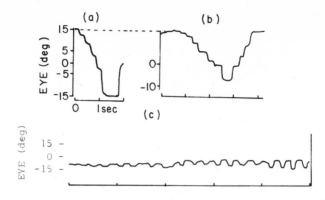

FIGURE 3.   Positive feedback and high negative feedback instabilities.

in target position can produce not only open loop, but any condition of variable feedback tracking. In particular, the use of a high-gain negative feedback loop can force
the saccadic eye tracking system into spontaneous oscillation of a limit cycle behavior
as shown in Figure 3C. Although the actual gain required to sustain oscillations varies
with instructions and training, the nature of the resulting oscillation is highly stereotyped. It consists always of a sequence of alternating saccadic eye movements separated
by intersaccadic intervals of no less than a minimum time equal to the psychological
refractory period of approximately 200 ms. Once again, this type of behavior is consistent with a discontinuous control system of which the sampled data system is a
common type.

D. Aliasing Peak in the Frequency Response

When the frequency response of the horizontal eye movement control system is calculated for a wide band pseudo-random continuous input signal, a relative peak in the
gain is often seen in the region of 2.0 to 2.5 Hz. This relative peak is not present when
either single-frequency sinusoidal stimulation is used or with low-frequency pseudo-
random stimulation. Several factors could be responsible for this relative peak, including the presence of a resonance in a continuous underdamped feedback system. The
lack of confirming sudden changes in the phase angle around this frequency does not
support the notion of resonance. This sampling peak is, however, consistent with the
effect of aliasing in a sampled data system with sampling rate between 200 and 250
ms. The effect of the sampling on the frequency response is to repeat the spectrum of
the unsampled frequency response about center frequencies corresponding to integral
multiples of the sampling frequency. If the original continuous spectrum contains frequencies above half the sampling frequency (the Nyquist frequency), then these signals
will be "folded over" and added to the signals at lower than the Nyquist frequency.
As a result, there will appear to be a relative peak in the apparent frequency response
and the irretrievable loss of not only the higher frequency information, but also the
lower frequency signals, which are thus masked. For a sampling rate of 200 to 250 ms,
for example, the Nyquist frequency is 2.0 to 2.5 Hz. This predicts the occurrence
of an increase in the apparent gain of eye tracking, peaking at 2.0 to 2.5 Hz for tracking signals whose bandwidth exceeds 2.0 to 2.5 Hz.

III. EVOLUTION OF THE SAMPLED DATA MODEL FOR THE
SACCADIC SYSTEM

As originally conceived, the sampled data model for saccade tracking ignored the details of the saccade itself. The time constants associated with the performance of the saccadic eye movement were such that the saccade was completed before any additional calculation in the planning of the next saccade took place. The earliest simple version is shown in Figure 4.[40,41] In its linearized version, with the foveal dead zone element and the saccade dynamics removed, the saccadic system was trivially simple, consisting merely of a sampler and a delay. To further simplify the calculations, the sampling interval was assumed constant and just equal to the delay, both being equal to 200 ms. It was recognized and pointed out in the early model that this would erroneously predict uniform reaction times to deterministic inputs and a completely stereotyped response.

As a result of the demonstration of the continuous nature of the pursuit tracking system, as well as the publication of more detailed work on the response to brief pulses and continuous pulses, a substantial revision of the original sampled data model was developed and published in 1968.[44] Although many further refinements are possible as a result of accumulating information about eye movement patterns in the vertical, as well as the horizontal plane and varying instruction sets, this will be used as the point of departure for the remainder of this discussion about the sampled data model's predictions and limitations.

The stochastic model is given in Figure 5, with the addition of an explicit indication of an efferent copy mechanism as the source of eye movement information necessary to provide the pursuit system with an estimate of target velocity relative to the head. The position of the sampler is also shown as just preceding the internal delay in the saccadic loop, although mathematically the function is unchanged, whether the sampler be before or after the dead zone or the delay. This is indicated merely as a reminder that the presence of the sampler does not imply that visual information is not taken in and processed between samples. The simple second order linear approximation to the ocular motor dynamics is retained for simplicity, since it produces adequate dynamic responses for the purposes of overall eye movement control modelling. We are fully aware of the pulse-step nature of the force commands for preemphasis to drive the actual long time constant eye dynamics in saccade-like responses consistent with the time-optimal control strategy.[9,28,30] In arriving at this random sampling formulation, we were cognizant of several experimental results on the apparent velocity sensitive nature of saccades. Zuber[47] had first shown that the size of a corrective saccade depended upon the velocity following a target step, as well as the step amplitude itself, in a series of ramp-step-ramp experiments. Fuchs[11] performed analogous experiments in monkeys with step-ramp targets and discussed the results of Lauringson and Shehedrovitskii[21] working in man, who also reported that the size of the saccade following a step-ramp depended upon the ramp velocity. There are obviously two ways to account for this effect in the sampled data model. One rather direct approach would be to provide some lead compensation to the saccadic controller, so that the subsequent saccade was not made equal to e, but rather to $e + k\dot{e}$, representing a weighted sum of the sampled retinal error and retinal velocity. This straightforward approach was used by Murphy and Deekshatulu[26] in their modification of the Young-Stark model. Fuchs[12] proposed, for discussion purposes only, a somewhat more complex version of the sampled data model to incorporate the velocity sensitivity of saccades by a velocity sensitive gain control and intersample interval variability. The model shown in Figure 5 is an attempt to account for the velocity sensitivity of the saccades by simple realization of the random nature of the sampling interval. Since samples are unlikely to occur exactly at the time of a step, but rather occur some time afterwards, it is clear that the sampled error magnitude will depend on both the post-step target velocity and the delay between a step and the subsequent sample.

Although single moving targets in the 1 to 30°/s range are normally followed pri-

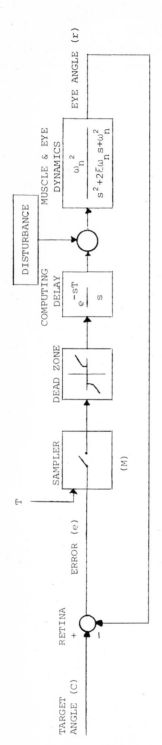

FIGURE 4.   Sampled data model — the saccadic system.

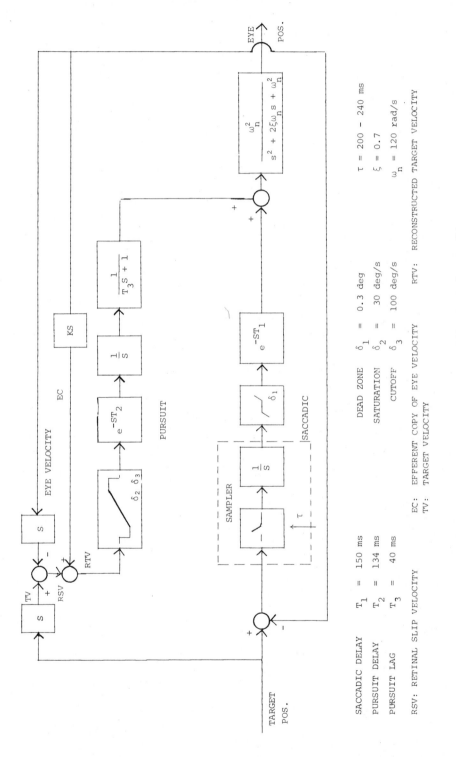

FIGURE 5. Stochastic model — showing efferent copy for pursuit loop.

marily by continuous pursuit eye movements, it is not unusual to see the underlying saccadic psychological refractory period in cases in which the target is pursued by a staircase of saccadic jumps. After administration of barbiturates,[27] the smooth pursuit system is essentially inactivated and tracking takes place with saccades separated by no less than 200 ms. Similar nonpursuit tracking has been reported in the case of schizophrenic patients, unless special care is taken to require accurate fixation of the moving target.[15] Recently, it has also been shown that infants, in their early weeks before developing smooth pursuit, will track continuously moving targets with a sequence of saccades separated by intersaccadic intervals of approximately 400 ms.[1]

The eye movement response to short pulses, mentioned earlier as one of the fundamental points of the sampled data model, was also one of the key issues in the restatement of it in terms of stochastic sampling intervals. Beeler,[5] Wheeless et al.,[37] Becker and Fuchs,[4] and Levy-Schoen and Blanc-Garin[22] all experimented with various combinations of the pulse duration and the direction and magnitude of the second part of the pulse. A principal result of these experiments was the finding that as the target-pulse width became significantly less than 200 ms, the probability increased that the primary saccade would go directly to the final target position, rather than proceeding first to the intermediate target position and remaining there for a full refractory period. This finding was adequately explained by the stochastic sampled data model, since the probability of an instantaneous or limited duration sample occurring during the pulse was inversely proportional to the pulse duration. On the other hand, a pulse which did not call forth any saccadic movement did, nevertheless, delay the average time of response to a subsequent step according to Wheeless et al.[37] One interpretation of this in the general context of the sampled data model is by the assumption that the system was able to cancel a programmed saccade at some time prior to the scheduled launch, but that the subsequent refractory period remained in effect.[16,40] More will be discussed about the relative timing of saccade amplitude, direction modification, and cancellation later in this Chapter.

Many other authors have examined the sampled data model, both in its original and revised stochastic version, over the two decades it has been in existence. Jury and Pavlidis[19] were the first to comment on its minor erroneous prediction of pursuit movement to very small steps. We now know that, in fact, small target displacements will at times be corrected by pursuit, rather than saccadic movements. This is particularly apparent in the smooth tracking of slightly off foveal after-images.[13,14,20,32,39] A number of authors have proposed other sampled data models with more than one sampling element. The first of these modifications was proposed by Johnson.[18] Vossius[35] suggested that the sampled data saccadic eye movement control system could be improved over the original version by association with a continuous pursuit system. Most of the models for the generation of vestibular nystagmus or optokinetic nystagmus employ some means of retinal error sampling or equivalent eye position sampling in the generation of their fast phase.[24,34,38]

IV. FREQUENCY RESPONSE OF THE SAMPLED DATA MODEL

The frequency response of the entire stochastic sampled data model, as shown by Young et al.[44] reflects two modes. Tracking is largely pursuit at low frequencies and largely saccadic at higher frequencies, as shown in Figure 6. The amplitude dependence of the model frequency response is shown in Figure 7 and the comparison with experimental findings of nonpredictive tracking is illustrated in Figure 8. Notice that Dallos and Jones,[10] Wheeless et al.,[37] and Young[40] all showed an "aliasing peak" in the region of 2.0 to 2.5 Hz.

Although these results provided general support for at least the aliasing aspect of

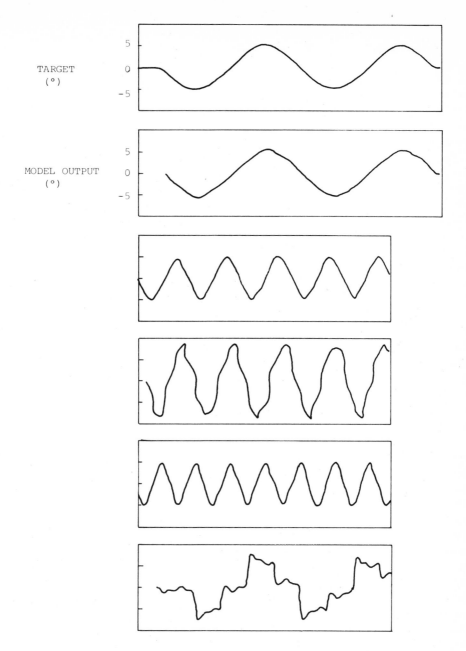

FIGURE 6. Model response to a single sinuosid (nonpredictive tracking) for three frequencies: $f = 0.194$ Hz (top left), $f = 1.04$ Hz (top right), and $f = 3.82$ Hz (bottom). The time scale is superimposed on the input (time between pulses is 200 msec).

the stochastic sampled data model, they could not provide a critical evaluation of either the saccadic or pursuit systems operating alone. Yasui[38] succeeded in obtaining the nonperiodic-input frequency response for the saccadic system alone. He devised a computational technique for eliminating the inherent influence of the pursuit system from the overall input-output frequency response to reveal the intrinsic saccadic frequency response.

His general concept of arriving at the intrinsic saccadic frequency response is shown

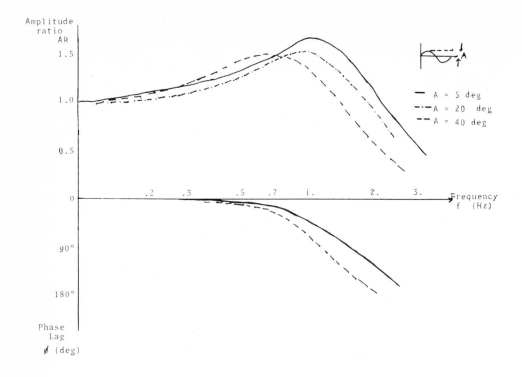

FIGURE 7.   Frequency response of plot of the model to various input amplitudes.

in Figure 9. It implies that although pursuit tracking clearly influences the retinal error sensed by the saccadic system, the converse is not true. (Robinson[29] reported an occasional effect of saccades in permitting discrete changes in pursuit velocity.) The intrinsic saccadic output is in response to the effective saccadic input which, in turn, is the target position minus the eye position attributable to the pursuit system. The apparent saccadic frequency response, $G_s(j\omega)$, is simply calculated as the vector difference (gain and phase at each frequency) between the composite frequency response ($G_C(j\omega)$) and the pursuit frequency response ($G_P(j\omega)$). The latter is easily computed by FFT from the eye movement signal from which all saccades have been removed and which represents cumulative pursuit or slow-phase position. The intrinsic saccadic frequency response is consequently given by

$$G_S^I\,(j\omega) \;=\; \frac{\theta_S(j\omega)}{\theta_{i_{eff}}(j\omega)} \;=\; \frac{G_C(j\omega) - G_P(j\omega)}{1 - G_P(j\omega)} \tag{1}$$

Yasui calculated G_i, G_P, G_S, and G_S' for several input spectra. For his medium bandwidth (B) input, cut off at 1.3 Hz, the composite pursuit and apparent saccadic frequency responses are shown in Figure 10. When the correction to G_s implied by Equation 1 is applied, the intrinsic saccadic frequency response $G_S^I(j\omega)$ is produced and is shown in Figure 11. Since this should correspond to the fundamental saccadic contribution to tracking, it was compared to the most elementary forms of the saccadic sampled data model shown in Figure 12b. For inputs less than 2.5 Hz and the sampling

55

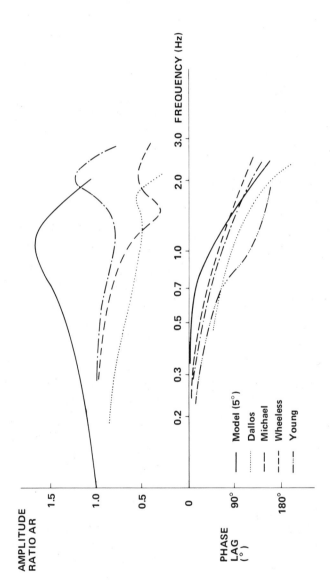

FIGURE 8. Frequency response of eye tracking movements (nonpredictive mode) established by several investigators and compared with model responses.

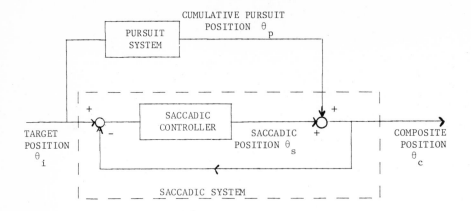

COMPOSITE SYSTEM,   EXPERIMENTAL DATA: $G_c(j\omega)$

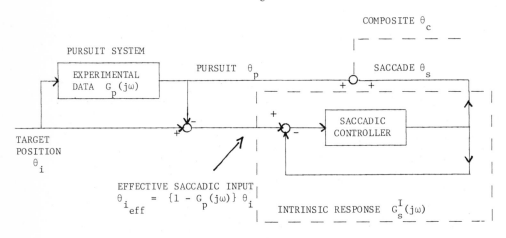

SACCADIC FREQUENCY RESPONSE

$G_c(j\omega) - G_p(j\omega)$ APPARENT

$\{G_c(j\omega) - G_p(j\omega)\}/\{ \ 1 - G_p(j\omega) \ \}$ INTRINSIC

FIGURE 9. Top: General organization of visual tracking system. Bottom: Decoupled diagram functionally equivalent to top figure.

rate interval (T) assumed equal to the dead time delay (T_o), the model frequency response is simply

$$G_S^T(j\omega) = \frac{\sin \dfrac{\omega T_0}{2}}{\dfrac{\omega T_0}{2}} \ \exp\left(-j \ \frac{3\omega T_0}{2}\right) \qquad (2)$$

By using the original model figures of $T_o = 0.2$ sec, the theoretical frequency response

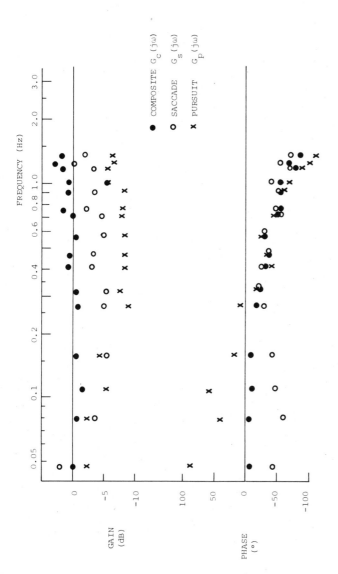

FIGURE 10. Frequency response results for composite, saccadic, and pursuit movements for pseudo-random input B. Note this saccadic result does not truly reflect the saccadic system itself due to the pursuit interference (average of four subjects).

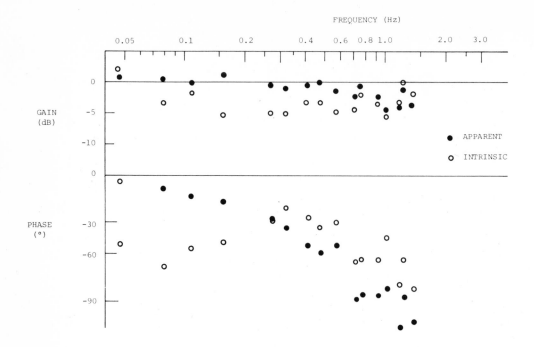

FIGURE 11.. Intrinsic and apparent nonperiodic-input saccadic frequency response results for pseudo-random input B (average of four subjects).

is as shown in Figure 13, and is compared with the intrinsic saccadic frequency response data from Figure 11, previously discussed. Yasui went on to examine the tracking records for the actual intersaccadic intervals during tracking of a pseudo-random continuous input. The composite intersaccadic interval histogram for his four subjects is shown in Figure 14a. This distribution has a mode of 200 to 300 ms, median of 300 to 400 ms, and an average interval of 510 ms with standard deviation of 100 ms. It is approximated by a Poisson process with most probable intervals from 200 to 300 ms. By way of comparison, Collewijn[7] published an intersaccadic interval histogram for the freely moving cat, shown in Figure 14b. The distribution shape is similar, but skewed toward shorter latencies in the cat, with mode of 200 ms and median of 270 ms. Yasui pointed out that while the mode might represent an average sampling interval, interval statistics cannot reveal samples which were below the saccadic dead zone and, consequently, produced no saccade.

Yasui explored the variable sampling rate model further, in an attempt to reconcile the observed intersaccadic intervals with the calculated gain and phase of the intrinsic saccadic loop. Assuming that the pure time delay (T_0) is less than the sampling interval (T_m) the calculated phase lag is given by

$$\phi(j\omega) = -(T_0 + T_m/2)\omega \tag{3}$$

and the gain is given by

$$G_S^T(j\omega) = \frac{\sin(\omega T_m/2)}{\omega(T_0/2)} \tag{4}$$

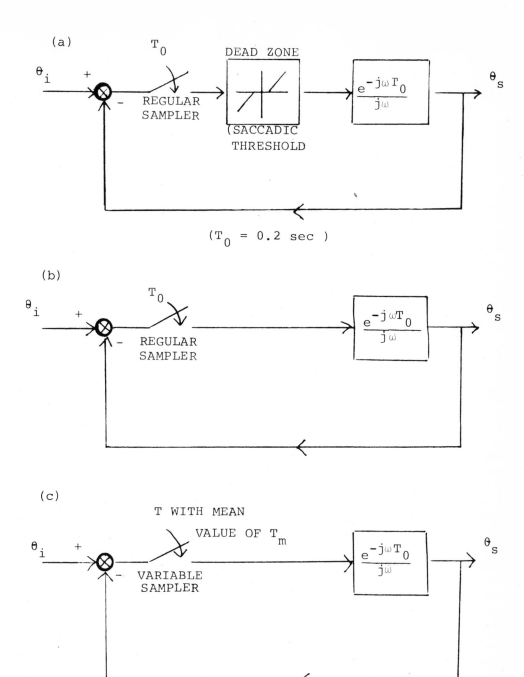

FIGURE 12.   Versions of sampled-data saccadic visual tracking model. (a) Young's original configuration; (b) Dead zone removed for linear analysis; (c) T_0 replaced by mean intersaccadic interval T_m, which turned out to be much greater than 0.2 sec ($T_m = 0.51$ sec) for the particular case being studied.

By choosing $T_m = 510$ ms as the average intersaccadic interval from Figure 14a and $T_0 = 45$ ms, he obtained the relatively good fit to the intrinsic saccade frequency response shown in Figure 15.

It is recognized that the mean intersaccadic interval is probably much larger than

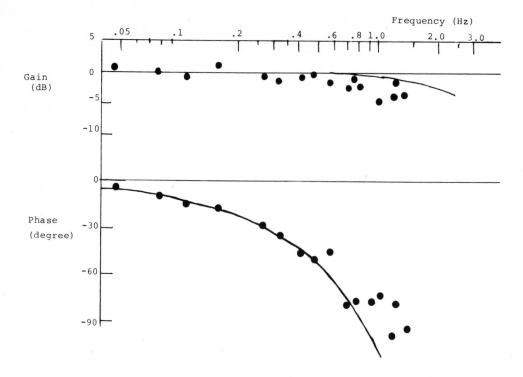

FIGURE 13. Intrinsic and extrinsic response result (with input B) as compared with prediction by Young's sampled-data model (saccadic dead zone ignored), where 0.2 sec is presupposed for the saccadic interval.

the median sampling interval, as calculated from the open loop experiments. Furthermore, 45 ms is shorter than the observed minimum saccadic reaction time delay. By using the usual minimum reaction time delay of $T_0 = 150$ ms, and the median intersaccadic interval of 300 ms for T_m, one computes exactly the same phase plot as in Figure 15, with quite similar gain.

The importance of these calculations performed by Yasui were in the separation of pursuit and intrinsic saccadic contributions to tracking of continuous wide-band signals. The consistency of the simple saccadic sampled data model with the intrinsic saccadic frequency response lends support, but not proof, to its applicability.

V. CORRECTIVE SACCADES

A large class of important experiments involve the need to correct an erroneous saccadic eye movement. The value of these tests lies in the *timing* information they afford concerning the generation and modification of saccades. Perhaps the simplest such experiment is the short pulse, discussed in the introduction. The fact that the target has returned to its origin before the saccade was launched implies that an erroneous saccade, once programmed, could not be *cancelled* by new visual information presented in the last 30 to 50 ms before movement. The length of time spent at the displaced position should also indicate the minimum sampling interval — under the assumption that the information processing for the return saccade did not begin until the first saccade was completed. The results of Beeler[5] and others showed occasional brief intervals between the two saccades. It seemed conceivable that the machinery for generating the second saccade was brought into play before the first saccade was completed — or even initiated. The observation that an increasing percentage of target

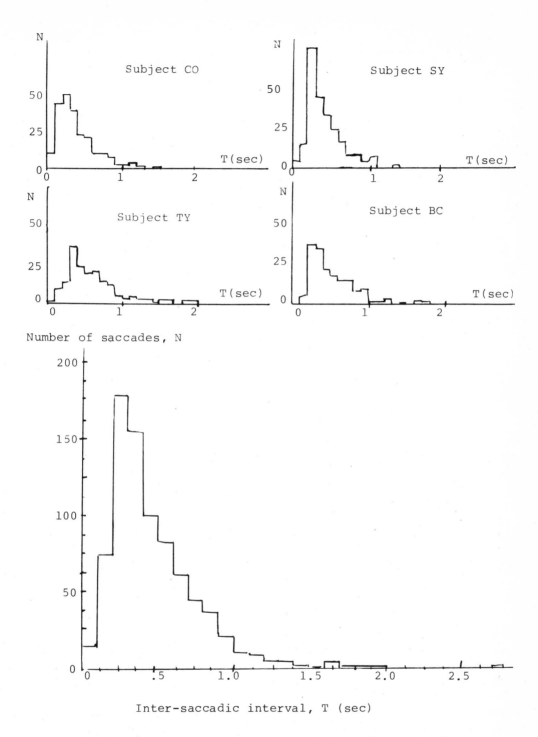

FIGURE 14a.   Histograms of inter-saccadic intervals with pseudo-random input B.

pulses elicited no saccadic response was consistent with the stochastic sampling model, since the probability of a sample falling within the target pulse is proportional to pulse width up to the intersample interval. Unfortunately, these pulse experiments could not distinguish between the cancellation of the first saccade or a new command to proceed

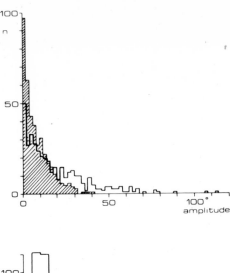

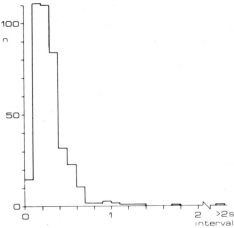

FIGURE 14b.   Histograms of the distribution of amplitude (above) and intersaccadic interval (below) for 400 saccades in a free cat in a period of active, exploratory behavior. Shaded: maximal deviation of eye in head; line: displacement of eye in space (gaze). (From Collewijn, H., Control of Gaze by Brain Stem Neurons, Baker, R. and Berthoz, A., Eds., Elservier, North Holland, Amsterdam, 1977. With permission.)

directly to the final position (which, in this case, was the original position). Considerable progress in this area resulted from the introduction of double-step experiments. The response to a continued step could either be a step directly to the final position, an extended (about 200 ms) rest at the first position before continuing or, on some occasions, a very brief pause of 50 ms or so at the intermediate position. In each case, the final saccade was made to the correct spatial position, regardless of the retinal error existing at the time it was planned.[22] These results support the concept of a spatiotopically organized system, with some ongoing means of accounting for the initial eye position. Only the first two of the double-step responses are accounted for by the stochastic sampling model. The brief pause at the intermediate position implies that the second saccade was programmed even before the first one was launched. Wheeless' pulse-step experiments, in which the final step was opposite to the initial pulse, showed

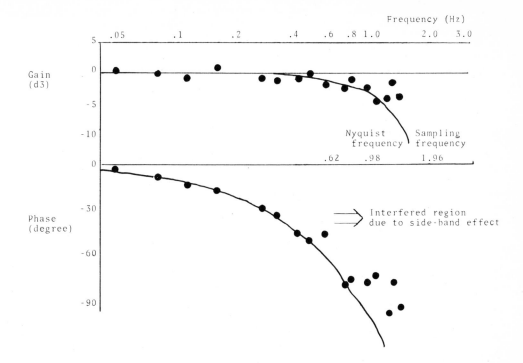

FIGURE 15. Intrinsic saccadic frequency response result (with input B) and corresponding theoretical prediction by Young's sampled data model with modified parameter values, T_m = 510 msec and T_d = 45 msec.

an increasing number of saccades going directly to the final position as the pulse width was reduced to less than 200 ms. This general trend is consistent with a stochastic sampler. However, the average latencies of these direct saccades to the final position was large — significantly longer than if the pulse and step were in the same direction. Young[40] and Horrocks and Stark[16] showed a higher probability of disregarding target position information appearing later than 80 ms prior to saccade initiation. Levy-Schoen and Blanc-Garin[22] attempted to distinguish between the timing programs for modulation of magnitude and direction of secondary saccades in a double-step stimulus experiment. They found, as did others, that a late appearance of the second stimulus decreases the likelihood of making a saccade directly to it. They also showed that a correct secondary response was more likely to a new target when the second stimulus was closer to the original fixation point than the first stimulus, regardless of whether or not a reversal of direction was required. On the other hand, a reversal of direction (opposite steps) was rarely achieved and subjects almost never jumped directly to a second target when it required a lengthening of the saccade beyond the initial one. These results do not completely pin down the relative timing mechanism in adjustment of saccade amplitude or direction, but they do point out the tendency to account for "easy modifications" which require less effort than the original saccade, at later times into the programming effort. We are led to the conclusion from these and other experiments that the timing decisions in the generation of a saccade are as follows:

Step 1   T = 0 ms   Sample the retinal error and begin a program after a rand — partly synchronized delay up to 50 ms

Step 2   T = 0 − 50 ms   Modify the direction or magnitude of the planned saccade

Step 3   T = 50 − 70 ms   Modify the magnitude, but not the direction, of the planned saccade on the basis of new visual information.

Step 4   T = 70 − 100 ms   Modify the magnitude only to reduce the planned saccade in the same direction.

Step 5   T = 100 − 150 ms   Cancel the planned saccade if appropriate and sample again to compute the next saccade in the next 50 to 100 ms.

Step 6   T = 150 − 200 ms   Proceed with the planned saccade and model the expected error at its end. If this error will be greater than 0.3°, begin parallel processing of the corrective saccade

Step 7   T = 200 ms   Initiate the saccadic jump

Step 8   T = 200 − 300 ms   If a parallel preprogrammed corrective saccade was planned, proceed to generate it. If not, sample the retinal error again as in Step 1.

This timing scheme is shown in Figure 16. The particular time intervals for the various phases of this timing scheme are highly speculative and presented only to stimulate research. It is interesting, however, to compare this timing scheme with the relative timing of unit activity in the visuo-oculomotor system. Carpenter's[8] recent compilation of the timing of activity in various neural centers, between the appearance of an off-foveal stimulus and the consequent saccade, is shown in Figure 17.

The notion of a parallel processing system, which can begin to process corrections of a future error — even before that error occurs, is an important outgrowth of the double-pulse experiments. This approach had been suggested by Johnson[18] as a way of accounting for corrective saccades. The actual proof of this important feature of saccadic control awaited two further observations — one very simple and the other quite complex. The simple experiment involved extinction of a displaced target within 50, 100, or 200 msec of the time it was stepped[3,47] The absence of a visible target during the saccade had no effect on the accuracy of the primary saccade, as expected from all other information concerning the lack of visual influence during a saccade. Furthermore, the blanking prior to the saccade also had no influence on the saccade magnitude. That is consistent with the timing scheme of Figure 16 and the previously discussed observations that the accuracy of a saccade to a remembered target position is not improved by the target's appearance any time later than 80 ms prior to the saccade. What was not evident was that a secondary and occasionally a tertiary corrective saccade would be made to correct the residual error made by the first saccade, even when no retinal error signal ever represented that error. These corrective saccades to blanked target locations were just as accurate as those to visible targets — an accuracy of 3.5% in Becker's experiment. In his paradigm, the corrective saccades in the dark differed only in their latency — which was nearly twice that observed when the target remained visible. It seems clear that the erroneous eye position was available to generate the saccade. (Although an efferent copy generation of this eye position signal seems parsimonious, afferent generation cannot be excluded.) It seems as though, in Becker's paradigm, the preprogrammed error correction was only implemented if no visual signal were present to confirm the target error. In the pulse-step experiments, on the other hand, the major preprogrammed error correction is based upon both a visual sample before the saccade is initiated (but after the pulse and step) and an internal model of where the eye was destined to be at the end of its first saccade.

The second element of the experimental proof rests on a recent experiment of Mays and Sparks[23] in monkeys. A target step was used to initiate a saccade. Before the

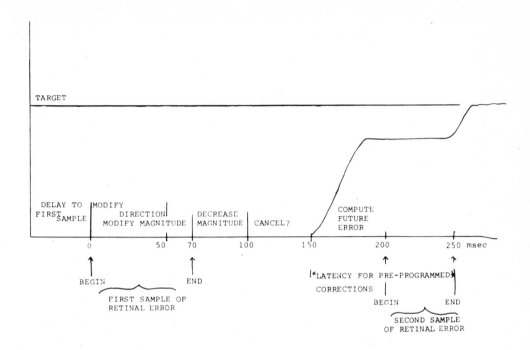

FIGURE 16.   Relative timing of events leading to saccades and saccadic corrections.

saccade began, however, the target was extinquished and the eye's starting position was driven to a new place by electrical stimulation of the superior colliculus. Even though no new visual information was available, the monkey made a subsequent saccade, after a short or zero latency, to the position in space corresponding to the original target location. Once again, the conclusion is that the saccades are spatiotopically, as opposed to retinotopically, organized. Furthermore, prior eye movements, even if erroneous, are taken into account by compensating the subsequent saccade for the previous electrically induced saccade.

In an attempt to pin down the relationship between sampling instants and the delay to corrective saccades in double-pulse experiments, we timed the second pulse to be synchronized to the first saccade.[44] Either a return or a continuing pulse occurred at a known time after the primary saccade initiation, and the latency to this second pulse was recorded, and is shown in Figure 18. We found, along with Beeler and Wheeless, that the latencies to return pulses took longer than those to continuing pulses. The return pulse results are consistent with a stochastic sampler run totally synchronized — so that pulses occurring just after a saccade must wait longer for the next sample to arrive — up to a maximum of the sampling interval. For a continuing pulse, on the other hand, the latency pattern lies closer to the predictions of a nonsynchronixed sampler in which the next sample can occur at any time from 150 ms to 250 ms after the previous sample or from 0 to 150 ms after the first saccade. These results are equivocal in deciding between the two extremes of synchronized vs. unsynchronized sampling. They do, however, support the notion referred to earlier in Figure 16, that magnitude corrections by corrective saccades or modifications of primary saccades, are performed up to a later presaccade moment than are direction changes. In view of the long time constant on-going mechanical activity in the motor system and the major reversal of innervation to the oculomotor nuclei required for a reversal, this extra delay does not seem unreasonable.

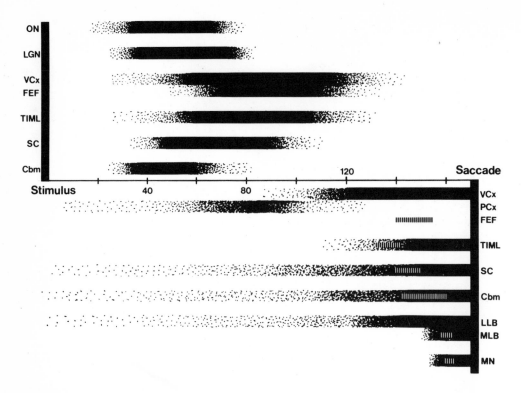

FIGURE 17.   Diagram showing the approximate timing of various events in the visuo-oculomotor system following appearance of a stimulus and preceding a saccadic eye movement. Upper portion of the diagram represents timing relative the stimulus and lower portion relative to the onset of the saccade. Data collected from many sources by Carpenter[8] See his paper for complete references.

ON: Optic nerve. LGN: Lateral geniculate nucleus.

VCx: Visual cortex FEF: Frontal eye fields. SC: Superior colliculus. Cbm: Cerebellum. PCx: Parietal cortex.

LLB: Long lead bursters. MLB: Medium lead bursters.

MN: Motor nuclei. TIML: Thalamic intermediary.

VI. SACCADIC DEAD ZONE

An essential element of not only the sampled data model, but nearly all models, is an element commonly referred to as the foveal dead zone. The idea is a simple one. A small target which is already imaged on the fovea doesn't *normally* call forth a saccade to recenter it.[27] Perhaps a better term would have been an "indifference threshold" as used in manual control to refer to small errors which are noticeable, but not normally corrected. Clearly, small target jumps — well under 0.3° — are easily detected and small saccades — including microsaccades — often occur. However, the demonstration by Steinman et al.[33] that trained subjects can make small saccades in response to small target displacements, in no way invalidates the need for a functional dead zone to describe normal tracking scanning.

The occurrence of a secondary corrective saccade depends primarily upon the steady state error remaining after the completion of the first saccade.* Errors on the order of 0.25 to 0.5° are often not corrected, which is consistent with the ability of the visual system to fuse disparate binocular images. The existence of uncorrected steady state errors indicates an accuracy specification of saccadic eye movements of some sizable

---

* This section is based on an earlier report.[46]

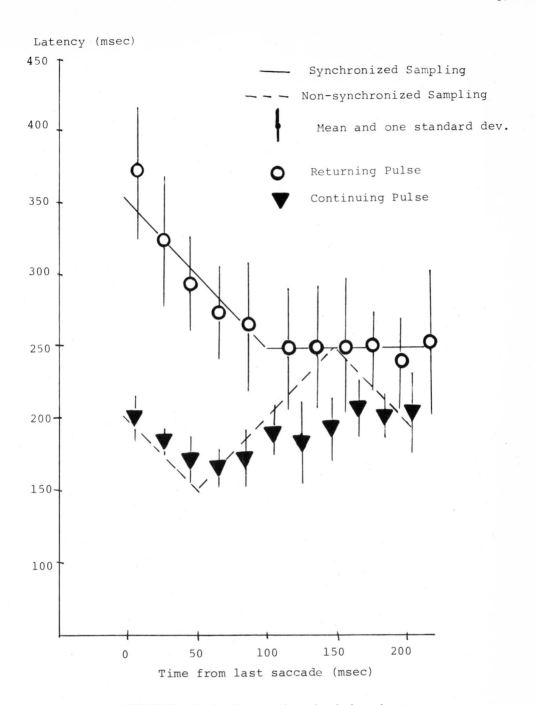

FIGURE 18.   Results of two saccade-synchronized experiments.

fraction of a degree. In addition, a threshold of response of the eye to target steps of small magnitudes was pointed out by Rashbass[27] and others.

Experiments on the saccadic dead zone conducted in 1962 and 1965 consisted of a random series of small horizontal target steps, all of magnitude less than 1°, presented to a subject. The time of occurrence of the saccadic eye movement or the failure of such a response to occur within one second following the stimulus were recorded. The data for this experiment, as shown in Figure 19, clearly indicates the tendency toward

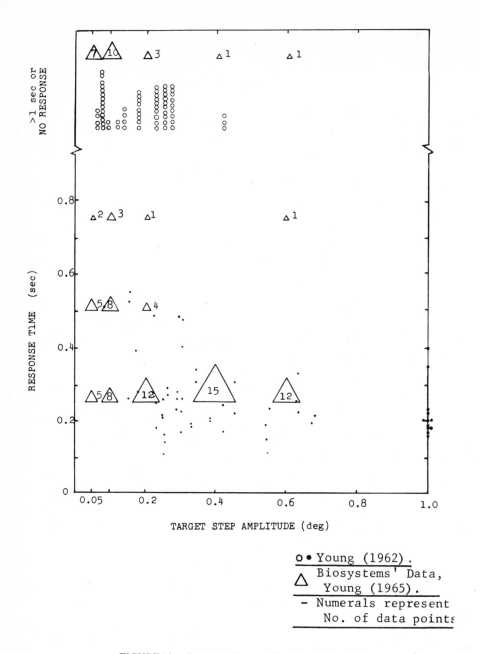

FIGURE 19.   Response time as a function of target step.

delayed response or no response at all for decreasing magnitude of the target step, and confirms the existence of a dead zone of sorts. The 1962 experiments were performed with a thin vertical line of light projected on a screen in a dark room. The 1965 experiments were performed with and without oscilloscope grid lines, but always with a rich visual field to eliminate the possibility of "no response" because the target was not *perceived* as moving relative to the background. The data show no apparent difference between the two sets of experiments.

The existence of a sizeable dead zone in the saccadic mechanism is paradoxical at first. The two-point resolution threshold for humans corresponds to the diameter of an individual cone on the retina. The cone diameter is about 1 μm, corresponding to a resolution limit of 1 arc min in the visual field, which is also approximately the diffraction limit imposed by the pupil aperture. Thus, a target step of 0.1 to 0.25° is certainly observed by the subject, and furthermore, microsaccades of less than 0.25° are frequently observed to occur spontaneously in correction of drifts, so that the quantization of saccadic corrections by the motor mechanism does not account for the observed threshold. It must be recalled, however, that the purpose of the eye movement control system is to position the eye so that the target image lies on the fovea, but not necessarily in the center of this high resolution area of the retina. The foveal diameter is about 50 μm, corresponding to less than 1° in the visual field. Thus, if the point target were initially at the center of the fovea, a step of less than half the foveal diameter would induce no immediate saccadic correction. Since the initial position of the image on the fovea is uncertain, it is seen that the occurrence of a response to any target step less than the foveal diameter can only be described statistically depending upon the magnitude of the steps. Furthermore, small random drifts always present during fixations are superposed on the image displacement due to the target step, and statistically might move the image off the fovea after some time and yield a delayed saccadic response. Thus, for any given magnitude small target step, the likelihood of a correction occurring should increase with the time following the stimulus, and by any given time exceeding one reaction time following the stimulus, the probability of a corrective saccade occurring should increase with the amplitude of the step.

A simple theory has been worked out to describe this phenomenon for a single axis. Assume that the initial fixation error (x degrees), before target motion, is uniformly distributed between the limits of the effective dead zone on the fovea ($\pm$e). Its probability density function is

$$f(x) = \begin{cases} 1/2e \text{ for } |x| \leq e \\ \\ 0 \quad \text{ for } |x| > e \end{cases}$$

Let the magnitude of the target step be y degrees. Assume the eye drift rate is constant during the period under consideration (D°/sec). The fixation error (z) at any time following the stimulus, assuming no corrective saccade has been made, is given by

$$z(t) = x + y + Dt$$

where the stimulus occurs at t = 0. Now, consider the probability density function of eye error *immediately following the next target step*. The uniform distribution of x will merely be shifted by the magnitude of the target step, and the error will be uniformly distributed between y − e and y + e.

$$f(z) = \begin{cases} 1/2e \quad \text{for } (y - e) < z < (y + e) \\ \\ 0 \qquad \text{for } z < (y - e) \text{ or } z > (y + e) \end{cases}$$

Assume further that a corrective saccade can occur one reaction time following the stimulus only if the poststimulus error [z(0)] exceeds the dead zone $|z(0)| > e$. The probability of z(0) exceeding e depends upon the step stimulus y, and is given by

$$P[z(0)] > e = \begin{cases} y/2e \ [P_{nt}(t_0)] \quad \text{for } y < 2e \\ \\ P_{nt}(t_0) \qquad\qquad \text{for } y > 2e \end{cases}$$

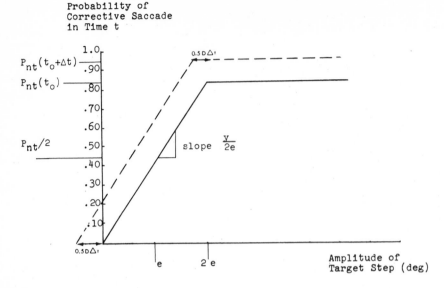

FIGURE 20.   Statistical model predictions of probability of corrective saccade. Solid line: predicted probability density of corrective saccade occurring in one reaction time. Dashed line: predicted probability density of corrective saccade occurring in one reaction time plus $\triangle$ sec. Slope: $y/2e$.

(The factor $P_{nt}(t_0)$ represents the nonthreshold-connected probability of eliciting a corrective saccade in a minimum reaction time t_0. Even with a large target step, a number of delayed responses are observed, and this factor is introduced to avoid confusion with the threshold phenomenon.) The probability density curve given by the above equation is the solid line in Figure 20. The probability of a corrective saccade occurring in one reaction time (approximately 250 msec) varies linearly with the amplitude of the target step from 0 up to a target step of 2e, or twice the dead zone angle, reaching a threshold probability $P_{nt}(t_0)$ for large target steps.

By waiting longer than one reaction time to observe a corrective saccade, one may include the statistical effects of the random drift. Assuming that a corrective saccade will be triggered if the error [z(t)] *ever* exceeds the dead zone e, it is clear that the effect of a constant velocity drift can only be to increase the probability of a corrective saccade by drifting the eye across the dead zone, but can never eliminate a corrective saccade by drifting the eye back into the dead zone once the error e had been exceeded. If the drift were always in the direction of increasing fixation error at D°/sec, then the effect of waiting an additional Δt seconds to observe a corrective saccade would be the same as adding a bias angle $D\Delta t$ to the target step. If the simple assumption is made that half the time the drift is in the direction of increasing error than this bias is 0.5 $D\Delta t°$, as is shown by the dashed line in Figure 20. An additional correction is necessitated by the fact that the nonthreshold probability of corrective saccade occurrence is increased with increasing time after the stimulus.

To check this formulation, the data of Figure 18 was replotted in terms of the probability of corrective saccades vs target step amplitude, as shown in Figure 21. Notice first the data represented by the solid circles over the single horizontal lines, representing for each target step amplitude range the probability of observing a corrective saccade within 250 msec following the stimulus. This might be called the *one reaction time probability density*, although it is considerably longer than the minimum reaction time which can be observed. The data follows roughly the form predicted by the simple

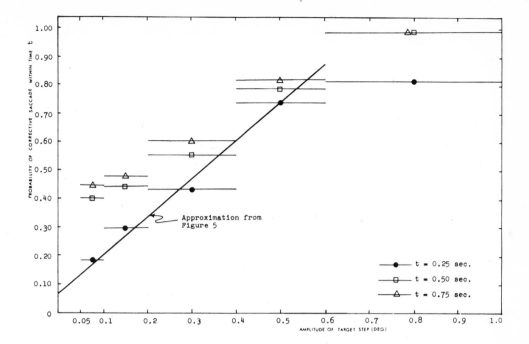

FIGURE 21.   Probability of corrective saccade within time versus target step amplitude.

statistical model illustrated in Figure 20, with the probability of a corrective saccade increasing linearly with target amplitude up to a certain angle and then leveling off. The straight line approximation to this data can be used to estimate the threshold level or the extent of the saccadic dead zone. The parameters describing this straight line approximation are

$$P_{nt}(0.25 \text{ sec}) = 0.82$$

$$\text{Probability density slope} = 1.35 \text{ (degrees}^{-1})$$

Probability density slope = 1.35 (degrees⁻¹)

The theory predicts:

$$\text{Probability density slope} = P_{nt}(t) [y/2e]$$

This data approximation yields a dead zone amplitude of

$$e \simeq 0.3 \text{ degrees}$$

Alternatively, if e is estimated from the fiftieth percent of asymptotic probability point, the curve yields

$$e \simeq 0.26 \text{ degrees}$$

The fact that the straight line approximation does not pass through the origin may be accounted for by the distribution of reaction times. Since reaction times shorter than 250 msec allow for the favorable influence of eye drift, the entire curve might be shifted upward slightly from the predicted curve.

Figure 21 also indicates the probability of a corrective saccade occurring in longer than one reaction time following the target step. The line indicated by open squares and those denoted by open triangles represent the probability of corrective saccades occurring within 500 and 750 msec respectively, following the target step. As predicted by the simple theory, the probability density curve is shifted to the left by waiting over increased intervals following the target step, and the nonthreshold probability also increases when longer time is permitted to observe a corrective saccade. This data is not sufficiently complete to make accurate quantitative estimates of high-drift rate to check the statistical model; however, an approximate calculation may be made as follows. Assume that the data of Figure 20 yields an average shift of the probability density curve to the left of approximately 0.1 deg for every 0.25 sec of additional time following one reaction time. Using the equation

$$Bias = 0.5d\Delta t$$

one calculates $D = 0.8$ deg/sec for the eye drift rate, which is quite consistent with the drift rate observed under normal fixation conditions.

In summary, these experiments on saccadic eye movement dead zone confirm a simple statistical theory for the probability of corrective saccades as a function of time and amplitude. The accuracy specifications on saccades, therefore, must be to keep the eye positioned within a dead zone of approximately ±0.3 deg, with corrective saccades occurring whenever the combination of initial fixation error, target movement, and eye drift move the eye out of the dead zone.

VII. CONCLUSIONS

A review of the evolution of the sampled data model and dead zone approximation for saccadic eye movements is presented, along with some of the principal experimental observations relevant to the model. Although no successful attempts have identified the "neurophysiological sampler", the model continues to serve a useful role for hypothesis generation and experiment interpretation. It is in this continuing process of model generation and of experiments, the results of which support or change the model, that the real value of all such quantitative theories resides.

REFERENCES

1. Aslin, R., Development of smooth pursuit in human infants, in Proc. Behav. Res. Dir., U.S. Army Human Engineering Laboratory's Conference on Eye Movements, February, 1980.
2. Baker, R. and Berthoz, A., Eds., Control of Gaze by Brain Stem Neurons, in *Developments Neurosci.*, Vol. 1, Elsevier, North Holland, 1977.
3. Becker, W., Control of eye movements in the saccadic system, *Bibliogr. Ophthalmol,* 82, 233, 1972.
4. Becker, W. and Fuchs, A. F., Further properties of the human saccadic system: eye movements and correction saccades with and without visual fixation points, *Vision Res.,* 9, 1247, 1969.
5. Beeler, G., Visual threshold changes resulting from spontaneous saccadic eye movements, *Vision Res.,* 7, 769, 1967.
6. Brodskey, J. S. and Stark, L., New direct evidence against intermittency or sampling in human smooth pursuit eye movements, *Nature,* 218, 273, 1968.
7. Collewijn, H., Gaze in freely moving subjects, in *Control of Gaze by Brain Stem Neurons,* Baker, R. and Berthoz, A., Eds., Elsevier/North Holland, Amsterdam, 1977.
8. Carpenter, R. H. S., The oculomotor procrastination, in Proc. Behav. Res. Dir. U.S. Army Human Engineering Laboratory's Conference on Eye Movements, February, 1980.

9. Clark, M. R. and Stark, L., Time optimal behavior of human saccadic eye movement, IEEE Trans. Autom. Control, June 1975, 345.

10. Dallos, P. J. and Jones, R. W., Learning behaviour of the eye fixation control system, IEEE Trans. Autom. Control, AC-8, 218, 1963.

11. Fuchs, A. F., Periodic eye tracking in monkey, J. Physiol., 193, 161-171, 1967.

12. Fuchs, A. F., The saccadic system, in The Control of Eye Movements, Bach-y-Rita, P., Collins, C. C., and Hyde, J. E., Eds., Academic Press, New York, 1971.

13. Grüsser, O. J. and Grüsser-Cornehls, U., Interaction of vestibular and visual inputs in the visual system, in Basic Aspects of Central Vestibular Mechanisms, Prog. Brain Res., Vol. 37, Brodal, A. and Pompieano, O., Eds., Elsevier, Amsterdam, 1972.

14. Heywood, S. and Churcher, J. H., Eye movements and the after-image. I. Tracking the after-image, Vision Res., 11, 1163, 1971.

15. Holzman, P. S., Kringlen, E., Levy, D. L., Proctor, L. R., Habermann, S. J., and Yasillo, N. J., Abnormal pursuit eye movements in schizophrenia, Arch. Gen. Psychiatr., 34, 802, 1977.

16. Horrocks, A. and Stark, L., Experiments on error as a function of response time in horizontal eye movements, Quarterly Progress Report, Res. Lab. Electron. Massachusetts Institute of Technology, 1964, 72, 267.

17. Hsu, F., Krishnan, V. V. and Stark, L., Simulation of ocular dysmetria using a sampled data model of the human saccadic system, Ann. Biomed. Eng. 4, 321, 1976.

18. Johnson, L. E., Human eye tracking of apreiodic target functions, Report 37-B-63-8, System Research Center, Case Institute of Technology, Cleveland, 1963.

19. Jury, E. I. and Pavlidis, T., Discussion of a sampled data model for eye tracking in 2nd Int. Conf. IFAC, Butterworths, 1963, 461.

20. Kommerell, G. and Taumer, R., Investigation of the eye tracking system through stabilized retinal images, Bibliogr. Ophthalmol., 82, 280, 1972.

21. Lauringson, A. and Shchedrovitskii, L., Certain information on the systems of tracking of the eye, Biofizika, 10, 137, 1965.

22. Levy-Schoen, A. and Blanc-Garin, J., On oculomotor programming and perception, Brain Res., 71, 443, 1974.

23. Mays, L. and Sparks, D. Interaction of saccades induced by visual stimuli and electrical stimulation of the superior colliculus, Soc. Neurosci. Abstr., 5, 377, 1979.

24. Meiry, J. L., The Vestibular System and Human Dynamic Space Orientation, Sc. D. Thesis, Massachusetts Institute of Technology, Cambridge, 1965.

25. Morrasso, P., Bizzi, E., and Dichgans, J., Adjustment of saccade characteristics during head movements, Exp. Brain Res. 16, 492, 1972.

26. Murphy, D. N. P. and Deekshatulu, B. L., A new model for the control mechanism of the human eye, Int. J. Control, 6, 263, 1961.

27. Rashbass, C., The relationship between saccadic and smooth tracking eye movements, J. Physiol. (London), 159, 326, 1961.

28. Robinson, D. A., The mechanics of human saccadic eye movement. J. Physiol., 174, 245, 1964.

29. Robinson, D. A., Mechanics of human smooth pursuit eye movements. J. Physiol., 180, 569, 1965.

30. Robinson, D. A., Models of the saccadic eye movement control system, Kybernetik 14, 71, 1973.

31. Selhorst, J. B., Stark, L., Ochs, A. L., and Hoyt, W. F., Disorders in cerebellar ocular motor control. I. Saccadic overshoot dysmetria: an oculographic, control system and clinico-anatomical analysis, Brain, 99, 497, 1976. II. Macrosaccadic oscillation: an oculographic, control system and clinico-anatomical analysis, Brain, 99, 509, 1976.

32. Steinback, M. J. and Pearce, D. G., Release of pursuit eye movements using after images, Vision Res., 12, 1307, 1972.

33. Steinman, R. B., Haddad, G. M., Skavenski, A. A., and Wyman, D., Miniature eye movements, Science, 181, 810, 1973.

34. Sugie, N. and Melvill Jones, G., A model of eye movements induced by head rotation, IEEE Trans. Syst. Man, Cybern., SMC-1:251, 1971.

35. Vossius, G., Der Kybernetische Aspekt der Willkurbewegung, Prog. in Biocybern. (Jpn.), 2, 111, 1965.

36. Westheimer, G., Eye movement with respect to a horizontally moving visual stimulus, Arch Ophthalmol., 52, 932, 1954.

37. Wheeless, L. L., Jr., Boynton, R. M., and Cohen, G. H., Eye movement responses to step and pulse step stimuli, J. Opt. Soc. Am., 56, 956, 1966.

38. Yasui, S., Nystagmus Generation, Oculomotor Tracking and Visual Motion Perception, Ph.D. Thesis, Massachusetts Institute of Technology, Cambridge, 1974.

39. Yasui, S. and Young, L. R., Perceived visual motion as effective stimulus to the pursuit eye movement system, Science, 190, 906, 1975.

40. **Young, L. R.,** A Sampled Data Model for Eye Tracking Movements, Sc.D. Thesis, Massachusetts Institute of Technology, Cambridge, 1962.
41. **Young, L. R.,** A sampled data model for eye tracking movements, Int. Fed. Autom. Control, Basel, Switzerland, September, 1963; *Automatic and Remote Control,* Butterworths, 1963.
42. **Young, L. R.,** Pursuit eye tracking, in *The Control of Eye Movements,* Bach-y-Rita, P., Collins, C. C., and Hyde, J. E., Eds., Academic Press, New York, 1971.
43. **Young, L. R.,** Pursuit eye movement — what is being pursued?, in *Control of Gaze by Brain Stem Neurons,* Baker, R. and Berthoz, A., Eds., Elsevier, North Holland, 1977.
44. **Young, L. R., Forster, J. D., and Van Houtte, N. A. J.,** A revised stochastic sampled data model for eye tracking movements, 4th Ann. NASA Univ. Conf. Man. Control, NASA SP-192, 1968.
45. **Young, L. R. and Stark, L.,** Variable feedback experiments testing a sampled data model for eye tracking movements, IEEE Trans. Hum. Factors Electron, HFE-4, 38, 1963.
46. **Young, L. R., Zuber, B. L. and Stark, L.,** Visual and Control Aspects of Saccadic Eye Movements, 1966, NASA CR-564.
47. **Zuber, B. L.,** Physiological Control of Eye Movements, Ph.D. Thesis, Massachusetts Institute of Technology, 1965.
48. **Zuber, B. L. and Djordjevich, D.,** Effective sampling time for saccadic eye movements from experiments utilizing a vergence input, *Am. J. Ophthalmol. and Physiol. Opt.,* 57, 595, 1980.

Chapter 4

TIME OPTIMAL SACCADIC TRAJECTORY MODEL AND VOLUNTARY NYSTAGMUS

Lawrence Stark, William Hoyt, Kenneth Ciuffreda, Robert Kenyon, and Frederick Hsu

TABLE OF CONTENTS

I. INTRODUCTION

The motivation for presenting this chapter is to demonstrate control modelling in bioengineering. Current theories for eye movement control are most often embedded in such quantitative mathematical models that use simulation on digital computers as the preferred means to "crank" the model and to produce model behavioral output. Besides an explicit presentation of the theory, a model ensures consistency among the physical, physiological, and anatomical components of the model. The behavior of the model can then be compared with known facts of eye movements and may even be used to discover new phenomena. Indeed, here we find clinical applications play a vital role in pure scientific research; often a puzzling clinical phenomenon can be used as a stringent clinical test of the model. The particular example this chapter provided us with was an exciting test for the reciprocal-innervation trajectory model that was developed over the years, first for arm movement,[1,2] and more recently for eye saccades by Cook and Stark[3] and Clark and Stark.[4-6]

The trajectory model is based upon the time optimal control theory.[7-10] It predicted higher-order controller signal switchings in the envelopes of nerve impulse firings that represent the neurological control signals for the eye saccade. These higher-order switchings account for the existence of dynamic overshoots in a majority of saccades — an important and successful prediction of the basic theory.[11] It also demonstrated the mechanisms underlying the main sequence relationships studied experimentally since the early studies of Dodge in 1901.[12,13] Simulation studies of the trajectory model clearly show that the saccade is a not "mechanically ballistic" movement, since muscular mechanical forces act during the entire saccadic trajectory. Contrariwise, a ballistic movement receives all of its impetus at the initiation of the trajectory, as is true for a baseball.

Neurological studies of movement are older than modern engineering control theory and are more intuitive than quantitative; they provide us with the concept of different levels in the Jacksonian sense of motor control. From this neurological point of view, the trajectory model is at the Jacksonian "lower level". A "higher level" control model for eye tracking movements using visual feedback was developed by Young and Stark.[14,15] This sampled data model captures important intermittent characteristics of saccades. After the neuronal signals for a saccade are preprogrammed, these signals are ordinarily not altered, and thus, we see the "neurologically ballistic" saccade eventuated. It may be helpful to use the term "neurologically ballistic" to clearly specify the intuitive understanding that neurophysiologists and neurologists have of the behavior results of this intermittent discontinuous control function. Finally, at the "highest level" of control, one might mention the scanpath model for visual recognition that incorporates saccadic movements along with sensory subfeatures as the internal components of memory traces of complex visual objects.[16] These "highest level" models, unfortunately, have not yet developed to the quantitative precision of the "higher level" sampled data model or the "lower level" trajectory model. They do, however, illustrate the role of multi-level control and of the necessarily different levels of models for different levels of control.

Those familiar with models in current scientific epistemology realize that models are not absolutely true and forever. They are rather a tool for thinking and especially for suggesting new experiments.[17] Indeed, Wilkie has proposed that there is an optimal lifetime for a model or theory — if too short, the model does not become well enough known to be useful; if too long, the model has not succeeded in generating enough new experiments to require further modification and change. Thus, models are not put forward as arrogant or presumptuous final statements, but rather as entry vehicles to explore further and to expand our knowledge in their particular area.

Neurological implications of voluntary nystagmus with its willfully evoked, short-lasting bursts of shimmering horizontal oscillations, occasionally exceeding 2000 cycles/min have puzzled clinicians for years. Many features of this ocularmotor phenomenon had been described,[18-33] but its saccadic compostion was established only recently by analysis of high resolution oculographic recordings.[34-36] From oculographic recordings and computer simulations, this chapter describes the critical role of temporal sequencing of saccades in production of voluntary nystagmus.

II. METHODS

Horizontal eye rotation was measured with an infrared photocell instrument having a bandwidth of 1 kHz and a noise level equivalent to 8 min of arc.[37] Frequent calibration guaranteed that recorded eye movements faithfully reflected retinal rotations. Measurements were linear over a range of 20 degrees. Accurate interrelationsips of position velocity, and acceleration could be displayed for both normal saccades and the voluntary nystagmus saccades, because we used digital computer sampling at 5000 times/sec and computer algorithms for differentiation and summing or smoothing with bandwidths of 250 Hz to eliminate phase distortion.

These eye movements were measured in six normal subjects who could initiate their voluntary nystagmus at will in various ways — convergence, intense staring at distance. They followed an ocularmotor testing protocol which included fixation, smooth pursuit, saccadic tracking, vergence, and optokinetic nystagmus.

Simulation studies were done using a computer model that encompasses reciprocal innervation, the nonlinear force-velocity relationship of muscle, and globe mechanics.[3,38,39] The control signals in the model were pulse-step envelopes that were first-order and time optimal[38] and in which the step was shortened or truncated to reproduce the high frequency of voluntary nystagmus. The model was simulated on a minicomputer using mixed FORTRAN II and assembly code. The computer displayed the behavior of the model graphically on a storage scope and listed quantitative parameters on a typing terminal. Since it was a digital simulation, internal parameters were easily varied and model responses were noise free.

III. OCULOGRAPHIC FINDINGS

Amplitudes of nystagmus and how long it could be maintained varied widely from time to time and from subject to subject. Eye position traces (Figure 1) showed the "pendular" quality of voluntary nystagmus even when unsmoothed and unfiltered by our high fidelity recording system. The velocity traces (Figure 1) documented the high velocity that defines saccades.

The velocity traces of high-frequency, low-amplitude forms of the nystagmus (Figure 1) showed pendular form, with decelerating velocity of one saccade smoothly continuing into accelerating velocity of the next. Velocity traces of low-frequency, high-amplitude forms of the nystagmus (Figure 2) appeared more saccadic than pendular and showed occasional shelving, indicating an intersaccadic period. The conjugate nature of voluntary nystagmus (Figure 2) was documented in simultaneous position and velocity traces from right and left eyes. Minor, nonconjugate differences were also present; these conformed in magnitude to differences found in normal conjugate saccades and considered as dynamic violations of Hering's law by Bahill, Ciuffreda, Kenyon, and Stark.[40]

Amplitude, and with it frequency, of the nystagmus could be altered at will by several of our subjects (Figure 2). These amplitudes and frequencies had an obligate and inverse relationship (Figure 3). In its most rapid form, nystagmus frequency approached 40 Hz; this means 80 saccades/sec or 12.5 msec/saccade.

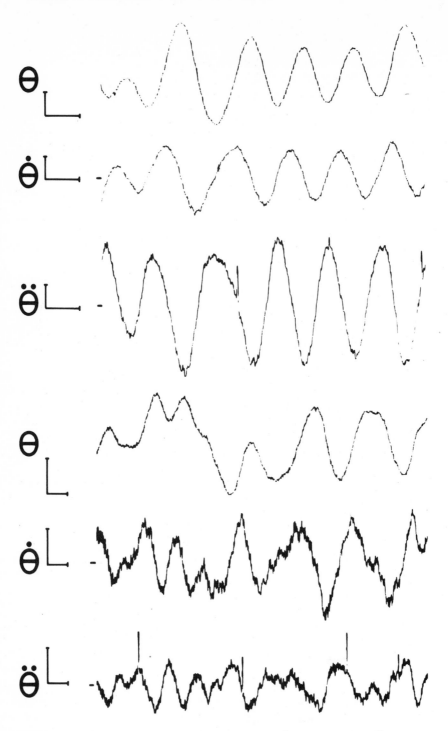

FIGURE 1.   Time functions of eye position, θ, velocity, $\dot{\theta}$, and acceleration, $\ddot{\theta}$, for two subjects. Note, especially, very high velocity which is defining feature of saccadic eye movements. Absence of zero velocity and zero acceleration regions appearing as "shelves" suggests some attenuation in duration of a least part of stepphase of normal pulse-step saccades. Acceleration trace also shows noise limitations in eye movement recording. Vertical calibration bars indicate 0.51 deg, 103 deg,/sec, and 20,000 deg,/sec/sec for upper traces and 0.57 deg, 62 deg,/sec, and 30,000 deg,/sec,/sec, for lower traces, and also zero levels of eye position velocity, and acceleration; horizontal calibration bars represent 100 msec.

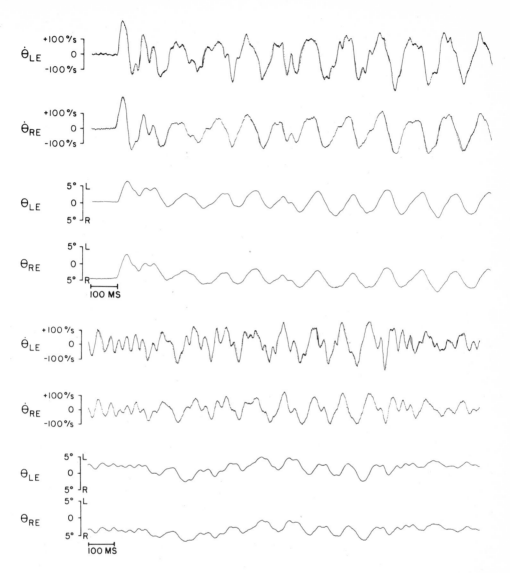

FIGURE 2. Hering's Law Conjugacy in Voluntary Nystagmus: Top four traces show conjugate eye movements occurring during voluntary nystagmus. Especially with velocity traces, one can see small dynamic violations of Hering's Law similar to those occurring with normal saccadic eye movements. Initiation of voluntary nystagmus is shown at beginning of trace. Lower four traces show another sequence of voluntary nystagmus and again conjugacy of these rapidly succeeding eye movements.

Peak accelerations, peak velocities and durations, as functions of amplitudes of eye movements, were plotted for ordinary refixation saccades and saccadic components of the nystagmus (Figure 4). Plots of the data from the refixation saccades fitted the main sequence relationship, first studied by Dodge.[12,41] Plots of peak velocity data from the saccades of voluntary nystagmus fell above the main sequence. Similarly, plots of peak acceleration data from the saccades of the nystagmus fell above the main sequence (Figure 4).

Two of our subjects could initiate and maintain voluntary nystagmus while performing saccadic tracking and smooth pursuit tasks. Oculographic recordings (Figure 5) during such tasks documented saccades of voluntary nystagmus superimposed upon refixation saccades and upon smooth pursuit movements.

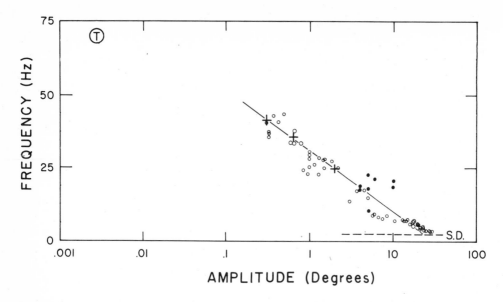

FIGURE 3.   Frequency-amplitude diagram for voluntary nystagmus. Open circles are values derived by us from our subjects. Filled circles are data from literature. Crosses show results of simulations. Lowest frequency approaches 2.5 Hz sampled data frequency (S.D.). At high frequency region, point "T" represents the 0.0027° amplitude of 70 Hz physiological microtremor. Main sequence position of the microtremor values supports our novel suggestion that this microtremor is saccadic.

Frequency-amplitude plot is determined both by dynamic and control characteristics of saccades as diagrammed on main sequence and also by overlapping of voluntary nystagmus saccades until synchronization and summation of successive acceleratory phases occurs.

IV. COMPUTER SIMULATION STUDIES

In simulating voluntary nystagmus, we used the reciprocal innervation model of extraocular muscles, globe dynamics, and pulse-step innervation. The model translates a sequential train of pulse-step innervations into a sequential train of alternating saccades so constructed that the initial amplitudes (1° (Figure 6) and 2.3° (Figure 7)) produced velocities corresponding to representative peak velocities from our subjects, voluntary nystagmus traces.

Spacing between the saccades in the model was gradually collapsed by truncating the step portions of the controller signals. Behavior of these simulated trains of saccades (Figures 6 and 7) was examined in terms of the acceleration time functions. As the pulse signals occurred closer together, the deceleration phase of one saccade approached the acceleration phase of the next, until close packing of these pulse signals produced superposition of successive decelerations and accelerations. At this point, the model reached "synchronization" frequency. At this frequency, saccades were overlapped and saccadic amplitudes truncated; peak accelerations, being superimposed, had values in excess of those for normal main sequence saccades. Peak velocity, because it occurs in mid-trajectory, is not altered by this close packing process. At synchronization frequency in our model, the data plots for peak acceleration, peak velocity, and duration closely fit plots from the parallel oculographic data of our subject's voluntary nystagmus (Figure 4). Also, at synchronization frequency, simulated voluntary nystagmus displayed the smooth pendular form documented in our oculographic recording and so often remarked upon by other investigators. For each amplitude, synchronization of the models' alternating opposed saccades (with superposition of acceleration phases) also determined a particular frequency. The frequency-amplitude

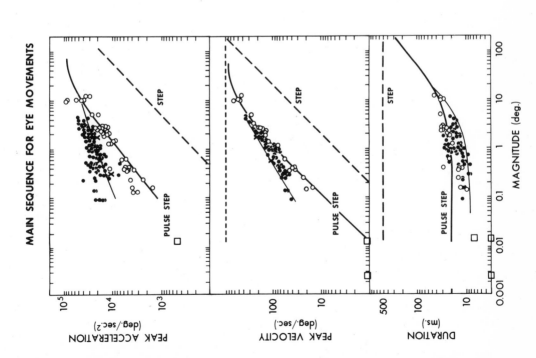

FIGURE 4. Main sequence of acceleration, velocity, and duration as functions of amplitude. Solid lines and x's represent simulation values for pulse-step controller and dashed lines values for step-controller. Refixation tracking saccades (open circles) of our subjects fit pulse-step controller lines, demonstrating normal controller signals, eye muscle contraction forces and patterns, and eyeball dynamics. Voluntary nystagmus saccades (solid circles) are clearly related to saccadic pulse-step controller lines, rather than to step-controller line for slower vergence and glissadic eye movements. Minor deviations with larger velocities and accelerations and shorter durations are understandable in terms of amplitude truncation produced by rapid succession of next alternating saccades seen in these high-frequency voluntary nystagmus saccadic trains and verified by simulations as in Figures 5 and 6.

Peak velocities and accelerations of the saccades of voluntary nystagmus are somewhat higher and the durations somewhat shorter than normal main sequence values, suggesting that succession of alternating saccades is so rapid that full amplitude of saccades are not achieved. Thus, peak velocities found are appropriate for larger saccades than occur and are larger than normal for saccadic amplitudes measured.

Also note six square boxes in small magnitude region of graph. The two leftward boxes represent amplitude, duration, and velocity for physiological microtremor.[47,48] The four rightward boxes are shifted to estimate unattenuated amplitude when fitted to main sequence velocity and acceleration curves for pulse-step control.

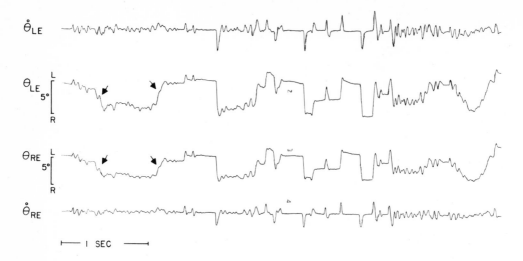

FIGURE 5.   Superpostion of voluntary nystagmus saccades onto 8° refixation tracking saccades (beginning of trace) and during smooth pursuit (end of trace). Note especially (arrows) summation of motoneuronal controller signals for voluntary nystagmus saccades and usual refixation tracking saccades, thus, indicating separate and independent saccadic generating mechanisms at some level of neurological control. Left eye velocity, left eye position, right eye position, and right eye velocity, from top to bottom, respectively, as functions of time, for subject D.T.

relationship of the model nicely fits the frequency-amplitude relationship found in our oculographic recordings (Figure 3).

V. DISCUSSION

A. Voluntary Nystagmus is Saccadic

Before starting these present oculargraphic and computer simulation studies, we knew that voluntary nystagmus is saccadic.[34-36] The motor definition of saccades rests on the very high velocity of these extraordinary movements. All saccades — schematic, refixational, corrective, and microfixational — share the defining velocity-amplitude relationship studied since the time of Dodge.[12-13,41,42]

B. Overlapping Produces Truncation

An apparent discrepancy in the velocities of voluntary nystagmus saccades is that they lie above the normal Main Sequence velocity-amplitude relationship (Figure 4); with our high resolution recordings, we established this apparent discrepancy. By means of our simulation studies, we showed it to be a consequence of truncation of amplitudes of voluntary nystagmus saccades, while velocities remain normal. These simulations demonstrated the mechanism for truncation, namely, overlapping of closely packed saccadic trajectories. Peak velocity, occurring in the middle of the trajectory, is unaffected by overlapping and truncation. According to the model, the width of the pulse envelope of neural firing is much less than the duration of these small saccades, thus, the high-frequency bursts of motoneural activity is also unaffected by overlapping and truncation.[43] An alternative explanation explored was that voluntary nystagmus subjects might have unusually strong, fast ocular muscles. However, parametric data of normal refixation saccades from our voluntary nystagmus subjects (open circles, Figure 4) lie right on the Main Sequence curves; this alternate hypothesis was discarded.

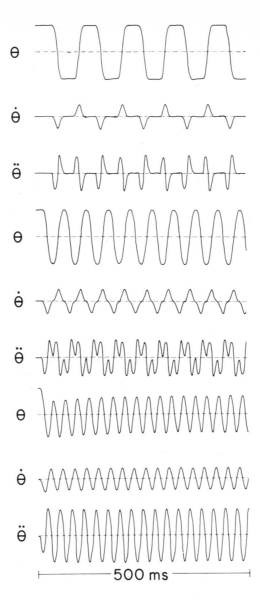

FIGURE 6. Simulation studies: Upper three traces show position, velocity, and acceleration of simulated successive closely-spaced, but not overlapping, saccades with 1° amplitude, 88°/sec peak velocity and 11,300°/sec/sec peak acceleration. Middle three traces represent compression of successive saccades, but still without overlapping or amplitude attenuation. Peak velocity and peak acceleration values remain the same. Note absence of intersaccadic interval and also two distinct acceleration phases for each saccade.

Bottom three traces show further compression of successive alternating saccades to produce overlapping saccades and attenuation of saccadic amplitude to 0.66°. Peak velocity remains approximately same value in center of saccadic trajectory. Deceleratory phase synchronous with following acceleratory phase produces large summation acceleration of 17,000°/sec/sec.

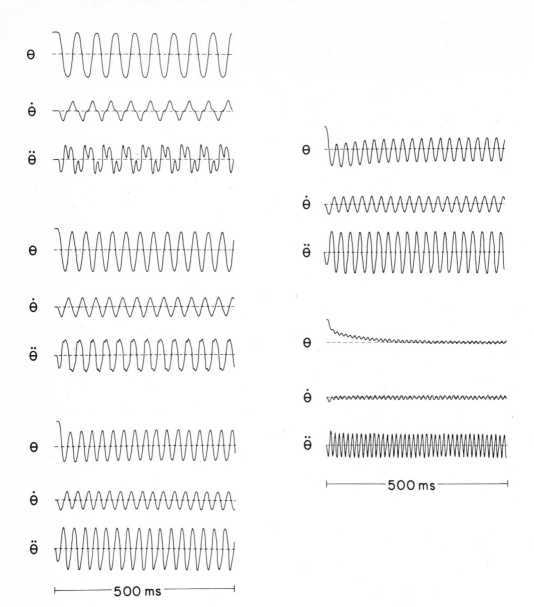

FIGURE 7. Simulation studies: Top left shows very closely spaced saccades almost with absence of inter-saccadic interval but without overlapping. Magnitude of 2.3°, peak velocity of 188°/sec, and peak acceleration of 23,500°/sec/sec. Middle left shows slightly overlapping saccades, with not quite synchronized phases of acceleration. Maximum velocity shows no decrement, but amplitude is attenuated about 10%. Bottom left shows accelerations now synchronized and summated with a high value of 35,000°/sec/sec. Maximum velocity is unchanged, but amplitude now reduced to 1.5° because of overlapping of saccades; frequency of simulated voluntary nystagmus is 33 Hz.

Upper right: Lateral compression of simulated voluntary nystagmus saccades is continued so that magnitude is now only 1.1° by virtue of overlapping. Maximum velocity negligibly affected and maximum acceleration still the large synchronized summated value; frequency 40 Hz. Lower right: Simulation now greatly oorcompressed beyond where the voluntary nystagmus frequency-amplitude is found experimentally.

C. "Synchronization" Determines the Frequency-Amplitude Relationship of Volunatary Nystagmus

Synchronization of acceleration phases with the preceeding deceleration phases provides qualitative explanation for one of the striking features of voluntary nystagmus, its pendular form (Figure 1). The resulting summation of acceleration phases provides a quantitative explanation for the increased acceleration values (Figure 4).

Synchronization frequency is analogous to the rhythmic rocking that a skilled driver produces by precisely timed shifting between first and reverse gears in working an automobile out of snow or sand. Apparently, subjects performing voluntary nystagmus pack saccades closely enough to obtain a similar synchronization.

This synchronization ties amplitude and frequency in an obligate relationship (Figure 3). We have a wide enough range of amplitudes (0.4 to 30 degrees) and frequencies (42 to 3 Hz) from our six subjects and from data in the literature[22,24,25,27,28,33] to confirm the validity and accuracy of the model. Our model of voluntary nystagmus successfully embodies both dynamics of normal saccades *and* close-packing to synchronization frequency of voluntary nystagmus saccades. Proposed neural models[44] should be tested to see if they can also predict these quantitative facts concerning voluntary nystagmus.

D. Microtremor Appears to be Saccadic

The wide range of amplitude and frequency evident in our measurements of voluntary nystagmus (Figure 3) documents a clear and inverse relationship — the smaller the amplitude, the higher the frequency. At the highest frequency, about 40 Hz, the nystagmus amplitude is less than ½ degree; at this level the shimmering of the eye is barely perceptible to the subject or the clinician.

This voluntary ocular tremor at 40 Hz approaches the 50 to 80 Hz tremor of 5 to 40 sec of arc recorded by optical lever techniques, during normal fixation.[45-48] We speculated that fixational microtremor lies at one extreme of the frequency-amplitude function for synchronized trains of alternating saccades (Figure 3). We calculated the velocity of the approximately sinusoidal 10 sec of arc, 70 Hz microtremor to be 1.2 degrees/sec, and the acceleration to be 50 degrees/sec/sec. By entering this data into the Main Sequence plot (Figure 4), we found support for our speculation, since the values fitted reasonably at the low magnitude extreme of the curves identifying saccades. Simulation of the microtremor confirmed our analyses and demonstrated absence of mechanical limitations to oscillation at this high frequency and low amplitude.

E. Independent Vs. Shared Mechanisms Suggest a Locus of Injection of Voluntary Nystagmus Control Signals

The saccades of voluntary nystagmus and of normal refixation have important differences in the neurological substrate for their command signals. It has been hypothocated that refixation saccades operate on a sampled data principle* using intermittent neurologically ballistic motor control and accomplish perceptual stabilization of visual space by employing efferent copy corollary discharge information.[49,50] The high-frequency and tight packing of voluntary nystagmus saccades precludes use of sampled data mechanisms. Oscillopsia, a sensory hallmark of voluntary nystagmus, also pre-

---

* The sampled data model captures the important intermittent characteristic of saccades.[14,15] After the neural signals for a saccade are preprogrammed, the signals are ordinarily not altered and we see the neurologically ballistic saccade eventuated. Since muscular mechanical forces act during the entire saccadic trajectory, it is clear that the saccadic eye movement is not mechanically ballistic, in the sense of receiving all of its impetus at the initiation of trajectory as would be true for a cricket ball!

cludes use of efference copy.* [22,34,36] This means that the command signals for voluntary nystagmus bypass these two supranuclear mechanisms, sampled data and efference copy, that participate in refixation saccades. In this study, we discovered that voluntary nystagmus saccades can be superimposed upon trajectories of refixation saccades (Figure 5). This is direct evidence that higher level, in the Jacksonian sense, mechanisms generating voluntary nystagmus and refixation saccades are independent.

Saccades of voluntary nystagmus and of normal refixation saccades have important similarities in the neurological substrate for their command signals at the brainstem level. Both kinds of saccades are conjugate, have pulse-step envelopes of neural firing, and employ reciprocal innervation. Impressive conjugacy of voluntary nystagmus is demonstrated in our high resolution records (Figures 1 and 2), but minor discrepancies exist in line with normal movements.[40] The time optimal control studies of the model and of normal saccades show the importance of the pulse-step envelope in generating saccadic movements. The pulse-step form of the neural controller signals provides for satisfactory simulation of voluntary nystagmus as it does for refixation saccades. The normal peak velocities of both types of saccades are evidence of normal reciprocal innervation. Furthermore, the synchronization of accelerations and the rapid alternation of saccades suggests that all of these lower level, in the Jacksonian sense, brainstem mechanisms for generation of saccades are present and normal.

Thus, the locus of injection of control signals for voluntary nystagmus saccades lies between the higher-level mechanisms for refixation saccades — and the shared lower-level mechanisms.

F. Initiation of Voluntary Nystagmus Remains Enigmatic

Voluntary nystagmus appears to be generated by exaggerated controller signal reversals; normal controller signal reversals are exemplified in microtremor and dynamic overshoot eye movements. Studies of reversing or "multiple pulse" control signals resulting in dynamic overshoots indicated that they achieve time optimal performance in a robust manner;[10] this suggests a physiological role for neurological signal reversals.

Subjects may initiate voluntary nystagmus by engaging a process that amplifies normal microfixational tremor, increasing its amplitude while decreasing its frequency, until oscillopsia is sensed and the oscillations can be observed clinically. This amplification process is accompanied by fixity of gaze and intensity of facial expression indicating obvious effort in this forced maneuver.

Similarly, conversion of the control signal reversals of dynamic overshoot into a postsaccadic, prolonged sequence may initiate and produce voluntary nystagmus. Indeed, one of our patients generated voluntary nystagmus for about 1 sec following each refixation saccade[34] (Figure 6). Often a forced convergence is an initiating maneuver by subjects producing voluntary nystagmus oscillation. Dynamic overshoot appears to be increased when fixational saccades superimpose onto ongoing vergence.[53] Thus, exaggeration of normal processes for neural signal reversal in dynamic overshoot may be another means to initiate the oscillations of voluntary nystagmus.

Some subjects produce nystagmus at several amplitudes, each with its own synchronization frequency. This ability to alter amplitude of nystagmus may be related to the ability to initiate nystagmus by exaggerating and modifying normal processes and normal eye movements such as microtremor and dynamic overshoot. Subjects may also produce apparently unsynchronized forms of voluntary nystagmus, subcomponents of which are an irregular mix of small and large saccades. In the appropriate clinical setting, involuntary movements of this type are called opsoclonus.

---

* During voluntary nystagmus, subjects do not perceive oscillopsia of after-images,[51] a finding that supports the Helmholtz outflow theory of stabilization of visual space.[52]

Voluntary nystagmus exemplifies elegantly neurological mechanisms for normal eye movements functioning at their limits. At a practical level, voluntary nystagmus, regardless of the patient's reason for initiating it, guarantees irrefutably the neural integrity of his brainstem. Its execution is equivalent to an olympic-style ocularmotor performance.

VI. SUMMARY

Voluntary nystagmus is saccadic as defined by the "main sequence" velocity-amplitude criterion — for any amplitude of a saccade there is a predictable maximum saccadic velocity. In this study, high fidelity recordings from six patients provided additional quantitative data indicating that the amplitudes of the saccadic subcomponents of voluntary nystagmus are truncated. Computer simulation studies using a reciprocal innervation model reproduced this truncation and the resulting overlap of successive saccades by means of close spacing of the neural bursts that are the control signals. As the neural control signals in the model were spaced more closely, a frequency of simulated voluntary nystagmus was achieved at which synchrony of acceleration phases with preceding deceleration phases occurred and the familiar pendular shape of voluntary nystagmus was reproduced. At synchrony, amplitude and frequency are tied in an obligate and inverse relationship. This demonstrated the critical role of temporal sequencing of neural control signals in the generation of voluntary nystagmus.

The same lower level supranuclear brainstem mechanism operates for saccades of voluntary nystagmus, as for saccades of normal refixation. Above this level in the brain, the generating processes are independent, as exemplified by the ability of some of our subjects to superimpose voluntary nystagmus upon refixation saccades.

ACKNOWLEDGMENTS

This investigation was supported by funds from Dean's Committee and Academic Senate, University of California, School of Medicine, San Francisco, to L.S. and W.F.H.; Neuro-Optometry Clinic grant from Professor K. Polse, Director of Clinics, University of California, School of Optometry, Berkeley, to L.S.; NIH Training Grant EY00076 to K.J.D. and R.V.K. We thank Professors A. T. Bahill, D. Fender, A. L. Ochs, and W. T. Schults, for helpful discussion, and D. Taylor for serving as a subject.

We would like to acknowledge partial support from NASA-Ames cooperative agreement NCC 2-86.

REFERENCES

1. Stark, L., *Neurological Control Systems: Studies in Bioengineering*, Plenum Press, N. Y., 1968.
2. Stark, L., Atwood, J., Elkind, J., Houk, J., King, M., and Willis, T., *Q. Prog. Rep., Res. Lab. Electr.*, 63, 215, 1961.
3. Cook, G. and Stark, L., Derivation of a model for the human eye-positioning mechanism, *Bull. Math. Biophys.*, 29, 153, 1967.
4. Clark, M. and Stark, L., Control of human eye movements. I. Modelling of extracular plant, *Math. Biosc.*, 20, 191-211. 1974.
5. Clark, M. and Stark, L., Control of human eye movements. II. A model for the extraocular plant, *Math. Biosc.*, 20, 213, 1974.
6. Clark, M. and Stark, L., Control of human eye movements. III. Dynamic characteristics of the eye tracking mechanism, *Math. Biosc.*, 20, 239, 1974.
7. Bellman, R., *Dynamic Programming*, Princeton University Press, Princeton, 1957.

8. Pontriagin, L. S., Boltyanskii, V. C., Camkrendze, R. V., and Mischenko, E. F., *The Mathematical Theory of Optimal Processes,* Translation by K. N. Trirogoff, Interscience, N.Y., John Wiley & Sons, New York, 1962.

9. Clark, M., Krishnan, V. V., and Stark, L., Inners and biocontrol models, *Bull. Math. Biol.,* 37, 161, 1975.

10. Lehman, S. and Stark, L., Simulation of linear and nonlinear eye movement models: sensitivity analyses and enumeration studies of time optimal control, *J. Cybern. Inf. Sci.,* 2, 21, 1979.

11. Bahill, T. A., Clark, M., and Stark, L., Dynamic overshoot in saccadic eye movements is caused by neurological control signal reversals, *Exp. Neurol.,* 48, 107, 1975.

12. Bahill, A. T., Clark, M., and Stark, L., The main sequence, a tool for studying human eye movements, *Math. Biosci.,* 24, 191, 1975.

13. Bahill, T. A. and Stark, L., Trajectories of saccadic eye movements, *Sci. Am.,* 240, 84, 1979.

14. Young, L. R. and Stark, L., A discrete model for eye tracking movements. IEEE Trans. Mil. Electron., MIL-7, 113, 1963.

15. Young, L. R. and Stark, L., Variable feedback experiments testing a sampled data model for eye tracking movements, IEEE Trans. Hum. Factors Electron., HFE-4, 38, 1963.

16. Noton, D. and Stark, L., Scanpaths in saccadic eye movements while viewing and recognizing patterns, *Vision Res.,* 11, 929, 1971.

17. Stark, L., Models of biocontrol systems, *Clinic All-Round,* 26, 9, 1977.

18. Elliot, R. H., A case of voluntary nystagmus, *Ophthalmoscope,* 10, 70, 1912.

19. Waddy, G., Voluntary nystagmus, *Opthlalmoscope,* 10, 316, 1912.

20. Friedenwald, H., Voluntary nystagmus, *Am. J. Ophthalmol.,* 9, 364, 1926.

21. Luhr, A. F. and Eckel, J. L., Fixation and voluntary nystagmus — a clinical study., *Arch. Ophthalmol.,* 9, 625, 1933.

22. Westheimer, G., A case of voluntary nystagmus, *Ophthalmol.,* 128, 300, 1954.

23. Friedman, M. W. and Blodget, R. M., Voluntary ocular fibrillation, *Am. J. Ophthalmol.,* 39, 78, 1955.

24. Goldberg, R. T. and Jampel, R. S., Voluntary nystagmus in a family, *Arch. Ophthalmol.,* 68, 62, 1962.

25. Wist, E. R. and Collins, W. E., Some characteristics of voluntary nystagmus, *Arch. Ophthalmol.,* 72, 479, 1964.

26. Rosenblum, J. A. and Shafer, N., Voluntary nystagmus associated with oscillopsia, *Arch. Neurol.,* 15, 560, 1966.

27. Blair, C. J., Goldberg, M. F., and von Noorden, G. K., Voluntary nystagmus — electro-ocular-graphic findings in four cases, *Arch. Ophthalmol.,* 77, 349, 1967.

28. Coren, S. and Komada, M. K., Eye movement control in voluntary nystagmus, *Am. J. Ophthalmol.,* 74, 1161, 1972.

29. Lipman, I. J., Voluntary nystagmus — ocular shuddering, *Dis. Nerv. Syst.,* 33, 200, 1972.

30. Blumenthal, H., Voluntary nystagmus, *Neurology,* 23, 223, 1973.

31. Keyes, M. J., Voluntary nystagmus in two generations, *Arch. Neurol.,* 29, 63, 1973.

32. Laux, U. and Krey, H., Der sogenannte willkurliche nystagmus, *Klin. Mbl. Augenheilk.,* 165, 936, 1974.

33. Aschoff, J. C., Becker, W., and Rettelbach, R., Voluntary nystagmus in five generations, *J. Neurosurg. Psychiatr.,* 39, 300, 1976.

34. Shults, W. T., Stark, L., Hoyt, W. F., and Ochs, A. L., Normal saccadic structure of voluntary nystagmus, *Arch Ophthalmol.,* 95, 1399, 1977.

35. Stark, L., Shults, W. T., Ciuffreda, K. J., Hoyt, W. F., Kenyon, R. V., and Ochs, A. L., Voluntary nystagmus is saccadic: evidence from sensory and motor mechanisms, *Proc. Assoc. Res. Vision Ophthalmol.,* p. 134, 1977a.

36. Stark, L., Shults, W. T., Ciuffreda, K. J., Hoyt, W. F., Kenyon, R. V., and Ochs, A. L., Voluntary nystagmus is saccadic: evidence from sensory and motor mechanisms, in Proc. Jt. Autom. Control Conf., San Francisco, 1410, 1977b.

37. Stark, L., Vossius, G., and Young, L. R., Predictive control of eye movements, *Inst. Radio Eng. Trans. Hum. Factors Electron,* 3, 52, 1962.

38. Clark, M. R. and Stark, L., Time optimal behavior of human saccadic eye movement, IEEE Trans. Autom. Control, AC-20, 345, 1975.

39. Hsu, F. K., Bahill, A. T., and Stark, L., Parametric sensitivity analysis of a homeomorphic model for saccadic and vergence eye movements, *Comput. Prog. Biomed.,* 6, 108, 1976.

40. Bahill, A. T., Ciuffreda, K. J., Kenyon, R. V., and Stark, L., Dynamic and static violations of Hering's Law of equal innervation., *Am. J. Opt. Physiol. Opt.,* 53, 786, 1976.

41. Dodge, R. and Cline, T., The angle velocity of eye movements, *Psychol. Rev.,* 8, 145, 1901.

42. Zuber, B. L., Stark, L., and Cook, G., Microsaccades and the velocity-amplitude relationship for saccadic eye movement, *Sciences,* 150, 1459, 1965.

43. Bahill, A. T. and Stark, L., The high frequency bursts of motoneural activity lasts about half the duration of saccadic eye movements, *Math. Biosci.*, 26, 319, 1975.

44. Zee, D. S. and Robinson, D. A., A hypothetical explanation of saccadic oscillations, *Ann. Neurol.*, 5, 405, 1979.

45. Ditchbourn, R. W. and Ginsborg, B. L., Involuntary eye movements during fixation, *J. Physiol. (London)*, 119, 1, 1953.

46. Matin, L., Measurement of eye movements by contact lens techniques, *J. Opt. Soc. Am.*, 54, 1008, 1964.

47. Ratliff, F. and Riggs, L. A., Involuntary motions of the eye during monocular fixation., *J. Exp. Psychol.*, 40, 687, 1950.

48. Riggs, L. A., Armington, J. C., and Ratliff, F., Motions of the retinal image during fixation, *J. Opt. Soc. Am.*, 44, 315, 1954.

49. von Holst, E. and Mittelstaedt, H., Reafferenzprinzip: Wechselwirkungen zwischen Zentralnervensystem und Periperie, *Naturwissenschaften*, 10, 464, 1950.

50. Sperry, R. W., Neural basis of the spontaneous optokinetic response produced by visual inversion, *J. Comp. Physiol. Psychol.*, 43, 482, 1950.

51. Nagle, M., Bridgeman, B., and Stark, L., Saccadic suppression during voluntary nystagmus, *Proc. Assoc. Res. Vision Ophthalmol.*, 107, 1977, Voluntary nystagmus, saccadic supression, and stabilization of the visual world, *Vision Res.*, 20, 717, 1980.

52. Helmholtz, H., *Physiological Optics,* Southhall, J. P. C., Translation published 1962 Dover Publications, Inc. 3, 242, 1866.

53. Kenyon, R. V., Ciuffreda, K. J., and Stark, L., Binocular eye movements during accommodative vergence, *Vision Res.*, 18, 345, 1978.

Chapter 5

THE ROLE OF INTEGRATION IN OCULOMOTOR CONTROL

Theodore Raphan and Bernard Cohen

TABLE OF CONTENTS

INTRODUCTION

The oculomotor system utilizes visual and vestibular information to maintain stable images on the retina. The vestibular system contributes to the stabilization by inducing compensatory eye movements in response to head movement. This occurs over the vestibulo-ocular reflex arc (VOR). The visual system generates slow eye movements that can either aid or suppress the VOR. This enables better matching between gaze and the visual surround when there is relative movement between the head and the environment. Three integrators play an important role in processing vestibular and visual signals. The purpose of this chapter is to describe these integrators and show how each functions. Some of the mathematical properties of an integrator are given first to clarify its role in oculomotor system modeling. In particular, the integrator's response to step, impulse, and sinusoidal functions will be considered. These inputs bring into evidence its behavior and are commonly used as stimuli in studying the oculomotor system.

II. PROPERTIES OF INTEGRATORS

By definition, an integrator is a system whose input-output relation is governed by the differential equation[1],

$$\dot{x} = -hx + u \qquad\qquad (1)$$

where x is the state of the integrator or its output, u is its input and i/h is its time constant (Figure 1). For a step in the input, u, i e, $u = rU(t)$ (Figure 2A), the output x rises exponentially until $x = r/h$ (Figure 2B). The time constant of the rise is l/h. As long as the stimulus persists, the integrator will maintain this level indefinitely. When the input goes to zero, the integrator dissipates its energy and the output decays to zero with its characteristic time constant l/h (Figure 2B). This system has been referred to as a "leaky" or "nonideal" integrator. If $h = 0$, the integrator is called "ideal" and its response to a step input is a linear rise or ramp whose slope is equal to the size of the input step (Figure 2C). For as long as there is an input, the output of the ideal integrator continues to rise. When the input goes to zero, the last level of output is maintained indefinitely (Figure 2C).

If the input is an impulse function (Figure 2D), the response of the nonideal integrator steps up to the value r (the strength of the impulse) and decays to zero with a time constant l/h (Figure 2E). The ideal integrator responds with a step r which is maintained for all time (Figure 2F). The impulse responses of the nonideal and ideal integrators (Figure 2E, F) are similar to the step responses for $t > t_1$, (Figure 2B, C). This is because the infinite power content of the impulse function charges the integrator in zero time and its characteristic source free behavior is seen following the impulse.

If the input u is a sinusoid, the integrator is characterized by its gain and phase as a function of frequency (Figure 3). For frequencies above $w = h$, the corner frequency (Figure 3A), the gain of the nonideal integrator drops at 20 db/decade, and the phase approaches −90 deg (Figure 3A, B). This asymptotic behavior of the nonideal integrator above the corner frequency is similar to the behavior of the ideal integrator (Figure 3C, D). Thus, the time constant of the nonideal integrator is important in determining both its time and frequency domain characteristics.

The most prominent aspect of an integrator is its ability to store information. This is best seen in its discharge characteristics in the time domain. After the input has gone to zero, there is still an output (Figure 2 B, C, E, F). The output of a nonideal integra-

INTEGRATOR

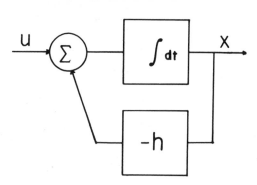

FIGURE 1.   Realization of an Integrator. x is the
state of the integrator or its output. u is the input.
The describing equation is $\dot{x} = -hx + u$. The time
constant of the nonideal integrator is l/h. When h
$= 0$, the realization is that of an ideal integrator.

tor decays to zero exponentially (Figure 2B, E). The effective length of time it can
store information is governed by its time constant: the larger the time constant, the
longer the storage. An ideal integrator stores information indefinitely (Figure 2C, F).
This corresponds to an infinite time constant, but it rarely occurs in nature.

The storage capability of an integrator determines its charge characteristics. The
ideal integrator has no mechanism for dissipating stored energy, and it accumulates
activity for as long as the stimulus persists (Figure 2C). During this time its output
rises linearly. The nonideal integrator has a loss of activity that is proportional to its
state or output: the greater the output, the greater the loss. For a step input, its output
rises exponentially to a steady level until the rate of loss of activity equals the input
(Figure 2B). At this point the rate of change of the state of the integrator is zero, i.e.,
$\dot{x} = o$ (Equation 1). This value is then held for as long as the input continues. For an
impulsive input, both the ideal integrator and nonideal integrator charge in the same
way (Figure 2E, F). This is in contrast to the difference in their discharge characteristics.

III. INTEGRATION IN THE PERIPHERAL VESTIBULAR SYSTEM

The first site of integration in the vestibulo-ocular reflex is the peripheral labyrinth.
Steinhausen[2,3] suggested that the semicircular canals behave as if they were torsion
pendulums. This implies that the cupula and endolymph respond to head rotation as
an overdamped, second order, linear system. The angular displacement of the cupula
$\xi(t)$ is related to the input angular acceleration $\alpha(t)$ by the differential equation

$$\theta\ddot{\xi} + \Pi\ddot{\xi} + \Delta\xi = \Delta\alpha \tag{2}$$

where θ is the moment of inertia, π the viscous damping coefficient and δ the elastic
restoring coefficient. The countertorque due to the moment of inertia is small compared to the viscous damping and elastic restoring torques.[4] Thus, if one neglects the
term $\theta\ddot{\xi}$ in Equation 2, the resulting equation describing the motion of the cupula is

$$\Pi\ddot{\xi} + \Delta\xi = \Delta\alpha \tag{3}$$

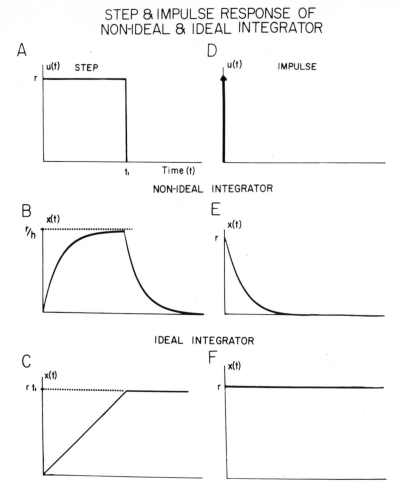

FIGURE 2.   (A) Step input, r, for 0<t<t₁, input steps back to zero for t>t₁; (B) step response of the nonideal integrator. The output, x, rises exponentially with time constant l/h to the asymptote r/h. When the input steps back to zero, the output declines to zero with the time constant l/h; (C) step response of ideal integrator. The output x rises linearly with a slope r for as long as the input is nonzero. When the input goes to zero, the output is maintained for all future time; (D) impulse functional. The functional goes to infinity at t = o but has a finite integral, r, called its strength; (E) impulse response of a nonideal integrator. The output, x, jumps to the value r (strength of impulse) and then decays to zero with a time constant l/h; (F) impulse response of ideal integrator. The output x jumps to the value r (strength of impulse). This value is maintained indefinitely.

By dividing Equation 3 by π and rearranging terms we get

$$\dot{\xi} = -(\Delta/_\Pi)\xi + (^\Delta/_\Pi)\alpha \tag{4}$$

Equation 4 is identical in form to that of Equation 1 describing the integrator. The time constant associated with the integration is $l/h = \pi/\Delta$ and the input $u = (\pi/\Delta)\alpha$ is proportional to the input angular acceleration. This simple analysis predicts that the labyrinth "integrates" angular acceleration.

GAIN & PHASE RESPONSE OF
NON-IDEAL & IDEAL INTEGRATOR

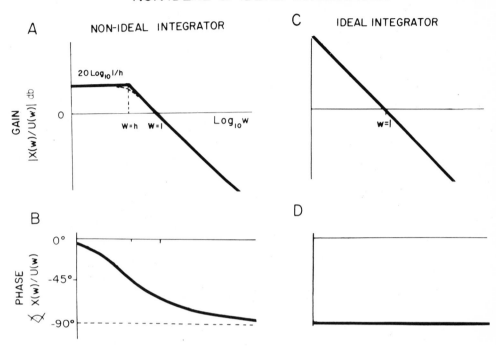

FIGURE 3. Gain and phase of nonideal and ideal integrator. (A) Gain of nonideal integrator as a function of radian frequency, w. For w<h, the gain is 20 log 1/h. For w>h, the gain drops at 20 db/decade. At w = h, the gain asymptotes intersect. This is called the break point or corner frequency. At w = 1, it crosses the zero db line. If h>1, the gain characteristic does not cross the zero db line and lies under it; (B) phase characteristics of nonideal integrator. At w = o, the phase is zero degrees. As w approaches infinity, the phase approaches −90 deg (90 deg lagging the input). At w = h, the phase is −45 deg (45 deg lagging the input); (C) gain characteristics of an ideal integrator. The gain falls at 20 db/decade with increasing w and crosses the zero db line at w = 1. The nonideal integrator gain (B) approaches that of the ideal integrator as h approaches zero; (D) Phase characteristics of an ideal integrator. It is −90 deg (90 deg lagging the input) for all frequencies, w. The phase characteristic of the nonideal integrator approaches the ideal integrator phase characteristic as h approaches zero.

Unit recordings in the eighth nerve support the theory that there is an integration of angular acceleration of the head by the semicircular canals. Afferent vestibular neurons have a resting discharge of about 50 to 100 spikes/sec. In response to head rotation, the frequency of firing is increased or decreased.[5-15] The modulation of the frequency of firing of units in response to a step of angular acceleration[9,10] (Figure 4A) is similar to the response of a nonideal integrator to a step (Figure 2B). When the input acceleration becomes zero, unit activity returns to resting levels over approximately the same time course (Figure 4B) as the discharge of the nonideal integrator (Figure 2B). The time constant associated with the rise and fall of the frequency of firing is about 3 to 5 sec (Figure 4A, B).

Some of the units show adaptative changes in firing rates (Figure 4A, right, Unit 73-21, closed circles). That is, during constant angular acceleration the neural activity approaches its resting level. When the acceleration goes to zero, the frequency of firing either undershoots or overshoots its resting level (Figure 4B, closed circles). The adap-

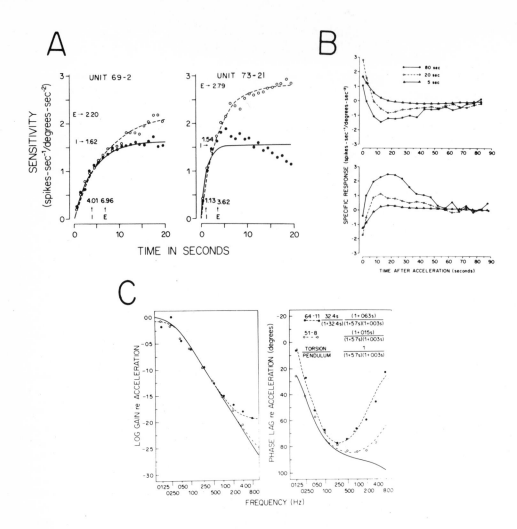

FIGURE 4.   (A) Time course of the excitatory response (open circles and inhibitory response (solid circles) of a horizontal canal unit (69-2) and a posterior canal unit (73-21). Curves, were fit with exponential approximations. The vertical arrows show the sensitivity factors of the excitatory, and inhibitory responses; (B) time course of recovery of a superior canal unit from excitatory accelerations (above) and from inhibitory accelerations (below). Each curve represents the response following an acceleration of specified duration. Accelerations were 80 sec at 3.75 deg/sec²; 20 sec at 15 deg/sec²; and 5 sec at 60 deg/sec²; (C) Bode plots (re acceleration) for two units. On the left are gain plots and the right, phase plots. The points are experimental values. The curves were calculated from the transfer functions. The log-gain at .25 Hz was arbitrarily set to the value expected from the torsion-pendulum model. Unit 64-11 was a posterior canal unit and 51-8, a horizontal canal unit. (From Goldberg, J. M. and Fernandez, C., *J. Neurophysiol.*, 34, 635, 1971; and Fernandez, C. and Goldberg, J. M., *J. Neurophysiol.*, 34, 661, 1971. With permission.)

tive changes occur over 40 to 80 sec. They are neglected here for simplicity. The underlying physical phenomena that account for adaptation in the signal processing at the peripheral level of the vestibulo-ocular reflex are still obscure. However, adaptation has been modeled by introducing an adaptation operator which is essentially an integrator with a time constant of about 80 sec.[14,16,17]

For sinusoidal stimuli up to 4 to 5 Hz, the gain and phase characteristics of the units in the vestibular nerve with regard to acceleration are similar to those of an integrator (Compare Figure 4C, 3A, and 3B).[10] This lends further support to the theory that the peripheral labyrinth approximates an integrator with head acceleration as its input.

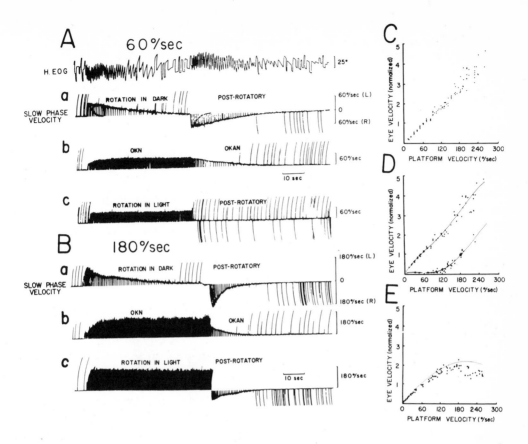

FIGURE 5.   (A) Nystagmus induced by a step of platform rotation in dark (a), by a step of surround rotation (b), and by a step of platform rotation in light (c). The top trace in A is the horizontal EOG. The other traces are slow phase velocity. The stimulus velocity was 60° in each instance. Note that when rotatory nystagmus and OKN were in the same direction, their after-responses were oppositely directed (a and b). Also note there was only a slight postrotatory response to the right after rotation in light (c); (B) nystagmus induced by steps of platform (a) and surround (b) rotation at 180°/sec. The buildup of steady state OKN in response to stimulation at 180°/sec was slower than for 60°/sec. At the end of OKN at 180°/sec, peak velocity of nystagmus was reached immediately and declined slightly as rotation continued. The oppositely directed postrotatory response was weaker than the postrotatory nystagmus after rotation in dark (a). Nystagmus eye velocity after rotation in light is approximately equal to the difference between postrotatory nystagmus and OKAN (b); (C) peak eye velocity (ordinate) induced by steps of platform velocity in darkness (abcissa). Eye velocity was normalized in relation to values recorded during 60°/sec rotation in light. Each dot is the peak velocity of one sample of per- or postrotatory nystagmus; (D) polynomial approximations of postrotatory slow phase eye velocity recorded in darkness after rotation in darkness (top points and curve) and in light (bottom points and curve); (E) Comparison of difference between polynomial curves of D (dotted line) with OKAN data from Figure 4C of Cohen et al.[22] (From Raphan, T., Matsuo, V., and Cohen, B., *Exp. Brain Res.*, 35, 229, 1979. With permission.)

IV. INTEGRATION IN THE CENTRAL VESTIBULAR SYSTEM

In response to an impulse of head acceleration, i.e., to a step in head velocity, the integrative function of the peripheral labyrinth would lead to modulation of firing rates of neurons of the eighth nerve as shown in Figure 2E. For rapid head movements, if the vestibular system gain (eye velocity/head velocity) were one, the compensatory eye velocity induced by this signal would be sufficient to maintain the gaze of angle in space. This is the case in the monkey[18] (Figure 5C). For a sinusoidal stimulus, the output from the peripheral vestibular system would have a phase lag relative to head acceleration of close to 90 deg for high-frequencies.[19,20] Again, if the gain were one, this would be sufficient for maintaining gaze fixed in space.

While the signal emanating from the semicircular canals appears to be sufficient as a velocity command signal to generate eye movements for short durations and at high-frequencies, the dynamics do not correspond to those of nystagmus induced by steps in velocity, i.e., by impulses in acceleration. The eighth nerve activity has a dominant time constant of 3 to 5 seconds, whereas vestibular nystagmus has a dominant time constant of about 12 to 20 sec over a wide range of species.[18,20,21] The difference between the time constant of the frequency change in the vestibular nerve activity and in eye velocity to a step in velocity is shown in Figure 5Aa. The exponential approximating the fall in eighth nerve activity is superimposed on the envelope of slow phase velocity. This indicates that activity coming from the end organ via the eighth nerve had been stored to be discharged over a longer period of time, i.e., that the dominant time constant of the velocity command signal had been lengthened centrally.

The simplest way to accomplish this would be to have the signal coming from the eighth nerve input to an integrator and to a direct pathway that extends around it. The eye velocity command would be a sum of these two signals. Initially, activity in the eighth nerve would drive the eyes via the direct pathway. It would also excite the integrator. Because of its longer time constant, the integrator would store the activity and continue to drive the oculomotor system after the eighth nerve signal had fallen to zero. Since the function of this integrator is to store velocity information from the eighth nerve and its output contributes to the command signal for eye velocity, it has been designated a "velocity storage" integrator.[18]

V. CENTRAL INTEGRATION IN VISUAL-OCULOMOTOR REACTIONS

Velocity storage is also utilized in visual-oculomotor responses. Evidence for this is found in the velocity characteristics of Optokinetic nystagmus (OKN) and Optokinetic After-nystagmus (OKAN).[22] In response to a step of visual surround velocity, there is an initial rapid rise in eye velocity during OKN and steady state values are reached over a time course of 5 to 10 seconds (Figure 5Ab, 5Bb). The steady state values are proportional to stimulus velocity up to about 180 deg/sec and are maintained for as long as the stimulus persists. At the end of stimulation, there is optokinetic after-nystagmus (OKAN) that lasts up to a minute in darkness (Figure 5Ab; Figure 5Bb). The persistance of nystagmus in darkness after the end of stimulation indicates that the nervous system had stored activity related to slow phase eye velocity during full field rotation that was subsequently used to drive the eyes during OKAN. This behavior is similar to the response of the integrator shown in Figure 2B.

The charge characteristics of the slow rise in OKN and the charge and discharge characteristics of OKAN indicate that integration is utilized in producing both responses.[22] Additional loops are used to modify the integration time constant during charge and discharge. The time constant of the integration is between 12 to 20 sec, and is reflected in the dominant time constant of OKAN in darkness. During OKN, the presence of light introduces a visual loop in the circuit that makes the effective charging time constant of the integrator about 3 sec in normal monkeys. During suppression of nystagmus, another loop causes the effective time constant to be about 1 sec. As with vestibular nystagmus, the output of the integrator and direct visual pathways form the velocity command signal that drives the eyes.

VI. CENTRAL INTEGRATION IN VISUAL-VESTIBULAR INTERACTIONS

It has been known since Ter Braak[21] that the postrotatory response is weaker after

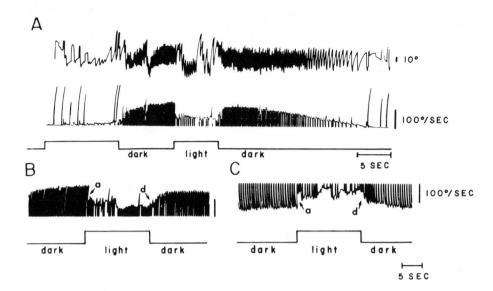

FIGURE 6. EOGs of 3 monkeys showing visual suppression of caloric nystagmus. The top trace in A is the horizontal EOG recorded bitemporally with DC coupling showing eye position. Upward trace deflections in the figures represent eye movements to the right. In A, the second trace is eye velocity. In A-C, the bottom two traces are slow phase velocity and a photocell recording showing light and darkness. Arrows show sudden drop in eye velocity at onset of period in light and much slower return of eye velocity when animals are put back into darkness. (From Takemori, S. and Cohen, B., *Brain Res.*, 72, 302, 1974. With Permission.)

rotation in light than in darkness. This occurs whether the postrotatory response is recorded in light[21] or in darkness (Figure 5Ac). At higher stimulus velocities, the after-nystagmus becomes more prominent (Figure 5Bc), but is never as strong as the after-nystagmus that follows rotation in darkness (Figure 5Ba). The difference between the peak after-response for rotation in light and dark (Figure 5D), lies along the peak response curve for OKAN that represents the velocity storage integrator (Figure 5E). This shows that the stored activity during rotation in light that was manifest as OKAN, had summed with the vestibular response.[18]

Additional evidence that this type of central integration exists in the vestibulo-ocular reflex comes from studies on visual-vestibular interactions during caloric nystagmus.[23] With the introduction of a caloric stimulus, there is a buildup of nystagmus (Figure 6A). When the lights are turned on, there is rapid suppression of the nystagmus (small a, Figures 6B and 6C). When the lights are turned off again, slow phase velocity rises more slowly than it fell (small d, Figure 6 B and C). This shows that in addition to the rapid suppression of eye velocity by the visual system during caloric nystagmus, there was also suppression of a more slowly activated mechanism that had participated in the response. Since eighth nerve activity is unaffected by the presence of vision or eye movements,[24] the slow rise in eye velocity must have been due to recharging the velocity storage integrator that had been suppressed during the period of visual fixation. The rapid drop in eye velocity when the lights are turned on is probably due to activation of direct pathways from the visual system. These pathways are also responsible for the rapid rise in eye velocity at the beginning of OKN and for the small rapid fall at the beginning of OKAN. The suppression of the integrator is due to additional loops that are brought in through vision to discharge the integrator. When the animal is put in darkness after the period of fixation, the direct visual pathways are inactivated and the integrator is slowly charged to the level of the eighth nerve activity induced by the caloric stimulus.

VII. MODEL OF VOR-OKN GENERATION AND OF VISUAL VESTIBULAR INTERACTION

A. Behavioral Characteristics of the Model

The preceding studies have led to the postulate that the velocity storage integrator superposes velocity signals from the visual system with those from the peripheral vestibular apparatus and outputs a velocity command. There is evidence that the same central integrator is used to store activity related to eye velocity during vestibular nystagmus, OKN and OKAN (Raphan et al.)[18] The time course of OKAN (Figure 5Ab) and per- and post rotatory nystagmus (Figure 5Aa) are similar, and both OKAN and vestibular nystagmus are affected in the same way by visual fixation. In support of this idea, a model that utilizes a common integrator and direct pathways from the visual and vestibular system predicts slow phase velocities of vestibular nystagmus, OKN, OKAN and the visual-vestibular interaction.

In the model, vestibular nystagmus and OKN are produced by combined activation of direct and indirect pathways (Figure 7). The indirect pathways include a velocity storage mechanism, represented by an integrator whose output is the VOR-OKAN state. Activity in the direct and indirect pathways summate to form the eye velocity signal (y) that drives the velocity to position integrator and motoneurons.

The inputs to the model are vestibular and visual signals representing head velocity r_v and surround velocity r_o. Presumably, surround velocity r_o is obtained by combining retinal error with an efference copy of eye velocity from the oculomotor system and a signal related to cupula deflection from the vestibular system.[25,26] In darkness, switch L opens, blocking the direct pathway, as well as the indirect pathway, from the visual system to the integrator. The system is then driven only by r_v, the eighth nerve signal. This signal is transmitted over the direct vestibular pathway and is also coupled to the integrator. Because the integrator has a longer time constant than the return of the eighth nerve activity to its resting level, it stores activity and effectively lengthens the dominant time constant of the VOR. Figure 8A shows the eye velocity predicted by the model in response to a step of vestibular excitation in dark. The overall characteristics are similar to those of vestibular nystagmus shown in Figures 5Aa and 5Ba. Figure 8B shows the predicted activity that would be induced in the eighth nerve (cupula) and integrator by a step of head velocity. This activity is combined to give slow phase eye velocity (S.P. Vel.). The inflection point in the response of Figure 8A simulates a plateau in eye velocity that occurs at the onset of vestibular nystagmus (Figure 5Aa). In the model, the plateau occurs because of the difference between the eighth nerve time constant T_c and the equivalent closed loop, charging time constant of the integrator T_r.[18] In accordance with the experimental data, the model predicts a longer plateau at lower velocities.

For a step in surround velocity during optokinetic stimulation, the eighth nerve signal r_v is zero and the model simulates OKN and OKAN (Figure 8C). Note the rapid and slow rise in velocity during stimulation, and the slight fall in velocity at the onset of OKAN. This is similar to a small drop in eye velocity at the onset of OKAN in the monkey[22] (Figure 5Ab). Figure 8D shows a comparison of the integrator response and the overall response. The difference between them is attributed to the contribution made by direct pathways from the visual system.

The response of the model to a step in head velocity in light is shown in Figure 8E. The direct vestibular pathway is activated and immediately drives the eyes to the velocity of the stimulus. The initial target velocity signal is approximately zero, since the eighth nerve signals that the head is turning and the environment, is stationary. As the cupula signal r_v decays, the environmental velocity signal r_o begins to excite the direct visual pathways, as well as the integrator. Consequently, head velocity becomes the

101

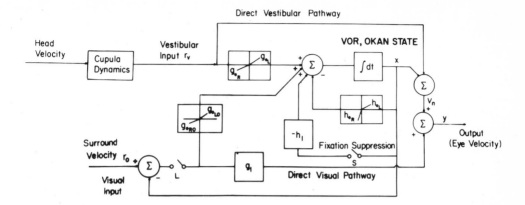

FIGURE 7. Model of OKN, OKAN, and vestibular nystagmus. Parameter values used in the model are $g_{olo} = 0.25$, $g_l = 0.6$, $= 0.85$, $h_l = 0.7$, $g_{ol} = 0.222$, $g_{oro} = 0.222$, $h_{or} = 0.111$. The cupula dynamics have been represented as having a dominant time constant $T_c = 4$ s. (From Raphan, T., Matsuo, V., and Cohen, B., *Exp. Brain Res.*, 35, 229, 1979. With permission.)

inertial frame of reference to which environmental motion is referenced. The slight decline in steady state velocity (Figure 8E) is due to a shift in dependence of the response from vestibular nystagmus with an initial gain of approximately 1 to OKN with a steady state gain of 0.92.[22] Data for steps of rotation in light show such a decline during perrotatory nystagmus, particularly at higher velocities (Figure 5Bc).[18]

Figure 8F shows the contribution of the integrator (Int.), the eighth nerve (Cup.) and the direct pathways to the total model response (S.P. Vel.). The step of velocity is in light, and the postrotatory response is in darkness, as in Figure 5 Ac. Because the eye velocity is low after rotation in light (Fig 8E), the plateau in eye velocity of the postrotatory nystagmus lasts longer than after rotation in darkness (Figure 8A). The model predicts that after-nystagmus following rotation in light in a stationary surround would always be in the postrotatory direction. This is because the response is dependent on a summation of activity in the direct vestibular pathway with that in the integrator. Since the direct pathway has a gain of 1, while the integrator can only be charged to about 0.85 of the total response,[22] an additional 15 to 20% of OKN would be necessary to abolish the postrotatory response.[18] Adding OKN to rotation in light would give proportional increments in the velocity of the after-nystagmus.

Fixation-suppression of nystagmus is accounted for by switches L & S (Figure 7). Switch L is open in darkness. When the visual environment is lighted after rotation or during OKAN, switch L closes. Because of the stationary surround, environmental velocity r_o is zero, but the state of the integrator is not zero due to its charge. This activates the fixation-suppression mechanism that discharges the integrator rapidly by closing switch S. Model predictions of suppression during postrotatory nystagmus and OKAN are shown in Figure 8G, H. The model predicts that vestibular nystagmus and OKAN would be discharged in a similar, but not identical fashion. For an equal starting velocity, vestibular nystagmus has a greater recovery velocity than OKAN and takes longer to disappear (Figure 8H). This is similar to findings in the monkey.[18]

The difference in recovery velocity of vestibular nystagmus and OKAN after fixation-suppression occurs because the integrator, but not the direct vestibular pathway, is susceptible to having its activity diminished by fixation suppression. During OKN, only the integrator is driving the eyes; consequently, its activity is discharged rapidly by fixation-suppression. However, during vestibular nystagmus, the eighth nerve activity continues to charge the integrator, making it less susceptible to suppression.

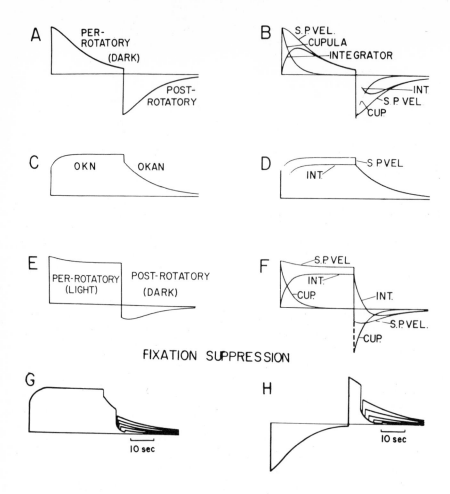

FIGURE 8.   Model predictions of slow phase eye velocity for a step of angular velocity in darkness (A), for a step of surround velocity (C) and for a step of angular velocity in light (E). B, D, F, Comparative changes in slow phase velocity, cupula deflection, and output of the integrator for the responses shown in A, C and E, respectively. G, H, Response of the model to varying periods of fixation suppression during OKAN (G) and post-rotatory nystagmus (H). The recovery velocity when put in darkness after being in light is higher in H than in G because of the contribution of the cupula. (From Raphan, T., Matsuo, V., and Cohen, B., *Exp. Brain Res.*, 35, 229, 1979. With permission.)

For sinusoidal vestibular inputs, the integrator would have the effect of extending the low-frequency phase characteristics of the vestibulo-ocular reflex. Figure 9 shows the phase characteristics that would be expected if only the direct path from the eighth nerve were present (Cupula). It can be compared to the phase characteristics of the VOR with the integrator (VOR). The integrator, plus the direct pathway, behave as a lag compensation network. This causes the VOR phase characteristics to be closer to zero over a wider range of frequencies than if it depended on the cupula dynamics alone (Figure 9).

Caloric nystagmus and the effects of fixation-suppression on caloric nystagmus can also be simulated by the model as shown in Figure 10. For this simulation, it was assumed that the eighth nerve activity (cupula deflection) rises rapidly and falls slowly. In response to this stimulus, eye velocity rises rapidly due to activation of the direct vestibular pathway and then more slowly due to activation of the integrator. When the lights are turned on in a stationary environment, eye velocity drops rapidly due to

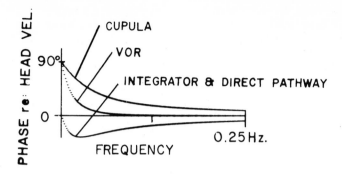

FIGURE 9. Model predictions of the phase response of eighth nerve activity (cupula) as a function of frequency. The integrator and direct pathway contribute a lag to compensate for the eighth nerve dynamics (cupula). This maintains the phase characteristics of the VOR at close to zero over a wide range of frequencies.

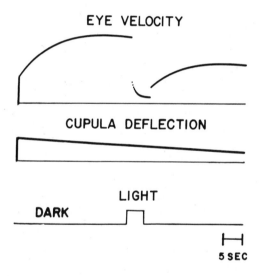

FIGURE 10. Model predictions of eye velocity during caloric stimulus. It is assumed that the eighth nerve activity (cupula) rises rapidly and declines linearly over a 60 sec time course. Eye velocity responds by jumping rapidly due to the direct vestibular pathway. It then rises slowly due to the contribution of the integrator. After reaching a peak, eye velocity begins to decline slowly. During fixation, eye velocity drops rapidly due to the activation of the direct visual pathway and the suppression of the integrator. When the lights are again turned off, the direct visual pathway to the integrator is inactivated, allowing the eighth nerve signal to recharge the integrator. Thus, the predicted eye velocity jumps slightly at the end of the period of fixation and then rises slowly as is observed in the monkey (Figure 6).

activation of the direct visual pathway and the discharge of the integrator. When the lights are turned off again, eye velocity jumps slightly due to inactivation of the direct visual pathway. It then rises slowly because the integrator is recharged by ongoing activity in the eighth nerve induced by the caloric stimulus (cupula deflection). This is qualitatively similar to the eye velocity waveforms shown in Figure 6. A quantitative study of the relationship between caloric nystagmus and the model predictions has not been done. Regardless, this simulation supports the contention that the integrator plays a role in producing the caloric responses.

B. The Model and its Relation to Unit Activity in the Vestibular Nuclei

It is not known how the visual system is coupled to the direct pathway and the integrator to generate the slow phases of nystagmus. Labyrinthectomy abolishes OKAN[27,28] and neurons in the vestibular nuclei respond to visual, as well as to vestibular stimulation. This suggests that the vestibular nuclei are important for realizing velocity storage integration. Consistent with this, frequencies of neurons in the vestibular nuclei are related to eye velocity during vestibular nystagmus and optokinetic after-nystagmus (OKAN).[29-31] However, during OKN, firing rates in the vestibular nuclei approximate the state of the integrator (Figure 8D) only up to saturation levels of about 60 deg/sec.[29,30] Vestibular nuclei unit activity during rotation in dark agrees more closely with slow phase velocity than with activity predicted for the integrator shown in Figure 8F. This suggests that the signal in the vestibular nuclei represents a summation of activity from the direct vestibular pathway and the integrator with the direct visual pathway being located elsewhere.

Other data support this view. Firing rates during rotation in dark were compared to firing rates during rotation in light where there was no relative movement between the monkey and the visual surround.[31] The relative stationary surround was achieved by rotating an animal and a surrounding OKN drum at the same velocity. The results of this experiment are shown in Figure 11A, B, and C. At low accelerations, (Figure 11A), unit activity in dark (closed circles) achieved higher frequencies of firing than during rotation in a relative stationary surround (open circles). As the acceleration increased, however, the unit activity with a relative stationary surround achieved peak frequencies that were closer to those found during rotation in dark (Figure 11 B and C).

If one considers the variable Vn, which is the summation of the direct vestibular pathway, and the integrator as the variable related to the unit activity, it is possible to predict the vestibular nuclei unit activity. Simulation of the experiment shown in Figure 11A-C is represented in Figure 11D-G. In each case, the lower trace represents unit activity that would be expected for rotation in light with a head fixed stationary environment and the upper trace, the response during rotation in dark.

The similarity of the experimental and model data suggests several organizational principles:

1. The peripheral vestibular system has a direct input to the vestibular nuclei, as well as to the velocity storage integrator. The integrator, in turn, inputs back to the vestibular nuclei. A summation of these two signals is observed in most vestibular neurons.[29-31]
2. The major visual input to the vestibular nuclei is through the velocity storage integrator. Thus, only slow changes in the visual input are represented there. Since the peripheral vestibular system has a direct pathway into the vestibular nuclei, vestibular excitation can elicit much faster responses in neural activity than the visual system.
3. For slow accelerations, the visual system keeps up with the vestibular drive and reduces the peak neural activity. As the acceleration increases, the vestibular drive on the neurons is too rapid to be affected by the visual system, and the neural activity approaches that found in darkness (Compare Figure 11 B and C to Figure 11 E-G). In the high acceleration condition with a head fixed surround,

UNIT ACTIVITY   MODEL PREDICTIONS

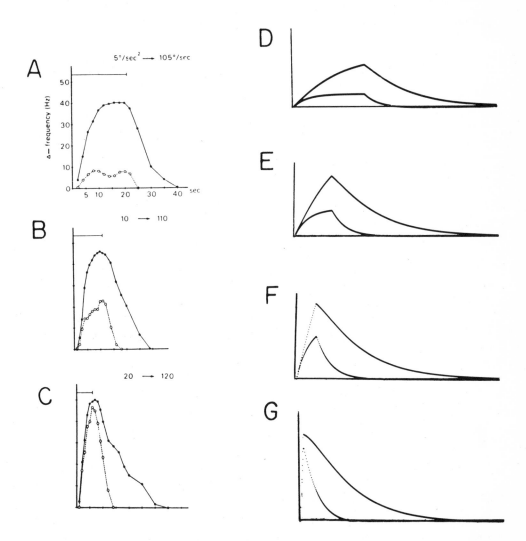

FIGURE 11. Comparison of unit activity recorded in medial vestibular nuclei with activity predicted by the model shown in Figure 7 for the variable Vn. A, At low accelerations (5 deg/sec²), unit activity in the dark (closed circles) reached higher frequencies than unit activity during rotation in a stationary surround relative to the monkey (open circles). B-C, Increasing rates of acceleration of rotation (10 deg/sec² and 20 deb/sec²) induced frequencies of firing in the stationary surround that were closer to frequencies of firing in darkness. (From Waespe, W. and Henn, V., *Exp. Brain Res.,* 30, 323, 1977. With permission.) D, E, F, G. Model predictions of the variable Vn for increasing accelerations of rotation in dark (upper trace) and in a lighted stationary surround relative to the subject (bottom trace).

the animal fixates and its eyes are stationary or move very little.[31] Consequently, eye velocity does not agree with vestibular nuclei activity. This can be explained as being due to the activity of direct visual pathways that extend around the vestibular nuclei and that are capable of reducing eye velocity even at the higher accelerations.

VIII. VELOCITY TO POSITION INTEGRATION DURING NYSTAGMUS

The model described above demonstrates how the velocity command signal to the eyes might be realized during nystagmus. Skavenski and Robinson[19] recorded from abducens motoneurons during sinusoidal vestibular nystagmus and found that the frequency of firing of the units was approximately in phase with eye position during slow phases of vestibular nystagmus. This suggested that there was a central integrator that had converted velocity signals to position signals that are needed to drive the eyes. A great deal of experimental evidence supports this view.[32,33] The velocity to position integrator functions to transmit position information to motoneurons to hold the eyes stationary at various points in the orbit.[32,34] It is utilized during slow eye movements, as well as during saccades and quick phases of nystagmus.[33,35-37] The time constant of this velocity-position integrator appears to be above 20 to 25 sec in man[38] and cat[33] and is capable of holding the eyes in eccentric positions of gaze for long periods of time even in darkness.

It should be emphasized that the velocity-position integrator is separate from the velocity-storage integrator. During nystagmus, the velocity-storage integrator is charged to approximately 85% of eye velocity and is independent of the quick phases. The velocity to position integrator, on the other hand, is reset by each quick phase. This implies that if the velocity-position integrator was not reset, it too would be charged to a steady state level and would hold the eyes in a deviated position. This is exactly what occurs after lesions in the PPRF that abolish the quick phase mechanism.[39] An example showing the effects of a PPRF lesion is shown in Figure 12. After a right PPRF lesion, saccades and quick phases of nystagmus could no longer be made to the right, and there was spontaneous nystagmus to the left (Figure 12A). Normal optokinetic nystagmus could be induced to the left, followed by leftward OKAN (Figure 12A). A stimulus that would induce right OKN failed to induce nystagmus (Figure 12B). Instead, the eyes deviated strongly to the left in the direction of the slow phases. At the conclusion of the optokinetic stimulus when the lights were turned off, the spontaneous nystagmus did not resume for about 15 to 20 sec, the duration of OKAN to the left side. This suggests that the velocity storage integrator had been charged during optokinetic stimulation to cancel the spontaneous nystagmus, even though no nystagmus was manifest.

There are other examples that show the separate functioning of the velocity-storage integrator and the velocity-position integrator. If vestibular nystagmus is induced in a monkey by a step of velocity in darkness, the envelope of the slow phase velocity declines over a regular course (Figures 5Aa and 13). If the monkey becomes drowsy during the period of nystagmus, slow and quick phase velocities decline and nystagmus disappears (Figure 13). If the animal is alerted, the slow phase velocity resumes the value it would have had, had the animal been alert throughout the nystagmus. This shows the independence of the two central integrators and the different functions performed by each in the control of eye movements.

IX. SUMMARY AND CONCLUSION

Evidence is presented in this chapter to show that integration is a basic process in oculomotor and vestibular organization. There is mechanical integration in the peripheral labyrinth and two central neural integrators. One stores information related to slow phase eye velocity, the other stores information about eye position. Using these integrators as fundamental components, slow phases of vestibular nystagmus, OKN

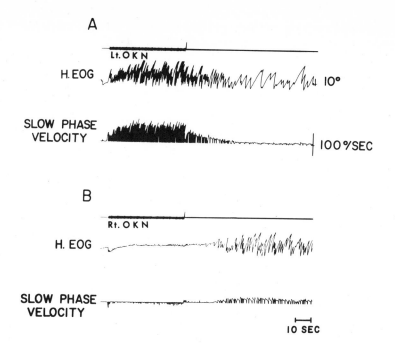

FIGURE 12.   OKN four days after a right PPRF lesion. During the recording, the eyes moved only in the left field of movement, and at rest they were strongly deviated to the left. The speed of surround rotation was 90°/sec. At the end of optokinetic stimulation, lights were extinguished and animal was in complete darkness for remainder of recording. Note the normal OKAN after left OKN (A). In B, only tonic deviation to left was induced by the stimulus. At the end of stimulation, there was a period before the spontaneous nystagmus began when the eyes were still. This time period was equivalent to the duration of left OKAN. (From Cohen, B., Komatsuzaki, A., and Bender, M. B., *Arch. of Neurol.*, 18, 78, 1968. With permission.)

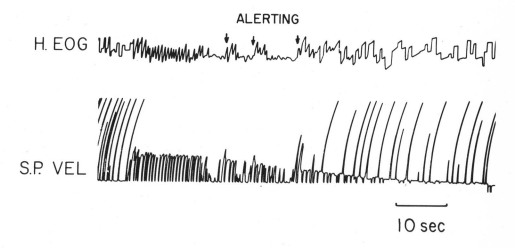

FIGURE 13.   Vestibular nystagmus of a drowsy monkey in response to a step in head velocity about a vertical axis. When the monkey becomes drowsy, slow phase eye velocity went to zero. Each time the monkey was alerted (downward arrows), slow phase eye velocity resumed a level consistent with the normal decline of eye velocity during vestibular nystagmus.

and OKAN are modeled. By relating the variables in the model to unit activity in the vestibular nuclei, an organizational scheme for generating the slow phases of nystagmus has been postulated. The model suggests that the signal in the vestibular nuclei is related to a summation of activity in the direct vestibular pathway and the integrator. The visual drive on the vestibular nuclei neurons is through the velocity storage integrator. The summation of the direct vestibular pathway, direct visual pathway and integrator forms the slow phase velocity command signal. A velocity to position integrator is then utilized to establish positional information that is used by motoneurons to drive the ocular plant. While the model utilizes integration as a basic element, its realization at the neuronal level is unknown. Therefore, a fundamental problem in understanding oculomotor control is to determine which brain structures are involved in realizing integration and how they work together to effect this realization.

REFERENCES

1. Zadeh, L. and Desoer, C., *Linear System Theory: The State Space Approach,* McGraw-Hill, New York, 1963.
2. Steinhausen, W., Uber den Nachweis der Bewegung der Cupula in der intakten Bogengangsampulle des Labyrinthes bei der Naturlichen rotatorischen und calorischen Reizung, *Pflugers Arch.,* 228, 332, 1931.
3. Steinhausen, W., Uber die Beobachtung der Cupula in den Bogengangsampullen des Labyrinthes des lebenden Hechts, *Pflugers Arch.,* 232, 500, 1933.
4. Oman, C. M. and Young, L. R., The physiological range of pressure difference and cupula deflections in the human semicircular canal, in *Basic Aspects of Vestibular Control Mechanisms,* Pompeiano, E. O. and Brodal, A., Eds., Elsevier Press, Amsterdam, 1972.
5. Lowenstein, O., The equilibrium function of the vertebrate labyrinth, *Biol. Rev.,* 11, 113, 1936.
6. Lowenstein, O., The effect of galvanic polarization on the impulse discharge from sense endings in the isolated labyrinth of the thornback ray (Raja Clavata), *J. Physiol (London),* 127, 104, 1955.
7. Lowenstein, O. and Sand, A., The mechanisms of the semicircular canal. A study of the responses of single-fibre preparations to angular accelerations and rotation at constant speed, *Proc. R. Soc.,* 129, 256, 1940.
8. Lowenstein, O. and Sand, A., The individual and integrated activity of the semicircular canal of the elasmobranch labyrinth, *J. Physiol. (London),* 99, 89, 1940.
9. Goldberg, J. M. and Fernandez, C., Physiology of peripheral neurons innervating semicircular canals of the squirrel monkey. I. Resting discharge and response to constant angular accelerations, *J. Neurophysiol.,* 34, 635, 1971.
10. Fernandez, C. and Goldberg, J. M., Physiology of peripheral neurons innervating semicircular canals of the squirrel monkey. II. Response to sinusoidal stimulation and dynamics of peripheral vestibular system, *J. Neurophysiol.,* 34, 661, 1971.
11. Goldberg, J. M. and Fernandez, C., Physiology of peripheral neurons innervating semicircular canals of the squirrel monkey. III. Variations among units in their discharge properties, *J. Neurophysiol.,* 34, 676, 1971.
12. Precht, W., Llinas, R., and Clarke, M., Physiological responses of frog vestibular fibres to horizontal angular rotation, *Exp. Brain Res.,* 13, 378, 1971.
13. Melvill Jones, G. and Milsum, J. H., Frequency response analysis of central vestibular unit activity resulting from rotational stimulation of the semicircular canals, *J. Physiol. (London),* 219, 191, 1971.
14. Goldberg, J. M. and Fernandez, C., Vestibular mechanisms, *Ann. Rev. Physiol.,* 37, 129, 1975.
15. Blanks, R. H. I. and Precht, W., Functional characterization of primary vestibular afferents of the frog, *Exp. Brain Res.,* 25, 369, 1976.
16. Young, L. R., Role of the vestibular system in posture and movements, in *Medical Physiology,* Vol. 1, Mouncastle, V. B., Ed., C. V. Mosby, St. Louis, 1974, 704.
17. Young, L. R. and Oman, C. M., Model for vestibular adaptation to horizontal rotation, *Aerosp. Med.,* 40, 1076, 1969.
18. Raphan, T., Matsuo, V., and Cohen, B., Velocity storage in the vestibulo-ocular reflex arc (VOR), *Exp. Brain Res.,* 35, 229, 1979.

19. Skavenski, A. A. and Robinson, D. A., Role of abducens motoneurons in the vestibulo-ocular reflex, *J. Neurophysiol.*, 36, 724, 1973.
20. Robinson, D. A., Adaptive gain control of vestibulo-ocular reflex by the cerebellum, *J. Neurophysiol.*, 39, 954, 1976.
21. Ter Braak, J. W. G., Untersuchungen Uber optokinetichen Nystagmus, *Arch. Neerl. Physiol.*, 21, 309, 1936.
22. Cohen, B., Matsuo, V., and Raphan, T., Quantitative analysis of the velocity characteristics of optokinetic nystagmus and optokinetic after-nystagmus, *J. Physiol. (London)*, 270, 321, 1977.
23. Takemori, S. and Cohen, B., Visual suppression of vestibular nystagmus in rhesus monkeys, *Brain Res.*, 72, 302, 1974.
24. Keller, E. L., Behavior of horizontal semicircular canal afferents in alert monkey during vestibular and optokinetic stimulation, *Exp. Brain Res.*, 24, 459, 1976.
25. Yasui, S. and Young, L. R., Perceived visual motion as effective stimulus to the pursuit eye movement system, *Science*, 190, 906, 1975.
26. Lanman, J., Bizzi, E., Allum, J., The coordination of eye and head movement during smooth pursuit, *Brain Res.*, 153, 39, 1978.
27. Uemura, T. and Cohen, B., Effects of vestibular nuclei lesions on vestibulo-ocular reflexes and posture in monkeys, *Acta Otolaryngol.*, 315, Suppl. 1, 1, 1973.
28. Uemura, T. and Cohen, B., Loss of optokinetic after-nystagmus (OKAN) after dorsal medullary reticular formation (Med-RF) lesions, *Pro. Barany Soc., Int. J. Equilibrium Res.*, Suppl. 1, 101, 1975.
29. Waespe, W. and Henn, V., Neuronal activity in the vestibular nuclei of the alert monkey during vestibular and optokinetic stimulation, *Exp. Brain Res.*, 27, 523, 1977.
30. Waespe, W. and Henn, V., Vestibular nuclei activity during optokinetic after-nystagmus (OKAN) in the alert monkey, *Exp. Brain Res.*, 30, 323, 1977.
31. Waespe, W. and Henn, V., Conflicting visual-vestibular stimulation and vestibular nucleus activity in alert monkeys, *Exp. Brain Res.*, 33, 203, 1978.
32. Robinson, D. A., Models of oculomotor organization, in *The Control of Eye Movements*, Bach-y-Rita, P., Collins, C. C., and Hyde, J. E., Eds., Academic Press, New York, 1971, 7.
33. Robinson, D. A., Cerebellectomy and vestibulo-ocular reflex arc, *Brain Res.*, 71, 215, 1974.
34. Henn, V. and Cohen, B., Quantitative analysis of activity in eye muscle motoneurons during saccadic eye movements and positons of fixation, *J. Neurophysiol.*, 36, 115, 1973.
35. Cohen, B., and Komatsuzaki, A., Eye movements induced by stimulation of the pontine reticular formation; evidence for integration in oculomotor pathways, *Exp. Neurol.*, 36, 101, 1972.
36. Robinson, D. A., Oculomotor control signals, in *Basic Mechanisms of Ocular Motility and Their Clinical Implications*, Lennerstrand, G. and Bach-y-Rita, P., Eds., Pergamon Press, Oxford, 1975, 337.
37. Raphan, T. and Cohen, B., Brainstem mechanisms for rapid and slow eye movements, *Ann. Rev. Physiol.*, 40, 527, 1978.
38. Becker, W. and Klein, H., Accuracy of saccadic eye movements and maintenance of eccentric eye positions in the dark, *Vision Res.*, 13, 1021, 1973.
39. Cohen, B., Komatsuzaki, A., and Bender, M. B., Electro-oculographic syndrome in monkeys after pontine reticular formation lesions, *Arch. Neurol.*, 18, 78, 1968.

Chapter 6

THE OPTOKINETIC SYSTEM

Han Collewijn

TABLE OF CONTENTS

I. INTRODUCTION

Eye movements elicited by moving visual patterns that are substantially larger than a single point target are usually called optokinetic. As we shall see, a more rigorous definition of the optokinetic system is desirable to sharply distinguish it from the smooth pursuit system.

The discovery of optokinetic nystagmus (OKN) or similar phenomena goes back to the nineteenth century. Purkinje reportedly[1] noticed OKN in 1825 in a crowd that watched a cavalry parade, and Helmholtz[1] mentioned in 1866 that such eye movements were most readily observed in train passengers that watched the moving landscape. For some time, "railroad nystagmus" was even the accepted term for OKN. The first (optical) recordings of the pursuit movements elicited by a series of moving objects were made by Dodge in 1903.[2] The credit for the introduction of optically elicited nystagmus as a clinical test should go to Bárány,[3] who studied it already in 1908 in connection with ocular palsies. As a stimulus he used a small, hand-held striped drum with a diameter of 20 cm, which was very convenient in a bedside test. Other investigators constructed their own versions of apparatus to generate moving patterns (for a survey see Ohm[4]), but all of these were of limited size and filled only a small part of the visual field. The very ease with which a nystagmus can be induced by such a stimulus in a cooperative human subject has been a source of confusion about the nature of OKN, which went so far as to deny the existence of OKN in the rabbit, while in fact, OKN is the only kind of visual tracking that this animal is capable of.

A great part of the older literature deals not with OKN in the strict sense, but with what we call nowadays smooth pursuit (SP). Even today the confusion between these two systems has not been completely resolved.

II. THE NATURE OF THE OPTOKINETIC RESPONSE

Ter Braak[5] was the first to recognize that the adequate stimulus for OKN is a relative movement of the visual surroundings *as a whole* with respect to the eye. He created such a stimulus using a large rotating striped drum, with the subject's head placed in the axis of rotation such that the drum filled the whole visual field. With such a full field stimulus, OKN was reliably elicited in the rabbit, and since then it has been found in any animal with spatially organized vision tested in a similar situation. The term "optokinetic" is usually reserved for the movements elicited of the eyes in the orbit. However, the responses often extend to the head, the trunk, the legs[6] and even the ears.[7] For these more generalized responses, the term "optomotor" is often used.

The essential optokinetic response is a smooth tracking of the visual surroundings by the eyes (sometimes assisted by head and trunk). The tracking movements of the eye in the orbit (and of the head on the trunk) are interrupted regularly by fast movements in the opposite direction. A unidirectional motion stimulus will cause a more or less regular sequence of smooth and fast movements, the classical optokinetic nystagmus. The fast movements are so easily observed (and recorded) that in the clinical convention the direction of the nystagmus has been defined as that of the fast phase. In reality, the fast component of the optokinetic response is secondary to the smooth component. The latter is seen in isolation when the stimulus is limited (e.g., a small sinusoidal oscillation) or when the animal is free to rotate all around during slow unidirectional stimulation. The smooth component reduces the velocity of a continuous motion of the retinal projection; it helps to stabilize the eye on the visual surroundings.

Rotating visual surroundings are, of course, laboratory artifacts which do not occur in nature; the only physiological source of such movements is rotation of the head.

Head rotations will also excite the labyrinths, in particular the semicircular canals, and give rise to vestibuloocular reflexes (VOR) which also essentially consist of compensatory smooth eye movements, opposite to the head movements. The VOR can be measured in isolation in absolute darkness, and since under such condition it has no physiological function, it also represents a laboratory artifact. Physiologically, OKN and VOR function always together and complement each other in the stabilization of the eye in the world. The intimate relation between OKN and VOR has been recognized long ago.[5] Thus, the OKN is part of a *postural* reflex system that is activated only when all or nearly all of an animal's surround moves en bloc. It has nothing to do with the voluntary pursuit of a moving target.

III. DISTINCTION OF OKN FROM SMOOTH PURSUIT SYSTEM

Whereas OKN is elicited by the movement of the whole background, SP is used to track a selected target that moves with respect to a stationary background. Human subjects are capable to smoothly pursue any real or perceived target independent of the background as long as velocity and bandwidth of the stimulus do not exceed certain limits. When the stimulus contains multiple target points or is repetitive (such as the Bárány drum), the SP will be interrupted by saccades in the opposite direction and a nystagmic pattern will result. The essence of SP is that the subject tries to keep or acquire a subjectively selected target (or part of the moving pattern) on the fovea. The SP velocity is usually inferior to that of the target[8] and, therefore, it will be assisted by saccades in the same direction as long as the same target point is pursued, and a saccade in the opposite direction when a new target point within the pattern is selected. SP only makes sense and, indeed, is only found in species with a fovea or area centralis, such as man and monkey, and to a certain extent the cat and dog. A further prerequisite for its occurrence is the active interest of the subject in the pursuit of the relevant target. This interest has to be secured by instructions or conditioning procedures. A rabbit has no fovea, but only a visual streak, and small targets on a stationary background are not pursued. This makes the rabbit an ideal animal to study OKN. A major problem with the study of OKN in foveate species is that any optokinetic stimulus will also excite the SP system, and some smooth pursuit targets may excite the OKN system. This has the following implications for some commonly used experimental situations.

1. Small targets moving on a stationary background. An example is a small striped drum in a hospital room or an oscilloscope spot in an illuminated laboratory. This is a SP stimulus. During pursuit, the background moves in the opposite direction; this would stimulate the OKN, but apparently any response to this peripheral stimulus is suppressed.

2. Rotation of the entire background, such as a drum that surrounds the subject, or the room when the subject is rotated. These stimuli excite the OKN system, but the subject may also use SP to track certain details in the pattern. Instructions to just look at the pattern and not voluntarily follow any detail are often given to diminish the contribution of smooth pursuit, but there is no real criterion for checking their efficacy.

3. Single targets with no background, such as a light spot on a screen in a dark room. Such a stimulus is often used to elicit SP but, of course, nothing will prevent the OKN system to participate in it. Even the rabbit shows OKN under such conditions.[5]

This survey shows that whenever the OKN system is stimulated in a foveate species, the SP system may also participate, dependent on instructions, interest and motivation of the subject.

The distinction between OKN and SP has been made in other terms. Ter Braak[5] defined them as "stare" and "look" types of optokinetic nystagmus ("Stier" and "Schau"-nystagmus) and later the terms "passive" and "active" optokinetic nystagmus have been used.[9]

On the basis of ablation experiments, Ter Braak[5] has attributed the "stare" OKN to subcortical circuits, while for the "look" OKN (SP) the visual cortex was deemed to be essential.

IV. INPUT-OUTPUT RELATIONS OF OKN

The properties of a pure OKN system without SP will be mainly illustrated with data from the rabbit, the best investigated representant of nonfoveate mammals. After the pioneering work by Ter Braak[5] measurements of the rabbit's OKN have been more recently resumed.[10-13] With the head restrained, most rabbits make very few spontaneous eye movements, even when it is tried to elicit them with "interesting" targets. All our measurements were made with the inductive scleral coil method.[14] The animal was surrounded by a drum lined with a grid or random dot pattern.

As shown in Figure 1A and B, the rabbit's eye does not move when the drum is abruptly displaced (position step), even though the steps were relatively small (0.5 to 4°) compared to the visual pattern (grid of 10° white and 10° black bars).[13] This shows that position of the pattern as such is not a relevant input to the OKN system. However, when the drum suddenly starts a continuous motion (velocity step), the eye will start to move in the same direction after a well-defined latency time of about 75 msec (Figure 1C).[13] If the drum continues to rotate in one direction, a regular nystagmus will develop. For slow steady drum velocities (up to a few °/sec), the slow phase (after the latency) immediately reaches a steady velocity, which is maintained as long as the drum moves (Figures 2A and 3A). For higher drum velocities (up to 30 to 60°/sec), the slow phase velocity is initially not higher than 1 to 2°/sec, and only when stimulation is continued slow phase velocity gradually increases to a maximum (Figures 2B and 3B). When the ratio *slow phase eye velocity/stimulus velocity (= gain)* is plotted as a function of stimulus velocity (Figure 4), we see that in the rabbit (Figure 4A) for relatively low stimulus velocities the gain is about 0.8, but for higher velocities it drops to negligible values, even though the maximally reached (steady state) eye velocities were used in the graph. Ter Braak[5] showed that a drum velocity as low as 6.4 sec arc/sec still elicited a regular, although extremely slow OKN.

For comparison, some gain — stimulus velocity relations for other species are also shown in Figure 4. They have been partly extracted from the literature, in which such data prove to be surprisingly scarce. Figure 4B shows some of our own (unpublished) data on cats with permanently implanted eye coils, recorded in the rotating magnetic field.[15] A major advantage of this recording method is the absolute calibration. Also plotted are data from Evinger and Fuchs,[16] recorded in a full-field drum when the cats also saw food, a condition that gave the best responses (calibration is approximate). Obviously, the cat's OKN is almost identical to that of the rabbit. This is probably because the cat has only a moderately developed central area and SP responses are poor.[16]

This is in sharp contrast with data obtained in humans. We show our own data (unpublished, calibration absolute, instructions not to pursue any details), those of Zee, Yee, and Robinson[17] (DC electrooculography), and old data extracted from Grüttner,[18] who was one of the first to give a complete and profound description of human OKN (Figure 4C). Clearly, the human gain is much better than of the rabbit and cat, especially for higher velocities. A quite similar picture is obtained for the monkey (Figure 4D) for which data are shown derived from Komatsuzaki et al.[19] (elec-

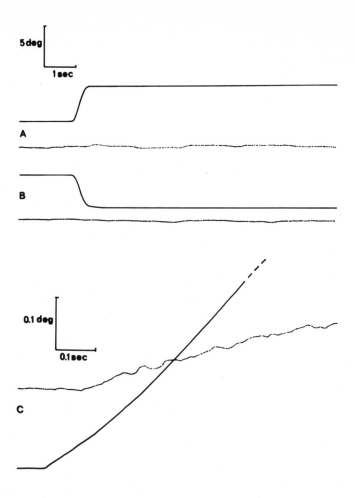

FIGURE 1. Responses of the rabbit's eye (dotted line) to step-wise changes in position (A,B) and velocity (C) of a full-field stimulus consisting of black and white bars, each 10° wide (solid line). Each record is the average of 25 responses. (From Collewijn, H., *Brain Res.*, 36, 59, 1972. With permission.)

trooculography, calibration approximate) and Igarashi et al.[20] (electrooculography, calibration procedure not mentioned.) A precise calibration is lacking in almost all monkey experiments, and often it is just assumed that the monkey OKN gain equals 1 at a stimulus velocity of 60°/sec.[21] In this light, the gain values higher than 1 in Figure 4D should be viewed with suspicion. Apart from this, the data for the monkey are remarkably similar to that of man. The monkey has a well-developed SP system,[22] and we may postulate that Figure 4C and D represent the combined OKN-SP response of foveate species, while Figure 4A and B represent the pure OKN response of afoveate species. To confirm this distribution, we need more data of different species. Although the spread of the data is not indicated in the average values of Figure 4, it should be realized that considerable intersubject variability is found in all species.

The data for the afoveate species show that during the slow phase of OKN, the eye tracks the stimulus with a velocity gain that may approach the ideal value of 1.0 for low velocities, but is relatively low for fast stimulus motion, especially if the stimulus lasts only short. Such properties would predict a poor response to high-frequency components of a stimulus. Indeed, with sinusoidal motion of the drum, it was found in

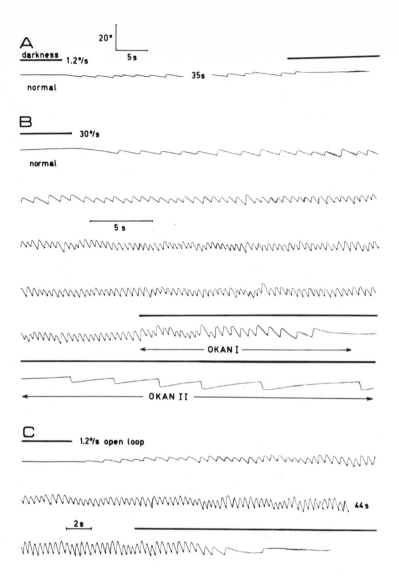

FIGURE 2.   Typical examples of OKN and OKAN in the rabbit. The horizontal
bars mark periods of darkness. (A) Stimulus velocity 1.2°/sec. Immediate and
sustained reaction, no after-nystagmus; (B) Stimulus velocity 30°/sec. Gradual
build-up of slow phase velocity; OKAN I and II in darkness. Continuous recording; (C) Open-loop conditions: seeing eye immobilized, moving eye covered.
Stimulus velocity 1 to 2°/sec in anterior direction. Gradual build-up of slow
phase velocity far in excess of stimulus velocity; after-nystagmus in darkness.
See Figure 3. (From Collewijn, H., *Exp. Neurol.*, 52, 146, 1976. With permission.)

the rabbit[10] that only very low-frequencies at low-amplitudes were followed faithfully
by the eye. At higher frequencies and amplitudes, the gain decreased very rapidly, and
the responses were distorted due to a number of nonlinearities. The first nonlinearity
is the introduction of fast eye movements. This does not really concern us, since the
function of OKN is the velocity compensation during the slow phase. Therefore, the
fast phase can be neglected and the cumulative slow phase (as defined by Meiry[23]) is
considered as the essential optokinetic response. (The same is true for vestibulo-ocular

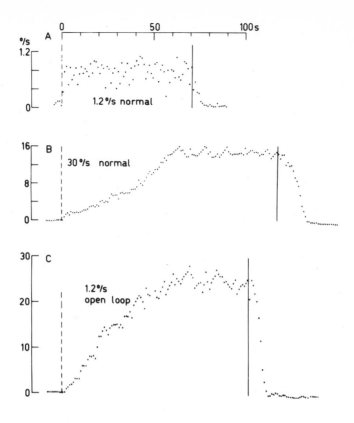

FIGURE 3. Time course of slow phase velocity of the same three recordings shown in Figure 2. Beginning and end of stimulation are marked by the interrupted and solid lines, respectively. (From Collewijn, H., *Exp. Neurol.*, 52, 146, 1976. With permission.)

responses). The second nonlinearity is the poor response of the system to velocities higher than 1 to 2°/sec, combined with a maximal acceleration on the order of 1°/sec². Unlike steady rotation, sinusoidal oscillation leaves the optokinetic system no time to build up a higher velocity in a period of seconds to minutes. These combined properties restrict the eye velocity in response to sinusoidal stimulation to about 1°/sec, and when gain is plotted as a function of maximal stimulus velocity (Aω), rather than of the frequency ω itself, the same straightforward relation as for continuous rotation is obtained.[10] The severe decrease in gain for higher frequencies is accompanied by an only mild increase in phase lag, which is largely accounted for by the delay (about 75 msec).[13]

The extremely low bandwidth and velocity range of the rabbit's OKN (the cat being hardly better) would seem to raise serious doubts about the functional relevance of the system. However, as stated before, OKN is a laboratory artifact and to see the real function of the system we should study the combined action of OKN and VOR due to head movements. To illustrate this point, Figure 5 shows gain as a function of frequency for the OKN alone (drum movements), the VOR alone (head movements in darkness), and the combination (head movements in the light) for the rabbit. While OKN performs poorly for the higher frequencies, the VOR is working well in that range, but not for the low frequencies, where the OKN response is superior. The combined systems show a remarkably good and flat gain over the frequency range tested.

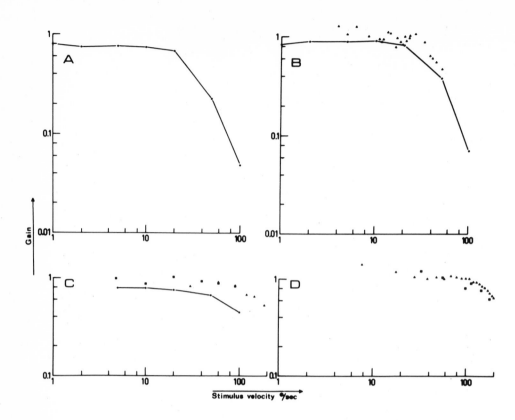

FIGURE 4.   Slow phase velocity gain of OKN as a function of stimulus velocity for different species. A. Rabbit;[119] B. Cat. Continuous line: Collewijn, unpublished data; triangles: after Evinger and Fuchs[16]; C. Man. Continuous line: Collewijn, unpublished data; squares: after Zee et al.[17]; triangles: after Grüttner.[18] D. Monkey. Triangles: after Igarashi et al.[20]; squares: after Komatsuzaki et al.[19]

V. OPEN-LOOP EXPERIMENTS

The findings described above suggest that movement of a pattern on the retina (= slip) elicits an eye movement in the same direction. This will decrease the slip velocity, and therefore the stimulus. Thus, the response immediately interacts with the stimulus and the OKN system forms a closed loop, such in contrast to the VOR, as eye movements are not fed back to the labyrinth. The feedback loop in combination with the nonlinearities makes the real stimulus-response relationship rather untransparent. A dissociation between the stimulus and response (open-loop conditions) could give a more direct insight in the optokinetic input-output relations. The classical approach to this problem has been through clinical cases with unilateral paralysis of the eye muscles, with intact vision, as first described by Ohm.[24] When a paralyzed eye with intact vision is stimulated with a moving pattern, optokinetic movements are elicited in the contralateral eye, even if the latter is covered. This phenomenon has been verified several times in patients,[25,26] and it has been noted that the slow phase eye velocity in this situation can surpass the stimulus velocity by a factor of 2 or more. However, no quantitative input-output studies have been reported for such cases.

Experimentally, the same situation can be achieved by paralyzing or mechanically immobilizing one eye. This was done by Ter Braak[5] and Collewijn[10] in the rabbit, and by Körner and Schiller[27] in the monkey. An example of such a recording in a rabbit is shown in Figure 2C, with the time course of slow phase velocity in Figure 3C. With a

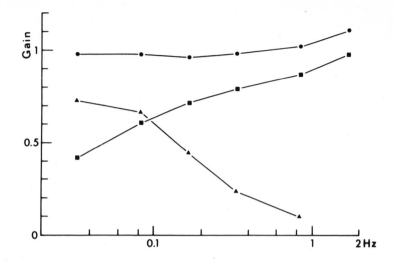

FIGURE 5. Gain of compensatory eye movements as a function of frequency for sinusoidal stimulation. Triangles: motion of drum only (OKN); squares: motion of rabbit in dark (VOR); dots: motion of rabbit in light (VOR + OKN). Stimulus amplitude 10° peak-to-peak, except for 0.83 Hz (5° p.p.) and 1.66 Hz (2.5° p.p.). Average values for eight rabbits with permanently implanted eye coils. (From Collewijn, H., unpublished data.)

steady stimulus of 1.2°/sec (about the optimal velocity) the slow phase velocity gradually accelerates to a maximum (in this case about 25°/sec), and when the lights are turned off, an after-nystagmus is seen. The overall course is rather similar to that elicited under normal conditions with a relatively high stimulus velocity (Figure 2B and 3B). Apparently, a high OKN slow phase velocity can be built up only gradually in the rabbit, either in normal or open-loop conditions.

More recently, a similar dissociation was achieved with normally moving eyes in rabbit[28] and man[29] by Dubois and Collewijn. A moving pattern was projected on a screen in an otherwise dark room, with two perpendicular servocontrolled mirrors in the light pathway. These mirrors were controlled by the horizontal and vertical eye position signal. In this way, the position of the moving pattern could be stabilized on the retina, independent of eye movements, and a very flexible stimulus condition was created. The effect of activation of the eye position-controlled mirrors (opening the OKN loop) in a human subject is shown in Figure 6A,[29] which demonstrates the runaway effect clearly. (Another effect is the deviation of the eye movements from the horizontal plane.[29]) One technical limitation is the restricted size of the stimulus pattern (diameter 30°). *Open-loop gain/stimulus velocity* relations obtained in this condition for man and rabbit are shown in Figure 6B.[28,29] The highest gain (on the order of 100) is reached for stimulus velocities in the range 0.01 to 0.1°/sec, with a drop to about 1.0 for stimuli around 10°/sec and a further drop for higher velocities. The relation is rather straight in the double logarithmic coördinates, and may be approached by a power function, at least for a certain range of stimulus velocities. The results for rabbit and man are remarkably similar. For the monkey with one paralyzed eye, a similar relationship has been found.[27,30] In rabbits with one eye fixed, the *gain/stimulus velocity* relation was somewhat steeper than with the eye free,[10,28] which may indicate an influence of extraretinal signals, e.g., extraocular stretch receptors.

The most parsimonious explanation of these phenomena is to consider the OKN as a velocity—compensating feedback system. In the normal situation, the OKN slow phase eye velocity is always a little lower than the stimulus velocity. The difference *stimulus velocity − eye velocity = slip velocity* maintains the response, and the internal gain of the system is equal to the quotient *eye velocity/slip velocity*. A great problem in the rabbit (for which these values have been measured most accurately) is that the latter quotient is rarely higher than 5 to 10, while in the open-loop situation, gains of 100 are no exception. The discrepancy is more than trivial and may indicate that the concept of OKN as a feedback system with only retinal slip velocity as the input, is too simple.

VI. TIME COURSE OF OKN AND AFTER-NYSTAGMUS

In the rabbit, it is very clear that OKN slow phase velocities faster than a few degrees per second are built up only slowly (Figures 2B and 3B).[10,31] In the open-loop situation, a similar gradual increase of eye velocity is seen when a steady, low velocity stimulus is presented (Figures 2C and 3C).[31] A gradual buildup has been observed also in the monkey under normal[21] and open-loop conditions,[27] as well as in cats and parrots.[1] Man seems to be an exception in generating high OKN velocities almost instantly.[1] This immediate response in man was found also under open-loop conditions.[29] For a clean recording of such buildup phenomena, it is, of course, necessary to present the stimulus at once at full speed.

The complementary phenomenon is found in optokinetic after-nystagmus (OKAN), the persistence of nystagmus when the stimulus is suddenly removed by turning the lights off. The primary after-nystagmus (OKAN I) is similar in direction to the preexisting OKN; when it wears off it is sometimes followed by a secondary after-nystagmus (OKAN II) in the opposite direction and even further successive phases in alternating directions have sometimes been seen. The time course and several phases of OKAN have been extensively studied in the monkey,[21,27,32-34] and in man[35-37] in which OKAN was first noticed in 1921 by Ohm.[38] In the monkey, OKAN is generally better developed than in man. Also, in the rabbit,[5,31,39] it is a very marked phenomenon (Figures 2B, C and 3B, C).

OKAN I has been related to the compensation of vestibular postrotatory nystagmus.[5,40,41] When an animal is rotated in the light, the OKAN I and postrotatory vestibular nystagmus will be opposite in direction and may cancel each other if they have a similar magnitude and time course. Thus, OKAN I may be considered as a meaningful contribution to ocular stability instead of a mere laboratory curiosity. Buildup and after-nystagmus in the monkey have been described as the charge and discharge of a central integrator.[21] Peak OKAN I slow phase velocities were linearly related to OKN velocities for stimulus velocities up to 90 to 120°/sec. The OKAN I mechanism charged in 5 to 10 sec and discharged over 20 to 60 sec in darkness. Short periods of visual fixation introduced during the OKAN I resulted in a rapid discharge of the OKAN. While OKAN I seems to be primarily a function of OKN velocity, OKAN II is strongly related to OKN duration. It is weaker than OKAN I, but can last much longer. With longer exposure times, the maximal slow phase velocity of OKAN II increased and the duration of OKAN I decreased.[33,34] Short periods of visual fixation during OKAN I inhibit OKAN I, but enhance OKAN II. Presumably, the visual suppression of OKAN exposes OKAN II at an earlier time. OKAN II depends not on the occurrence or strength of OKAN I, but mainly on parameters of the preceding nystagmus.[34,37]

In normal animals, a strong convergence of visual direction-selective and vestibular inputs upon single cells in the vestibular nuclei has been demonstrated in the goldfish,[42,43] rabbit,[44] and monkey.[45] The vestibular nuclear activity has been recorded in the monkey during OKN[46] and OKAN I[47] and a close parallel between the time

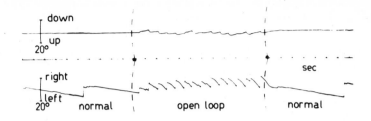

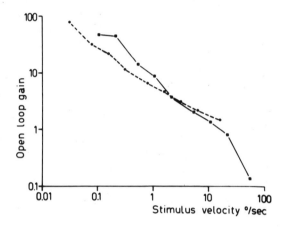

FIGURE 6. Open-loop OKN. Above: effect of opening the loop in a human subject, by activating an eye-position controlled mirror system that stabilized the stimulus outline centrally on the retina. Stimulus velocity 1.6°/sec. Below: open-loop gain as a function of stimulus velocity measured with this system in man (circles) and rabbit (squares). (From Dubois, M. F. W. and Collewijn, H., *Vision Res.*, 19, 9, 1979. With permission.)

courses of OK(A)N velocity and single-unit discharge frequency has been found. These findings support the concept of OKN as a postural reflex and its tight functional relationship with the VOR. Probably, the vestibular nuclei are shared by both systems. The relationship between the VOR, OK(A)N and circularvection is further supported by the finding that all of these phenomena are strongly affected or even abolished by bilateral labyrinthectomy in monkey,[48] rabbit,[31,49] and man.[17] The effect of labyrinthectomy is primarily a very strong reduction of the basic activity of vestibular neurons, which may block the function of these units in the build-up of OK(A)N. Interestingly, the immediate OKN response to stimuli up to 1 to 2°/sec was maintained in labyrinthectomized rabbits,[31] but OKN never reached any higher velocities. In man[17] and monkey,[48] OKN was depressed but not absent in long-standing cases, while OKAN remained absent. Possibly, the OKN in these foveate species was actually generated by the smooth pursuit system. It is important to note that SP apparently never causes circularvection or after-nystagmus.

The functional meaning of OKAN II probably reflects a long-term adaptation of the neuronal circuitry. Physiologically, a long lasting nystagmus indicates that the system is unbalanced, e.g., due to some injury. In such a case, the nervous system will generate a bias that tends to offset the unbalanced input that generates the nystagmus. Such a function has been discussed by Robinson.[50]

VII. THE FUNCTION OF DIFFERENT PARTS OF THE VISUAL FIELD IN OKN

The description given above of OKN as a global visual stabilizing system for which whole field motion is the adequate stimulus might suggest equipotentiality of the whole visual field in eliciting OKN. Actually, not all parts of the retina are equally sensitive to a moving stimulus, and also the sensitivity to different directions of movement may be distributed inhomogeneously. The rabbit has no fovea, but it has a visual streak, which is normally kept aligned with the horizon. In this streak, the density of photo-receptive and neuronal elements is much higher than in the periphery.[51] Recently, it has been shown that in the rabbit the area of maximal optokinetic sensitivity is coextensive with the visual streak.[28] The total sensitive area is extended between 50° superior, 10° inferior, 75° posterior, and 100° anterior in the visual field of one eye. Beyond this area, no OKN could be elicited even with very large stimuli. In this investigation, relatively small stimuli (30 × 30°) had, of course, to be used to map OKN sensitivity, but as the rabbit has no SP, confusion with that system was impossible.

The other inhomogeneity in the rabbit is the strong preference of each eye to respond to movement of the visual surroundings in an anterior direction (temporal to nasal).[5,10] With one eye covered, the horizontal OKN responses, therefore, are very asymmetrical in the two directions. The rabbit shares this property with many other animals, such as the pigeon[52] and the guinea pig.[53] An interesting question, investigated by Tauber and Atkin,[54] is whether such a directional preference is associated with laterally directed eyes and (almost) complete crossing of optic nerve fibers in the chiasm, or with afoveate organization of the retina. From observations on a great number of mammals, birds, and reptiles, Tauber and Atkin[54] concluded that in all cases unidirectional responses in monocular vision correlated with the absence of a fovea, and bidirectional responses with the presence of a fovea, irrespective of the proportion of crossing optic nerve fibers. The monocular preferred direction was always from temporal to nasal. The cat's monocular OKN responses, which are normally bidirectional (in agreement with the presence of an area centralis), become asymmetric (preference temporal to nasal) when the visual cortex is removed[55] and also when the cats are reared from birth under monocular visual deprivation.[56] Strange enough, the asymmetry was not only seen in the deprived eye (after reversal of lid closure), but also in the nondeprived eye during the deprivation period, which lasted 8 to 10 months. Thus, the deprivation of binocularity appeared to be the crucial factor. Most interestingly, Atkinson[57] has recently found that asymmetric monocular OKN is also present in infant monkeys and humans for several months after birth, after which OKN becomes symmetrical. Possibly, this is related to the maturation of the fovea and/or binocular vision. In cases of acquired central scotomata in man reported so far,[58-60] OKN elicited from the diseased eye was weakened, but not overtly asymmetrical. Dubois and Collewijn,[29] in their study on human open-loop OKN, introduced artificial central scotomata (deletions from the stimulus pattern, the location of which was stabilized on the retina). Scotomata, as such, did not introduce asymmetries in monocular OKN. However, to compare a human subject with a rabbit, it seemed more logical to search for asymmetries between the two hemifields of vision, rather than the two eyes. It was found[29] that a peripheral moving pattern elicited stronger responses when the movement was centrifugal (away from the fovea) than when it was centripetal. Thus, a stimulus in the right hemifield elicited the strongest open-loop OKN when it was moving to the right. The differences were most marked when the stimuli fell entirely outside the central area. Körner and Schiller[27] did not find a similar direction preference in their open-loop experiments in monkeys. The preference found in man[29] seems of functional interest, since the responses would favor foveal acquisition of the target. However, this explanation may indicate that the effect is more related to SP than to OKN.

Another problem is the relative importance of central and peripheral parts of the retina in eliciting OKN. Although the mixing of OKN and SP cannot be avoided when this question is investigated in foveate species, at least the overall quantitative relations can be assessed. On one hand, there is evidence that the central parts of the retina are the most powerful in eliciting OKN. Körner and Schiller[27] found in the monkey that field size diameter necessary for eliciting OKN increased as an exponential function of excentricity. Cheng and Outerbridge[61] deleted central parts of a computer-generated stimulus pattern and found in humans a marked decrease of OKN gain for deletions larger than 5° in diameter. Dubois and Collewijn,[29] also in man, found a similar and quantitatively even stronger effect. A decrease of the stimulus diameter with maintained stimulation of the center on the other hand caused comparatively little decrease of OKN. In the three investigations quoted, the stimulus positions on the retina were sufficiently controlled to obtain unambiguous results. Most of the older work on central vs. peripheral stimuli is of little significance now, since it was not controlled for the inhibitory effects of stationary visual contrasts and the effects of eye movements on retinal stimulus position. On the other hand, a dominant role of the peripheral retina has been claimed. Hood[60,62] reported that a subject with a unilateral central scotoma showed a better OKN (especially for higher stimulus velocities) with the scotomatous than with the normal eye when exposed to a full field stimulus. In normals, a strong decrease of OKN gain was found when the periphery was progressively restricted by masks. A related experiment was reported by Dichgans, Nauck, and Wolpert.[63] A horizontally moving stripe pattern was presented with variable restrictions of the size in horizontal or vertical dimension. Vertical reductions of pattern size (down to 2°) hardly affected OKN slow phases, but horizontal reductions progressively reduced OKN gain, especially for higher stimulus velocities. One limitation of the experiments of Hood and Dichgans is that the reduction in stimulus size was paralleled by a reduction in the number of visible contrasts. In discussing the role of central and peripheral retina, Dichgans[64] concludes that OKN can be elicited from both, but that in man, simultaneous stimulation of center and periphery is necessary for an optimal gain at higher stimulus velocities. Clearly, more investigations will be needed for a complete understanding of these relations. A problem with peripheral stimuli in general is that they are easily neglected by the subject and a special effort ("attention") is required to insure that the peripheral stimulus is used as input to the oculomotor system.[29,61] This problem is undoubtedly related to the selective processes involved in smooth pursuit.

On the other hand, the dominating role of the periphery in circularvection seems to be quite clear. Circularvection can be easily dissociated from eye movements by offering a stationary fixation point to a subject seated in a full-field drum. Under such conditions, OKN is suppressed by fixation, but circularvection is maintained.[44] When the lights are extinguished after such a stimulus, an OKAN is generated in agreement with the peripheral stimulus.[37] It is even possible to generate eye movements and circularvection in mutually conflicting directions. When a central pattern (diameter 30°) moved in a direction opposite to that of the full-field background, OKN followed the central stimulus, but circularvection was determined by the peripheral motion.[65] One might speculate that in this case the eye movements were controlled by smooth pursuit, with suppression of the OKN induced by the periphery, as is usual in SP. The actual direction of gaze is controlled by the voluntary SP system, which is hierarchically superior to the global OKN system. If the whole surroundings move, the eye must follow, since the SP system has lost the option to select a target that moves differently from the background. Of course, the selective fixation—SP system can still be used to look at different parts of the full-field stimulus. However, the postural responses associated with a full-field stimulus (such as circularvection) remain determined by the motion of the background, whatever the eye may look at. This arrangement seems very meaningful for a subject that is moving actively through its environment and, at the same time, looking at different targets.

VIII. SOME ASPECTS OF THE NEUROPHYSIOLOGY OF OKN

An extensive treatment of the neuronal circuitry involved in OKN is beyond the scope of this Chapter, and only a few relevant aspects will be discussed. Obviously, parts of the OKN pathway are shared by other oculomotor systems. For recent reviews of oculomotor neurophysiology see References 50, 66, and 67.

A. Visual Motion Detection

In the rabbit, a neuronal substrate for visual motion detection was discovered by Barlow and Hill[68] at the level of the retinal ganglion cells, about a quarter of which proved to be direction-selective. Such neurons respond maximally to movement in a particular ("preferred") direction, but not to movement of the same stimulus in the opposite ("null") direction. These direction-selective cells have been divided into on-off and on type units, which differ in receptive field maps, but also in the movement velocity range to which they respond best.[69] The distribution of the preferred directions among these retinal cells was then investigated, and on the basis of a coincidence between a clustering found in these directions and the pulling directions of the eye muscles, a role of these units in OKN was postulated.[70,71] The discharge frequency of these units as a function of stimulus velocity was then determined more precisely and compared to the slow phase velocities elicited by a similar stimulus in the rabbit under open-loop conditions.[72] It was concluded, that input-output relations of the combined units could account for that of open-loop OKN. Retinal direction-selective ganglion cells have also been described in many other species but, of course, there is no direct proof that retinal direction-selective units are instrumental in OKN.

An important center of convergence for direction-selective visual information has been identified in the pretectal nucleus of the optic tract (NOT) in the rabbit[73] and the cat.[74] The NOT seems to contain almost exclusively direction-selective units that are highly similar in both species. These units in the rabbit typically had a high resting discharge (25 to 50 action potentials/sec) and large, horizontal receptive fields of up to $40 \times 150°$ in the visual streak area of the contralateral eye. They were excited by motion of a (preferably large) visual pattern in one direction (usually anterior) and inhibited by motion in the opposite direction. Many units reacted to a wide range of velocities (0.01 to 20°/sec), with a peak sensitivity often for about 10°/sec, but sometimes for lower velocities. Their latency for visual motion detection was about 60 msec, which would account for most of the OKN latency (about 75 msec).[13] All these properties make the role of NOT units in OKN very plausible. Further evidence for this function of the NOT has been provided by experiments with electrical stimulation in the meso-diencephalic area of the rabbit.[75] The NOT proved to be a circumscript and specific trigger zone for horizontal nystagmus (slow phase to the ipsilateral side), especially after degeneration of the optic tract.

While the NOT seems to represent mainly horizontal direction-selectivity, the medial terminal nucleus (MTN) of the posterior accessory optic tract has been recently[76] identified as a center of direction-selective units oriented mainly in vertical direction, but otherwise similar in properties to the NOT units. The efferent pathways from MTN and NOT that may mediate OKN have still to be identified.

B. The Role of Higher Visual Centers

In the rabbit, the essential OKN circuits seem to be wholly subcortical and even subtectal. Decortication in the rabbit has very little effect on OKN,[5] even immediately after the operation.[77] In rabbits with a complete ablation of the superior colliculi and no significant lesions of the pretectum, OKN is also preserved.[75] The cat's OKN after removal of the visual cortex develops a direction-specific deficit in monocular vision[55] and becomes similar to the OKN of the rabbit. Also, in the dog,[5] OKN was still present after bilateral ablation of the hemispheres, but the maximal drum velocities (normally 400°/sec) that still elicited OKN were lowered to 40°/sec. The same was found when only the visual cortex was removed. Smooth pursuit (called "Schaunystagmus" by Ter Braak) which can be elicited with some difficulty in the dog, was abolished by these cortical lesions.[5] A monocular asymmetry of OKN was probably not looked for. After unilateral hemispherectomy, OKN (presumably elicited binocularly) was permanently asymmetrical, in the sense that OKN with the smooth phase in the direction of the lesion could only be elicited with low stimulus velocities, while in the opposite direction it was normal.

Ter Braak[5] also investigated the effect of cortical lesions on OKN of the monkey (Macacus rhesus). After bilateral ablation of the striate area, and even after bilateral hemispherectomy, a vivid OKN could still be elicited with a full-field motion stimulus, although the animal appeared otherwise to be totally blind and, as expected, had no smooth pursuit. This result has been challenged by Pasik, Pasik, and Krieger[78] who were unable to elicit OKN in the monkey after a histologically confirmed complete removal of both striate cortices. However, Ter Braak and Van Vliet[79] later confirmed the earlier results[5] with histological verification of completeness of the lesion. Thus, a subcortical OKN in the monkey appears to exist. After unilateral lesions of the striate cortex, both groups agree that OKN remains essentially symmetrical, in contrast to the dog, although a hemianopsia was, of course, present.

Our knowledge of the circuits involved in human OKN depends completely on clinical cases. Many cortical or brainstem lesions may cause abnormalities in OKN, in particular directional asymmetries. This kind of symptomatology will not be discussed here and can be found in the clinical literature.[80,81] However, it is important to discuss the relatively few cases that have been reported of complete visual cortical lesions, since in all other species examined so far a subcortical OKN has been demonstrated.

In man, the findings in this respect have been negative except in one case. Ter Braak, Schenk, and Van Vliet[82] describe a case of long lasting, apparently complete cortical blindness due to a cerebral vascular accident in which a rudimentary OKN could be elicited for the first time 4 months after admission to the hospital. Apart from the pupil reflex, the OKN remained the only response to visual stimulation. The patient denied any perception of light or movement. This is important, since in all other reported cases of cortical blindness a return of OKN has been accompanied by return of some visual perception in a part of the visual field. Necropsy revealed practically total destruction of both striate areas and degeneration of both lateral geniculate bodies. Similar cases described by Velzeboer[83] and Brindley and coworkers[84,85] failed to supply evidence for a subcortical OKN in man. Needless to say, only very careful investigations with full-field stimuli and optimal conditions can furnish admissable evidence in this argument. For the moment, the existence of subcortical OKN in man must be considered doubtful at best, in contrast to all other species where it is almost certainly present. A difficulty in the interpretation, as always in the absence of a function after a lesion, is that the visual cortex sends massive descending projections back to the lower visual centers, and that the degeneration of those connections may profoundly disorganize the function of subcortical circuits that normally are operative. The permanent abolition of OKAN after bilateral labyrinthectomy is an example of such a phenomenon.

Unilateral lesions of the occipital (and also parietal and temporal) cortex generally result in a reduced OKN response when the drum is moved towards the side of the lesion.[80,81] This characteristical asymmetry was already reported by Bárány.[86] However, this asymmetry is by no means absolute and even homonymous hemianopsias with macular involvement may occur with normal symmetric OKN.[64,80] In one unique case[87] of a longstanding left hemispherectomy, smooth pursuit of a small target was deficient (but not absent) to the left side. The clinical consensus about the direction of asymmetries cannot be related to the preference for centrifugal motion found by Dubois and Collewijn.[29]

C. Function of the Cerebellum in OKN; Adaptive Functions

The function of the cerebellum in the control of eye movements has been investigated intensively in recent years, and the following aspects can now be recognized:

1. Vermal lobules VI and VII seem to be involved in the regulation of the amplitude of saccades.[88,89]
2. The flocculus has been implicated in both short and long-term interaction between the visual and vestibular system, in smooth pursuit and in the maintenance of excentric gaze.

In cerebellectomized rabbits, the smooth component of OKN remained relatively intact,[90] but the fast phases were deficient, especially with higher slow phase velocities, so that the eyes reached extreme deviations (up to 40°) from the midposition. Possibly, this effect was due to the absence of the regulatory influence of the vermis on saccades.

The VOR elicited by head movements is normally strongly influenced by vision: a stationary visual world enhances the VOR (and ocular stability in space), while visual patterns rotating with the head will reduce the VOR. With a full-field stimulus, this phenomenon is quite clear in the rabbit.[91] In the albino rabbit, a similar effect, obtained with a single light slit, was abolished by destruction of the flocculus.[92] A similar defect has been described in the monkey after flocculus lesions[93] and in human cerebellar disfunction.[94,95]

In humans, specifically the suppression of the VOR by fixation of a target that moves with the head is defective. Also smooth pursuit of small targets on a stationary background is disturbed in monkey[96,97] and man[94,95] by cerebellar pathology. In SP, a suppression of OKN caused by the relative motion of the background is normally required and one might speculate that this is a cerebellar function, analogous to the suppression of the VOR while following a moving target with the head.

In addition to the severe defects of SP after flocculus lesions, there is also a relatively milder deficiency of full-field OKN.[93-95] OKAN is preserved after cerebellar lesions,[50,93] although it may be reduced commensurately with OKN.

Finally, the long-term recalibration of the VOR in response to changes in the quantitative relation between head movements and retinal image slip appears to be abolished by cerebellar and particularly floccular lesions.[98,99]

All these recent findings indicate a subtle role of vestibulo-cerebellum in the adjustment of the gain of visual and vestibular oculomotor responses and their mutual interaction. Although OKN in its pure form, as well as the isolated VOR, seem to be relatively preserved after cerebellar lesions, the normal physiological situation will always require an adequate interaction between these two systems for optimal visual function, and therefore, the cerebellar modulation is essential in the function of OKN.

Details of the relevant cerebellar circuits have been mainly investigated in the rabbit and the monkey. An important efferent cerebellar pathway consists of Purkinje cell axons that project on the vestibular nuclei, and have been shown to modulate the

VOR.[100] Among the afferent pathways, the inferior olive—climbing fiber system has been especially investigated in the rabbit. The NOT seems to project directly on the dorsal cap of the inferior olive[101-103] which, in turn, projects to the flocculus.[104] The direction-selectivity of this pathway was demonstrated by Simpson and Alley[105] at the climbing fiber level and by Barmack[106] in the dorsal cap. Destruction of this pathway interferes with the long-term visual adaptation of the VOR[107] and also reduces the gain of OKN in the rabbit.[106] The existence of a projection of direction-selective NOT cells to the inferior olive has also been demonstrated electrophysiologically[108] and neuroanatomically[109] in the cat.

The rabbit's flocculus also receives a mossy fiber visual projection[110] which conveys rather complicated signals, such as a integrated eye velocity signal.[111]

Another powerful mossy fiber input to the rabbit's flocculus consists of vestibular afferents. The modulation of Purkinje cell activity by vestibular stimuli (head oscillation) and their changes in short and long-term adaptation have been discussed by Ito and colleagues[112-114] who have postulated that the climbing fiber signals on retinal slip cause a long-term change in the conduction of mossy fiber signals through the Purkinje cells. Finally, it is very probable that eye movements as such also are relayed by a nonvisual mossy fiber signal to the rabbit's flocculus.[115]

The activity of Purkinje cells of the monkey's flocculus during head and eye movements has been investigated by Lisberger and Fuchs.[116,117] Purkinje cells were activated both during SP and during visual suppression of the VOR, but only moderately when the VOR was elicited in darkness. A head velocity signal reaches these Purkinje cells through vestibular afferents (mossy fibers) and an eye velocity signal, which essentially represents a corollary discharge, probably is conveyed from the brainstem nuclei controlling eye movement, also through mossy fibers. Both signals are added at the Purkinje cell level and cancel when eye and head movements are opposite, i.e., when the VOR is working. Lisberger and Fuchs[116,117] propose that the output of these Purkinje cells sustains SP and suppression of the VOR during visual fixation. However, it is still unclear how such a mechanism is visually activated. The function of climbing fibers in the monkey's flocculus has still to be described.

The intimate linkage between OKN and VOR predicts that many of these findings will prove to be important for the understanding of OKN. The plasticity of OKN alone has been rarely investigated. In the rabbit, it has been recently demonstrated that the OKN responses to sinusoidal oscillation of a large drum are capable of considerable adaptation: the gain of such reactions improved very much during a few hours of sustained stimulation.[118] Such a gain increase of OKN for sinusoidal stimulation is illustrated in Figure 7. Moreover, this improvement transferred to the VOR, tested at the same stimulus frequency.[119] A decrease of OKN gain in dark-reared rabbits, with partial recovery in the light, has also been found.[120] The effects of dark-rearing in cats[56] were already mentioned. In man, a positive learning effect with increase in OKN gain due to repetitive stimulation has also been reported.[121]

IX. MODELS OF THE OKN SYSTEM

Attempts to model the OKN system have been relatively rare. A number of properties of the rabbit's OKN system have been simulated some years ago[122] in a simple analog model which treated the OKN as a simple velocity feedback loop (Figure 8A). The nonlinear characteristics of the retinal direction-selective cells were used to shape the velocity input signal, obtained by differentiation of retinal image position. The velocity signal was then integrated to produce eye position. A second integrator, which was leaky and had a long time constant (30 sec), was introduced to simulate the slow build-up of OKN and the OKAN. The model simulated many of the known input-

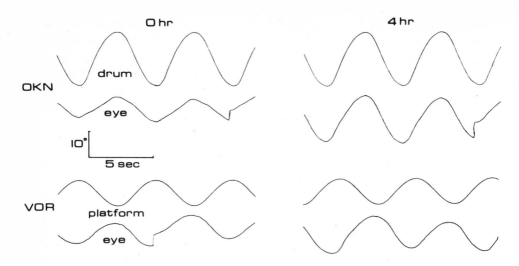

FIGURE 7.   Improvement of OKN and VOR gain in the rabbit due to four hr continuous stimulation with sinusoidal movement (0.16 Hz, 20° peak-to-peak) of a full-field visual stimulus. The VOR was tested only briefly in darkness once an hour; otherwise the rabbit's head was stationary. Visual input was never combined with a labyrinthine stimulus. (From Collewijn, H., unpublished data.)

output relations for unidirectional and sinusoidal stimuli. On the other hand, it did not explain the nature of the postulated integrators, the origin and control of the fast phase, the interaction with the vestibular systems or any type of variability or adaptation.

A conceptually related model accounting for the build-up and OKAN phenomenon was recently proposed by Cohen et al.[21] Robinson[123] introduced a model in which OKN and VOR are integrated (Figure 8B). A major difference with Collewijn's model is the replacement of the integrator with a long time constant by an internal positive feedback loop with eye velocity (efference copy) as the input. This loop, which should have a gain slightly smaller than unity to prevent instability, could account for many properties of OKN, VOR, OKAN, and circularvection.

Such models are extremely useful in conceptualizing the signal flow patterns that are minimally required to explain the input-output relations of a system, and Robinson[124] has succesfully applied his model to data of Waespe and Henn[46] to show a linear addition of optokinetic and vestibular signals in the vestibular nucleus. On the other hand, they suggest a rigidity and machine-like performance which is often at odds with the capricious behavior of the living system. Also, the incredible complexity of the neuroanatomical substrate revealed by modern neuroanatomical methods seems to make the achievement of more perfect models somewhat illusory.

X. SOME SPECIAL FORMS OF OKN

A. Nonhorizontal OKN

Vertical OKN is rarely investigated and torsional OKN almost never, largely due to technical difficulties in recording such eye movements. Both types can be easily elicited in the rabbit with appropriate full-field stimuli.[125] They are highly similar to horizontal OKN except that for stimulus velocities above 1°/sec gain remains very low and no buildup of slow phase velocity is seen. This may be related to the recent description of vertically oriented direction-selective units in the MTN[76] which have a maximum sensitivity to velocities around 1°/sec. In contrast to horizontal OKN, each eye re-

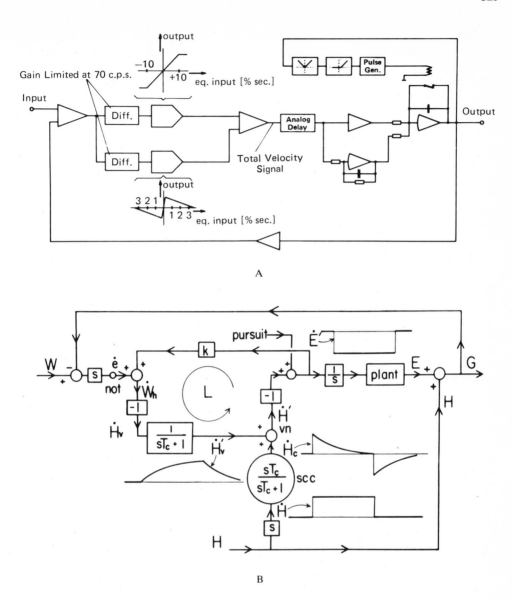

FIGURE 8.(A).   A simple model (Collewijn[122]) of the rabbit's OKN as a feedback system with retinal slip as the input. Slip velocity is coded by differentiating circuits with a transfer function similar to that of the two types of retinal direction-selective elements. After a time delay, the total velocity signal is passed through a proportional plus integrating (long time constant) network which simulates build-up and OKAN, and finally a pure integrator which recreates position out of the velocity signal. The last integrator is reset to zero after reaching a certain threshold voltage, as a crude equivalent to the fast phase; (B) Robinson's[123] model of the optokinetic system and vestibulo-ocular reflex. Head velocity $\dot{H}$ is transduced by the semicircular canals, scc, into $\dot{H}_c$, the canals' best estimate of head velocity which is correct only transiently. When its sign is changed, it becomes an eye velocity command $\ddot{E}$ which is integrated and sent to the eye muscles (plant) to create eye position in the head E. This is a simplified description of the vestibuloocular reflex. Eye position in space, gaze G, is the sum of E and head position H. The retina compares the relative motion $\dot{e}$ of the gaze axis with respect to the seen world W. This signal appears in the nucleus of the optic tract, NOT. An efference copy of eye velocity $\ddot{E}$ is added to $\dot{e}$ to reconstruct the motion of the world with respect to the head W_h. Since the seen world never moves, this is the negative of $\dot{H}_v$, the visual system's estimate of head velocity in space. The high frequencies are filtered out and the low frequency version $\dot{H}'_v$ is added to $\dot{H}_c$ in the vestibular nucleus vn. Their sum, $\dot{H}$ is the brain stem's best estimate of the velocity of selfrotation based on both visual and vestibular information. ((A) From Collewijn, H., *Brain Res.,* 36, 74, 1972; (B) from Robinson, D. A., Control of Gaze by Brain Stem Neurons, Baker, R. and Berthoz, A., Eds., Elsevier/ North Holland, Amsterdam, 1977, 49.)

sponds symmetrically for vertical and torsional stimuli in both directions. Vertical OKN has also been recently investigated in open-loop conditions in rabbit[28] and man.[29] In man, the input-output relations for vertical OKN were almost identical to those for horizontal OKN, except that the average vertical gain was slightly smaller. Systematic directional preferences were not found, but individuals showed very marked ideosyncratic asymmetries, particularly in the nonhorizontal directions.

Cycloversion induced in man by a pattern rotating around the visual axis was demonstrated by Brecher[126] in man. It consisted either of a tonic deviation or a regular torsional nystagmus. The potential interest of this type of OKN might be the essentially nonfoveal nature of the stimulus, which might circumvent any SP response. Crone[127] obtained only the tonic deviation in similar experiments, and also Hass[128] rarely saw a true rotatory nystagmus. The dynamic properties of human torsional OKN have not been measured.

B. Unconventional Stimuli

Traditionally, OKN is induced by real, continuous movement of a real pattern. Smooth pursuit of a target that is perceptually reconstructed from a stimulus configuration, but does not exist as a projection on the retina, has been described.[129] Also, OKN can be induced by an apparent, rather than a real, target movement. Ter Braak[130] projected two identical patterns alternatingly with a spatial shift of 0.5 to 1° and a frequency of 6 to 15 Hz. With similar exposure times for both projections, the shifting image can be easily perceived as a continuously moving pattern (often called phi-movement) the direction of which is ambivalent. Such patterns elicit a well-developed nystagmus, the direction of which corresponds to that of the perception. Reversals of this direction regularly occurred and could be influenced by the subject. It appeared that movement perception preceded eye movements, rather than vice versa. The structure of the patterns was immaterial and could consist of stripes or visual noise. Dichoptic presentation of the patterns abolished the phenomenon in all but one of the subjects.

In this type of experiment, the movement perception is not dependent on the eye movements. However, if the eyes move at an adequate velocity across one intermittently illuminated, stationary pattern which contains a certain amount of spatial periodicity, a sustained pursuit movement of a perceived motion (sigma-movement) can also be elicited.[131] In this case, the eye movements are necessary to elicit the motion perception, and it has been postulated[131] that the internal feedback of the efferent oculomotor signals is instrumental in this phenomenon.

Another recent experiment[132] has shown that OKN can be induced by a moving bar pattern coded as a disparity in two random dot patterns (Julesz patterns). The pattern could only be perceived by binocular stereopsis. A vigorous nystagmus was induced in human subjects. Interestingly, the latency of this OKN was about 70 msec longer than for nystagmus induced by physical contours. The method is proposed as a possible test for stereopsis in humans and animals.

All these conditions seem to involve fairly complex levels of perceptual processing, and it remains to be seen whether they can be applied to nonhuman primates and a fortiori, nonprimates. In this context, it should be kept in mind that nystagmus has been induced in the rabbit[133] and monkey[134] by simple visual flicker (stroboscopic flashes at a rate of 10 to 20/sec). For man, the existence of this phenomenon has been denied.[135]

C. Inverted OKN

Inversion of OKN (slow phase motion opposite in direction to the stimulus motion) has been described in the clinical literature in association with certain pathological conditions such as congenital nystagmus[26,80] and ocular albinism.[136] Obviously, an inversion of OKN would create a positive feedback loop with disastrous consequences for the stability of the eye. The classical demonstration of this principle can be found in the experiments of Sperry[137,138] in which one eye of newts and fishes was rotated through 180°. With the other eye covered, these animals persisted in forced circling for the rest of their life. Although corollary discharge (equivalent to efference copy) was invoked by Sperry, the concept of retinal direction-selective motion detection as the input to a velocity feedback loop offers a sufficient and more parsimonious explanation.

Recently, it was discovered[139] that in albino rabbits, OKN is inverted in the anterior sector (90 to 180°) of the visual field, but normal in the posterior visual field. With the whole visual field exposed, the normal sector usually prevails and the eye and head are marginally stable, with OKN of normal direction. With the posterior visual field masked, eye and head are unstable and OKN is in the wrong direction. These effects are illustrated in Figure 9. The inversion could be due to erroneous connections of direction-selective fibers originating in the temporal part of the retina, analogous to the several other aberrant crossings and connections discovered in recent years in albinos. The inversion of OKN is associated with similar aberrations in the direction-selective receptive fields of single units in the nucleus of the optic tract.[140]

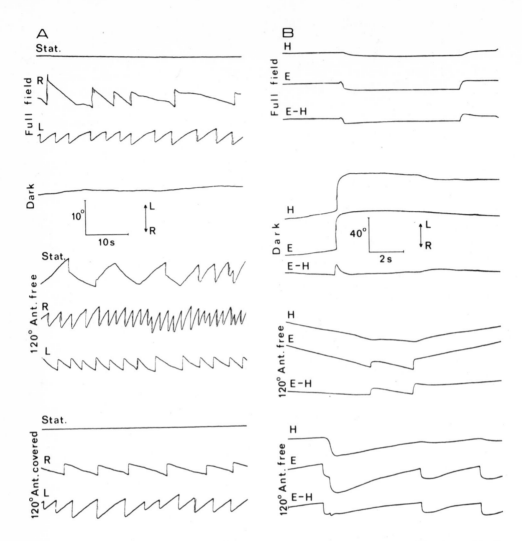

FIGURE 9.   Typical eye and head movements of albino rabbits. (A) Angular eye position in optokinetic drum with full visual field (full field), 120° anterior sector visible (120° Ant. free), and 120° anterior sector covered and posterior field visible (120° Ant. covered) to a stationary drum (Stat.), to rotation of the drum to the right (R) and left (L) at 1.2° per second, and in darkness (Dark); (B) Angular position of the head in space (H), eye in space (E), and eye in the head (E-H) in freely moving, but quiet animals with full visual field (full field), in darkness (Dark), and when 120° anterior sector was free (120° Ant. free). The rabbit's cubicle (80 × 80 cm) was draped with black and white gingham (elements 1 cm). (From Collewijn, H., Winterson, B. J., and Dubois, M. F. W., *Science*, 199, 1351, 1978. With permission.)

REFERENCES

1. Collins, W. E., Schroeder, D. J., Rice, N., Mertens, R. A., and Krantz, G., Some characteristics of optokinetic eye-movement patterns: a comparative study, *Aerosp. Med.,* 41, 1251, 1970.
2. Dodge, R., Five types of eye movement in the horizontal meridian plane of the field of regard, *Am. J. Physiol.,* 8, 307, 1903.
3. Bárány, R., Die Untersuchung der optischen und vestibulären reflektorischen Augenbewegungen in einem Falle von einseitigen Blicklähmung, *Mtschr. Ohrenheilk.,* 42, 109, 1908.
4. Ohm, J., Neue Vorrichtungen zur Auslösung des optischen Drehnystagmus, *Klin. Mblt. Augenheilk.,* 77, 14, 1926.
5. Ter Braak, J. W. G., Untersuchungen über optokinetischen Nystagmus, *Arch. Neerl. Physiol.,* 21, 309, 1936.
6. Thoden, U., Dichgans, J., and Savidis, T., Direction-specific optokinetic modulation of monosynaptic hind limb reflexes in cats, *Exp. Brain Res.,* 30, 155, 1977.
7. Schaefer, K. P., Meyer, D. L., and Schott, D., Optic and vestibular influences on ear movements, *Brain, Behav. Evol.,* 4, 323, 1971.
8. Kowler, E., Murphy, B. J., and Steinman, R. M., Velocity matching during smooth pursuit of different targets on different backgrounds, *Vision Res.,* 18, 603, 1978.
9. Scala, N. P. and Spiegel, E. A., Subcortical (passive) optokinetic nystagmus in lesions of the midbrain and of the vestibular nuclei, *Confin. Neurol.,* 3, 53, 1941.
10. Collewijn, H., Optokinetic eye movements in the rabbit: input-output relations, *Vision Res.,* 9, 117, 1969.
11. Collewijn, H., The normal range of horizontal eye movements in the rabbit, *Exp. Neurol.,* 28, 132, 1970.
12. Collewijn, H. and Van der Mark, F., Ocular stability in variable visual feedback conditions in the rabbit, *Brain Res.,* 36, 47, 1972.
13. Collewijn, H., Latency and gain of the rabbit's optokinetic reactions to small movements, *Brain Res.,* 36, 59, 1972.
14. Robinson, D. A., A method of measuring eye movement using a scleral search coil in a magnetic field, *IEEE Trans. Biomed. Electron.,* BME-10, 137, 1963.
15. Collewijn, H., Eye and head movements in freely moving rabbits, *J. Physiol. (London),* 266, 471, 1977.
16. Evinger, C. and Fuchs, A. F., Saccadic, smooth pursuit, and optokinetic eye movements of the trained cat, *J. Physiol. (London),* 285, 209, 1978.
17. Zee, D. S., Yee, R. D., and Robinson, D. A., Optokinetic responses in labyrinthine-defective human beings, *Brain Res.,* 113, 423, 1976.
18. Grüttner, R., Experimentelle Untersuchungen über den optokinetischen Nystagmus, *Z. Sinnesphysiol.,* 68, 1, 1939.
19. Komatsuzaki, A., Harris, H. E., Alpert, J., and Cohen, B., Horizontal nystagmus of rhesus monkeys, *Acta Otolaryngol.,* 67, 535, 1969.
20. Igarashi, M., Takahashi, M., and Homick, J. L., Optokinetic nystagmus and vestibular stimulation in squirrel monkey model, *Arch. Oto-Rhino-Laryng.,* 218, 115, 1977.
21. Cohen, B., Matsuo, V., and Raphan, T., Quantitative analysis of the velocity characteristics of optokinetic nystagmus and optokinetic after-nystagmus, *J. Physiol. (London),* 270, 321, 1977.
22. Fuchs, A. F., Periodic eye tracking in the monkey, *J. Physiol. (London),* 193, 161, 1967.
23. Meiry, J. L., Vestibular and proprioceptive stabilization of eye movements, in *The Control of Eye Movements,* Bach-y-Rita, P. and Collins, C. C., Eds., Academic Press, New York, 1971, 483.
24. Ohm, J., Ist der optische Drehnystagmus von einem unbeweglichen Auge auslösbar? *Klin. Mbtl. Augenheilk.,* 77, 330, 1926.
25. Körner, F. and Dichgans, J., Bewegungswahrnehmung, optokinetischer Nystagmus und retinale Bildwanderung, *v. Graefes Arch. Opthalmol.,* 174, 34, 1967.
26. Hood, J. D. and Leech, J., The significance of peripheral vision in the perception of movement, *Acta Otolaryngol,* 77, 72, 1974.
27. Körner, F. and Schiller, P. H., The optokinetic response under open and closed loop conditions in the monkey, *Exp. Brain Res.,* 14, 318, 1972.
28. Dubois, M. F. W. and Collewijn, H., The optokinetic reactions of the rabbit: relation to the visual streak, *Vision Res.,* 19, 9, 1979.
29. Dubois, M. F. W. and Collewijn, H., Optokinetic reactions in man elicited by localized retinal motion stimuli, *Vision Res.,* 19, 1105, 1979.
30. Körner, F., Untersuchungen über nichtvisuelle Kontrolle von Augenbewegungen, *Adv. Ophthalmol,* 31, 100, 1975.

31. Collewijn, H., Impairment of optokinetic (after-) nystagmus by labyrinthectomy in the rabbit, *Exp. Neurol.,* 52, 146, 1976.

32. Krieger, H. P. and Bender, M. B., Optokinetic after-nystagmus in the monkey, *Electroencephalogr. Clin. Neurophysiol.,* 8, 97, 1956.

33. Büttner, U., Waespe, W., and Henn, V., Duration and direction of optokinetic after-nystagmus as a function of stimulus exposure time in the monkey, *Arch. Psychiatr. Nervenkr.,* 222, 281, 1976.

34. Waespe, W., Huber, T., and Henn, V., Dynamic changes of optokinetic after-nystagmus (OKAN) caused by brief visual fixation periods in monkey and in man, *Arch. Psychiatr. Nervenkr.,* 226, 1, 1978.

35. Mackensen, G. and Wiegmann, O., Untersuchungen zur Physiologie des optokinetischen Nachnystagmus. I. Mitteilung. Die Abhängigkeit des optokinetischen Nachnystagmus von der Winkelgeschwindigkeit des Reizmusters, *v. Graefes Arch. Ophthalmol.,* 160, 497, 1959.

36. Mackensen, G., Kommerell, G., and Silbereisen, D., Untersuchungen zur Physiologie des optokinetischen Nachnystagmus. II. Mitteilung. Individuelle Unterschiede des Nachnystagmus, die Abhängigkeit des optokinetischen Nachnystagmus von der Reizdauer, *v. Graefes Arch. Ophthalmol.,* 163, 170, 1961.

37. Brandt, T., Dichgans, J., and Büchele, W., Motion habituation: inverted self-motion perception and optokinetic after-nystagmus, *Exp. Brain Res.,* 21, 337, 1974.

38. Ohm, J., Die klinische Bedeutung des optischen Drehnystagmus, *Klin. Mblt. Augenheilk.,* 68, 323, 1921.

39. Neverov, V. P. and Kissljakov, V. A., The reversive postoptokinetic nystagmus — an experimental model of the oculomotor centres automatic activity, in *Visual Information Processing and Control of Motor Activity,* Bulgarian Academy of Sciences, Sofia, 1971, 229.

40. Mowrer, O. H., The influence of vision during bodily rotation upon the duration of post-rotational vestibular nystagmus, *Acta Otolaryngol.,* 25, 351, 1937.

41. Igarashi, M., Takahashi, M., and Homick, J. L., Optokinetic after-nystagmus and postrotatory nystagmus in squirrel monkeys, *Acta Otolaryngol.,* 85, 387, 1978.

42. Dichgans, J., Schmidt, C. L., and Graf, W., Visual input improves the speedometer function of the vestibular nuclei in the goldfish, *Exp. Brain Res.,* 18, 319, 1973.

43. Allum, J. H. J., Graf, W., Dichgans, J., and Schmidt, C. L., Visual-vestibular interactions in the vestibular nuclei of the goldfish, *Exp. Brain Res.,* 26, 463, 1976.

44. Dichgans, J. and Brandt, T., Visual-vestibular interaction and motion perception, *Bibl. Ophthalmol.,* 82, 327, 1972.

45. Henn, V., Young, L. R., and Finley, C., Vestibular nucleus units in alert monkeys are also influenced by moving visual fields, *Brain Res.,* 71, 144, 1974.

46. Waespe, W. and Henn, V., Neuronal activity in the vestibular nuclei of the alert monkey during vestibular and optokinetic stimulation, *Exp. Brain Res.,* 27, 523, 1977.

47. Waespe, W. and Henn, V., Vestibular nuclei activity during optokinetic after-nystagmus (OKAN) in the alert monkey, *Exp. Brain Res.,* 30, 323, 1977.

48. Cohen, B., Uemura, T., and Takemori, S., Effects of labyrinthectomy on optokinetic nystagmus (OKN) and optokinetic after-nystagmus (OKAN), *Equilibrium Res.,* 3, 88, 1973.

49. Gutman, J., Zelig, S., and Bergmann, F., Optokinetic nystagmus in the labyrinthectomized rabbit, *Confin. Neurol.,* 24, 158, 1964.

50. Robinson, D. A., Oculomotor control signals, in *Basic Mechanisms of Ocular Motility and Their Clinical Implications,* Lennerstrand, G. and Bach-y-Rita, P., Eds., Pergamon Press, Oxford, 1975, 337.

51. Hughes, A., Topographical relationships between the anatomy and physiology of the rabbit visual system, *Doc. Ophthalmol. (Den Haag),* 30, 33, 1971.

52. Mowrer, O. H., A comparison of the reaction mechanisms mediating optokinetic nystagmus in human beings and in pigeons, *Psychol. Monogr.,* 47, 294, 1936.

53. Smith, K. U. and Bridgman, M., The neural mechanisms of movement vision and optic nystagmus, *J. Exp. Psychol.,* 33, 165, 1943.

54. Tauber, E. S. and Atkin, A., Optomotor responses to monocular stimulation: relation to visual system organization, *Science,* 160, 1365, 1968.

55. Wood, C. C., Spear, P. D., and Braun, J. J., Direction-specific deficits in horizontal optokinetic nystagmus following removal of visual cortex in the cat, *Brain Res.,* 60, 231, 1973.

56. Van Hof-Van Duin, J., Early and permanent effects of monocular deprivation on pattern discrimination and visuomotor behavior in cats, *Brain Res.,* 111, 261, 1976.

57. Atkinson, J., The development of optokinetic nystagmus in the human infant and monkey infant: an analogue to development in kittens, in *Developmental Neurobiology of Vision* Freeman, R. H., Ed., NATO Advanced Study Institute Series, Plenum Press, New York, 1979, 277.

58. Ohm, J., Zur Augenzitterkunde. III. Mitteilung. Über den optischen Drehnystagmus, *v. Graefes Arch. Ophthalmol.*, 117, 174, 1926.

59. Dodge, R. and Fox, J. J., Optic nystagmus, *Arch. Neurol. Psychiatr.*, 20, 812, 1928.

60. Hood, J. D., Observations upon the neurological mechanism of optokinetic nystagmus with especial reference to the contribution of peripheral vision, *Acta Otolaryngol.*, 63, 208, 1967.

61. Cheng, M. and Outerbridge, J. S., Optokinetic nystagmus during selective retinal stimulation, *Exp. Brain Res.*, 23, 129, 1975.

62. Hood, J. D., Observations upon the role of the peripheral retina in the execution of eye movements, *ORL*, 37, 65, 1975.

63. Dichgans, J., Nauck, B., and Wolpert, E., The influence of attention vigilance and stimulus area on optokinetic and vestibular nystagmus and voluntary saccades, in *The Oculomotor System and Brain Functions*, Zikmund, V., Ed., Butterworths, London, 1973, 281.

64. Dichgans, J., Optokinetic nystagmus as dependent on the retinal periphery via the vestibular nucleus, in *Control of Gaze by Brain Stem Neurons*, Baker, R. and Berthoz, A., Eds., Elsevier, Amsterdam, 1977, 261.

65. Brandt, T., Dichgans, J., and Koenig, E., Differential effects of central versus peripheral vision on egocentric and exocentric motion perception, *Exp. Brain Res.*, 16, 476, 1973.

66. Baker, R. and Berthoz, A., Eds., *Control of Gaze by Brain Stem Neurons*, Elsevier, Amsterdam, 1977.

67. Raphan, T. and Cohen, B., Brain stem mechanisms for rapid and slow eye movements, *Ann. Rev. Physiol.*, 40, 527, 1978.

68. Barlow, H. B. and Hill, R. M., Selective sensitivity to direction of movement in ganglion cells of the rabbit retina, *Science*, 139, 412, 1963.

69. Barlow, H. B., Hill, R. M., and Levick, W. R., Retinal ganglion cells responding selectively to direction and speed of image motion in the rabbit, *J. Physiol. (London)*, 173, 377, 1964.

70. Oyster, C. W. and Barlow, H. B., Direction-selective units in rabbit retina: distribution of preferred directions, *Science*, 155, 841, 1967.

71. Oyster, C. W., The analysis of image motion by the rabbit retina, *J. Physiol. (London)*, 199, 613, 1968.

72. Oyster, C. W., Takahashi, E., and Collewijn, H., Direction-selective retinal ganglion cells and control of optokinetic nystagmus in the rabbit, *Vision Res.*, 12, 183, 1972.

73. Collewijn, H., Direction-selective units in the rabbit's nucleus of the optic tract, *Brain Res.*, 100, 489, 1975.

74. Hoffmann, K. P., and Schoppmann, A. Retinal input to direction-selective cells in the nucleus tractus opticus of the cat, *Brain Res.*, 99, 359, 1975.

75. Collewijn, H., Oculomotor areas in the rabbit's midbrain and pretectum, *J. Neurobiol.*, 6, 3, 1975.

76. Simpson, J. I., Soodak, R. E., and Hess, R., The accessory optic system and its relation to the vestibulo cerebellum, in Reflex Control of Posture and Movement, Granit, R. and Pompeiano, O., Ed., *Progress in Brain Research*, Vol. 50, Elsevier, Amsterdam, 1979, 715.

77. Hobbelen, J. F. and Collewijn, H., Effects of cerebro-cortical and collicular ablations upon the optokinetic reactions in the rabbit, *Doc. Ophthalmol.*, (Den Haag), 30, 227, 1971.

78. Pasik, P., Pasik, T., and Krieger, H. P., Effects of cerebral lesions upon optokinetic nystagmus in monkeys, *J. Neurophysiol.*, 22, 297, 1959.

79. Ter Braak, J. W. G. and Van Vliet, A. G. M., Subcortical optokinetic nystagmus in the monkey, *Psychiatr. Neurol. Neurochir.*, 66, 277, 1963.

80. Jung, R. and Kornhuber, H. K., Results of electronystagmography in man: the value of optokinetic, vestibular, and spontaneous nystagmus for neurologic diagnosis and research, in *The Oculomotor System*, Bender, M. B., Ed., Harper & Row, New York, 1964, 428.

81. Hoyt, W. F. and Daroff, R. B., Supranuclear disorders of ocular control systems in man, in *The Control of Eye Movements*, Bach-y-Rita, P. and Collins, C. C., Eds., Academic Press, New York, 1971, 175.

82. Ter Braak, J. W. G., Schenk, V. W. D., and Van Vliet, A. G. M., Visual reactions in a case of long-lasting cortical blindness, *J. Neurol. Neurosurg. Psychiatr.*, 34, 140, 1971.

83. Velzeboer, C. M. J., Bilateral cortical hemianopsia and optokinetic nystagmus, *Ophthalmologcia*, 123, 187, 1952.

84. Brindley, G. S., Gauthier-Smith, P. C., and Lewin, W., Cortical blindness and the functions of the non-geniculate fibres of the optic tracts, *J. Neurol. Neurosurg. Psychiatr.*, 32, 259, 1969.

85. Brindley, G. S. and Janota, I., Observations on cortical blindness and on vascular lesions that cause loss of recent memory, *J. Neurol. Neurosurg. Psychiatr.*, 38, 459, 1975.

86. Bárány, R., Zur Klinik und Theorie des Eisenbahnnystagmus, *Acta Otolaryngol.*, 3, 260, 1920.

87. Troost, B. T., Daroff, R. B., Weber, R. B., and Dell'Osso, L. F., Hemispheric control of eye movements. II. Quantitative analysis of smooth pursuit in a hemispherectomy patient, *Arch. Neurol.*, 27, 449, 1972.

88. Llinás, R. and Wolfe, J. W., Functional linkage between the electrical activity in the vermal cerebellar cortex and saccadic eye movements, *Exp. Brain Res., 29*, 1, 1977.

89. Ritchie, L., Effects of cerebellar lesions on saccadic eye movements, *J. Neurophysiol., 39*, 1246, 1976.

90. Collewijn, H., Dysmetria of fast phase of optokinetic nystagmus in cerebellectomized rabbits, *Exp. Neurol., 28*, 144, 1970.

91. Baarsma, E. A. and Collewijn, H., Vestibulo-ocular and optokinetic reactions to rotation and their interaction in the rabbit, *J. Physiol. (London), 238*, 603, 1974.

92. Ito, M., Shiida, T., Yagi, N., and Yamamoto, M., Visual influence on rabbit horizontal vestibulo-ocular reflex presumably effected via the cerebellar flocculus, *Brain Res., 65*, 170, 1974.

93. Takemori, S. and Cohen, B., Loss of visual suppression of vestibular nystagmus after flocculus lesions, *Brain Res., 72*, 213, 1974.

94. Zee, D. S., Yee, R. D., Cogan, D. G., Robinson, D. A., and Engel, W. K., Ocular motor abnormalities in hereditary cerebellar ataxia, *Brain, 99*, 207, 1976.

95. Dichgans, J., Von Reutern, G. M., and Römmelt, U., Impaired suppression of vestibular nystagmus by fixation in cerebellar and noncerebellar patients, *Arch. Psychiatr. Nervenkr., 226*, 183, 1978.

96. Westheimer, G. and Blair, S. M., Oculomotor defects in cerebellectomized monkeys, *Invest. Ophthalmol., 12*, 618, 1973.

97. Westheimer, G. and Blair, S. M., Functional organization of primate oculomotor system revealed by cerebellectomy, *Exp. Brain Res., 21*, 463, 1974.

98. Ito, M., Shiida, T., Yagi, N., and Yamamoto, M., The cerebellar modification of rabbit's horizontal vestibulo-ocular reflex induced by sustained head rotation combined with visual stimulation, *Proc. Jpn. Acad., 50*, 85, 1974.

99. Robinson, D. A., Adaptive gain control of vestibuloocular reflex by the cerebellum, *J. Neurophysiol., 39*, 954, 1976.

100. Ito, M., Nisimaru, N., and Yamamoto, M., Specific patterns of neuronal connexions involved in the control of the rabbit's vestibulo-ocular reflexes by the cerebellar flocculus, *J. Physiol., 265*, 833, 1977.

101. Mizuno, N., Mochizuki, K., Akimoto, C., and Matsushima, R., Pretectal projections to the inferior olive in the rabbit, *Exp. Neurol., 39*, 498, 1973.

102. Mizuno, N., Nakamura, Y., and Iwahori, N., An electron microscope study of the dorsal cap of the inferior olive in the rabbit, with special reference to the pretecto-olivary fibers, *Brain Res., 77*, 385, 1974.

103. Takeda, T. and Maekawa, K., The origin of the pretecto-olivary tract: a study using the horseradish peroxidase method, *Brain Res., 177*, 319, 1976.

104. Alley, K., Baker, R., and Simpson, J. I., Afferents to the vestibulo-cerebellum and the origin of the visual climbing fibers in the rabbit, *Brain Res., 98*, 582, 1975.

105. Simpson, J. I. and Alley, K. E., Visual climbing fiber input to rabbit vestibulo-cerebellum: a source of direction-specific information, *Brain Res., 82*, 302, 1974.

106. Barmack, N. H., Visually evoked activity of neurons in the dorsal cap of the inferior olive and its relationship to the control of eye movements, in *Control of Gaze by Brain Stem Neurons*, Baker, R. and Berthoz, A., Eds., Elsevier, Amsterdam, 1977, 361.

107. Ito, M. and Miyashita, Y., The effects of chronic destruction of the inferior olive upon visual modification of the horizontal vestibulo-ocular reflex of rabbits, *Proc. Jpn. Acad., 51*, 716, 1975.

108. Hoffmann, K. P., Behrend, K., and Schoppmann, A direct afferent visual pathway from the nucleus of the optic tract to the inferior olive in the cat, *Brain Res., 115*, 150, 1976.

109. Itoh, K., Efferent projections of the prectectum in the cat, *Exp. Brain Res., 30*, 89, 1977.

110. Maekawa, K. and Takeda, T., Afferent pathways from the visual system to the cerebellar flocculus of the rabbit, in *Control of Gaze by Brain Stem Neurons*, Baker, R. and Berthoz, A., Eds., Elsevier, Amsterdam, 1977, 187.

111. Simpson, J. I. and Hess, R., Complex and simple visual messages in the flocculus, in *Control of Gaze by Brain Stem Neurons*, Baker, R. and Berthoz, A., Eds., Elsevier, Amsterdam, 1977, 351.

112. Ghelarducci, B., Ito, M., and Yagi, N., Impulse discharges from flocculus Purkinje cells of alert rabbits during visual stimulation combined with horizontal head rotation, *Brain Res., 87*, 66, 1975.

113. Ito, M., Neuronal events in the cerebellar flocculus associated with an adaptive modification of the vestibulo-ocular reflex of the rabbit, in *Control of Gaze by Brain Stem Neurons*, Baker, R. and Berthoz, A., Eds., Elsevier, Amsterdam, 1977, 391.

114. Dufossé, M., Ito, M., Jastreboff, P. J., and Miyashita, Y., A neuronal correlate in rabbit's cerebellum to adaptive modification of the vestibulo-ocular reflex, *Brain Res., 150*, 611, 1978.

115. Llinas, R., Simpson, J. I., and Precht, W., Nystagmic modulation of neuronal activity in rabbit cerebellar flocculus, *Pflügers Arch., 367*, 7, 1976.

116. Lisberger, S. G. and Fuchs, A. F., Role of primate flocculus during rapid behavioral modification of vestibuloocular reflex. I. Purkinje cell activity during visually guided horizontal smooth-pursuit eye movements and passive head rotation, *J. Neurophysiol.*, 41, 733, 1978.

117. Lisberger, S. G. and Fuchs, A. F., Role of primate flocculus during rapid behavioral modification of vestibuloocular reflex. II. Mossy fiber firing patterns during horizontal head rotation and eye movement, *J. Neurophysiol.*, 41, 764, 1978.

118. Collewijn, H. and Kleinschmidt, H. J., Vestibulo-ocular and optokinetic reactions in the rabbit: changes during 24 hours of normal and abnormal interaction, in *Basic Mechanisms of Ocular Motility and Their Clinical Implications*, Lennerstrand, G. and Bach-y-Rita, P., Eds., Pergamon Press, Oxford, 1975, 477.

119. Collewijn, H. and Grootendorst, A. F., Adaptation of optokinetic and vestibulo-ocular reflexes to modified visual input in the rabbit, in *Reflex Control of Posture and Movement,* Granit, R. and Pompeiano, O., Eds., Progress in Brain Research, Vol. 50, Elsevier, Amsterdam, 1979, 771.

120. Collewijn, H., Optokinetic and vestibulo-ocular reflexes in dark-reared rabbits, *Exp. Brain Res.*, 27, 287, 1977.

121. Miyoshi, T., Pfaltz, C. R., and Piffko, P., Effect of repetitive optokinetic stimulation upon optokinetic and vestibular responses, *Acta Otolaryngol.*, 75, 259, 1973.

122. Collewijn, H., An analog model of the rabbit's optokinetic system, *Brain Res.*, 36, 71, 1972.

123. Robinson, D. A., Vestibular and optokinetic symbiosis: an example of explaining by modelling, in *Control of Gaze by Brain Stem Neurons,* Baker, R. and Berthoz, A., Eds., Elsevier/North-Holland, Amsterdam, 1977, 49.

124. Robinson, D. A., Linear addition of optokinetic and vestibular signals in the vestibular nucleus, *Exp. Brain Res.*, 30, 447, 1977.

125. Collewijn, H. and Noorduin, H., Vertical and torsional optokinetic eye movements in the rabbit, *Pflügers Arch.*, 332, 87, 1972.

126. Brecher, G. A., Die optokinetische Auslösung von Augenrollung und rotatorischen Nystagmus, *Pflügers Arch.*, 234, 13, 1934.

127. Crone, R. A., Optically induced eye torsion. II. Optostatic and optokinetic cycloversion, *v. Graefes Arch. Ophthalmol.*, 196, 1, 1975.

128. Hass, H. D., Untersuchungen über die Erzeugung der rotatorischen optokinetischen Nystagmus, *v. Graefes Arch. Ophthalmol.*, 174, 186, 1967.

129. Steinbach, M. J., Pursuing the perceptual rather than the retinal stimulus, *Vision Res.*, 16, 1371, 1976.

130. Ter Braak, J. W. G., Ambivalent optokinetic stimulation and motion detection, *Bibl. Ophthalmol.*, 82, 308, 1972.

131. Behrens, F. and Grüsser, O. J., Bewegungswahrnehmung und Augenbewegungen bei Flickerbelichtung unbewegter visueller Muster, in *Augenbewegungsstorungen, Neurophiologle und Klinik,* Kommerell, G., Ed., Bergmann, Munchen, 1978, 275.

132. Fox, R., Lehmkuhle, S., and Leguire, L. E., Stereoscopic contours induce optokinetic nystagmus, *Vision Res.*, 18, 1189, 1978.

133. Costin, A., Chaimovitz, M., and Bergmann, F., Nystagmus evoked by intermittent photic stimulation of the rabbit's eye, *Experientia,* 21, 167, 1965.

134. Pasik, P. and Pasik, T., A comparison between two types of visually-evoked nystagmus in the monkey, *Acta Otolaryngol. Suppl.*, 330, 30, 1975.

135. Keane, J. R., Flash-evoked nystagmus: absence in man, *Neurology,* 22, 551, 1972.

136. Wildberger, H. and Meyer, M., Zur augenmotorischen Störung des Albino, *Klin. Mbl. Augenheilk.*, 172, 487, 1978.

137. Sperry, R. W., Effect of 180 degree rotation of the retinal field on visuomotor coordination, *J. Exp. Zool.*, 92, 263, 1943.

138. Sperry, R. W., Neural basis of the spontaneous optokinetic response produced by visual inversion, *J. Comp. Physiol. Psychol.*, 43, 482, 1950.

139. Collewijn, H., Winterson, B. J., and Dubois, M. F. W., Optokinetic eye movements in albino rabbits: inversion in anterior visual field, *Science,* 199, 1351, 1978.

140. Winterson, B. J. and Collewijn, H., Beyond the looking glass: direction sensitivity to frontal fields is inverted in units in the nucleus of the optic tract in albino rabbits, *Invest. Ophthalmol., (ARVO Abstract Suppl.)* 1979, 102.

Chapter 7

REFLEXIONS ON THE CONTROL OF VERGENCE

Cyril Rashbass

TABLE OF CONTENTS

I. DEFINITIONS

A single eye that is able to move freely within its ill-fitting socket has six degrees of freedom, and requires the specification of six coordinates to define its position in the head. Two eyes capable of independent movement would require 12 coordinates to specify their joint position. However, by making some approximations and by taking account of the natural constraints that are imposed on the movements of the eyes, a simpler coordinate system can be adopted.

Definition: The line of sight of an eye is the locus of points whose images, brought about by the eye's dioptrics, are concentric with the fovea.

Approximation: The center of rotation of an eye is a point fixed relative both to the eye and to the head.

Definition: The line of centers is the line that passes through the centers of rotation of the two eyes.

Approximation: The center of rotation of an eye lies on its line of sight.

Definition: Cycloversion is the rotational position of an eye about its line of sight, the zero of cycloversion being arbitrary.

Constraint: The changes in the cycloversion of one eye are equal to the changes in the cycloversion of the other eye[1].

Definition: The face plane is the plane tangent to the eyebrows and the chin.

Definition: The elevation of an eye is the angle between two planes through the line of centers, the one containing the line of sight and the other perpendicular to the face plane.

Constraint: The elevations of the two eyes are the same. This constraint is not absolute. Helmholtz[2] has shown that, with appropriate visual stimuli, the eyes can be made to assume different elevations. Under normal binocular or monocular viewing, the constraint applies.

Corollary: The line of centers and both lines of sight are coplanar.

Definition: The plane of sight is the plane containing the lines of sight.

Definition: The point of regard is that point in the plane of sight where the two lines of sight intersect.

Definition: The lateral direction of each eye is the angle its line of sight makes with a plane perpendicular to the line of centers, taking the rightward direction as positive.

With these simplifications, four coordinates suffice to define the joint position of the two eyes: cycloversion common to both eyes, elevation common to both eyes, and the lateral direction of each eye. It is possible to transform the two coordinates representing the lateral direction of each eye into two other coordinates of greater physiological utility.

Definition: Vergence is the lateral direction of the left eye minus the lateral direction of the right eye.

Corollary: Vergence is the angle at the point of regard subtended by the centers of rotation.

Definition: Lateral version is the mean of the lateral directions of the two eyes.

Henceforth, all consideration will be restricted to the plane of sight. "Lateral version" will be referred to as "version".

The point of regard is unambiguously defined in the plane of sight by the two coordinates, vergence and version. All points whose vergence is the same as that of a given point lie on a circle passing through that point and the centers of rotation. All points having the same version as that of a given point lie on a rectangular hyperbola passing through that point and through the centers of rotation, and centered at the point midway between the centers of rotation. When the head and body are free to move, version is rarely very large. For small angles of version, the circles of equal vergence do not deviate significantly from circles concentric with the point midway between the centers of rotation. Under the same restriction and with vergence restricted to realizable values, the hyperbolas of equal version do not deviate significantly from straight lines radiating from that midpoint. Thus, version is approximately the lateral direction of an hypothetical "cyclopean" eye situated in the midsaggital plane, and vergence is approximately a measure, albeit nonlinear, of the distance of the point of regard from the center of rotation of such an eye.

Version and vergence together define the position of the point of regard in the plane of sight. All points in the plane of sight can be assigned two coordinates having the values that version and vergence would have if that point were the point of regard. The position of a target point can be specified by these two coordinates.

Definition: Target version and target vergence are the version and vergence of a point of regard situated at the target point.

Definition: Disparity is target vergence minus vergence.

The choice of vergence and version to specify the position of the point of regard, rather than its Cartesian coordinates or the lateral directions of the two eyes, depends on the observation of Rashbass and Westheimer[3] that version and vergence are independently controlled. Changes in target version evoke responding changes in version, and changes in target vergence evoke responding changes in vergence. The temporal characteristics of these two sorts of response are different, and neither response interacts with the other.

When vergence changes, the eyes move.

Definition: A vergence movement is the time course of changing vergence, with the zero of movement arbitrarily defined as the vergence at the beginning of the epoch under consideration.

Version movement, target vergence movement, and target version movement can, mutatis mutandis, be similarly defined.

Synonyms: Version movement is sometimes called conjunctive or conjugate movement; vergence movement is sometimes called disjunctive movement.

Definition: Convergence is a vergence movement as a result of which vergence increases.

Definition: Divergence is a vergence movement as a result of which vergence decreases.

II. GENERAL PROPOSITIONS

The number of systematic experimental studies of the control of vergence is quite small.[4-8] The subject has been well-reviewed.[9,10] This Chapter will therefore, be restricted to a bare statement of a series of propositions defining the general properties of the vergence control system, followed by a discussion of some of the more puzzling outstanding problems, and of the most promising lines of future investigation. Most of these propositions are demonstrably untrue in particular circumstances. Each is, therefore, followed by a discussion of its limitations and implications.

A. Proposition 1
"The dominant input to the vergence control system is disparity."

Vergence movements are known to result from other inputs, in particular, accommodative stimuli. Covering one eye, or distorting the vision in it by means of a Maddox rod, makes what is seen by the two eyes so dissimilar that disparity becomes an unmeasurable, indeed an undefinable, quantity. In these circumstances, changes in the accommodative requirement of the unimpeded eye evoke vergence movements. This proposition asserts that when disparity is present, accommodation is ignored as an input to the vergence system. This is stated by Alpern,[9] and confirmed by Clark and Crane.[11]

The obvious target to use in the experimental study of vergence control is a single spot of light, so that target vergence is unambiguously specified, and so too is disparity. In normal viewing conditions, the two eyes see aspects of the world that differ only slightly. Apart from the rare cases of periodic patterns that occur sometimes in wallpaper and similar designs, the unambiguous identification of a target point is not difficult. Westheimer and Mitchell[12] have shown that vergence movements may be evoked by the relative positions of somewhat dissimilar figures seen by the two eyes, provided that the dissimilarity is not gross. This suggests that the identification of a target point is not necessary in order to stimulate vergence movements, and a quantity equivalent to disparity can be extracted from the statistical properties of the relationship between what is seen by the two eyes.

B. Proposition 2

"When, from an initial equilibrium state of constant target vergence, target vergence is abruptly changed, a period of about 160 ms elapses before any responding vergence movement starts."

This is shorter than the 200 to 250 ms reaction time that precedes a saccade, but is comparable to that preceding a smooth-tracking version movement.

It is tempting to extend the power of this proposition by suggesting that the system contains a pure time-delay element, such as conduction delay, constant at about 160 ms. This would be a valid extension if the assumption of linearity could be made with any confidence. However, under Proposition 6, the linearity of the system, particularly with respect to its temporal properties, will be seriously challenged. The present proposition cannot, therefore, be safely extended beyond the simple statement of observable fact.

C. Proposition 3

"A period of constant disparity evokes a period of vergence movement that has a velocity that is constant and increases monotonically with the disparity."

This proposition is based on the observations of Rashbass and Westheimer.[6] Periods of constant disparity occur during the reaction time that precedes the response to a step change of target vergence. Longer periods of constant disparity can be produced by contriving that the target vergence movement is a step added to a signal that is itself equal to the vergence movement of the eye — the open-loop condition (see Figure 1). In either case, the response consists of a period of vergence movement that has constant velocity. The extent of this movement is limited only by the ultimate positional extremes of convergence or divergence that the eyes can achieve. For small disparities in the range $\pm 0,2°$, the velocity of vergence is approximately proportional to disparity with a constant of proportionality of $10s^{-1}$ (i.e., deg/sec velocity per degree disparity) in one subject, and $7s^{-1}$ in another. At greater disparities, the ratio of velocity to disparity is somewhat smaller (see Figure 2).

Two implications of this proposition are of interest. The first is that, at least when disparity is small, there is no asymmetry between the velocity of convergence and that of divergence. Although large asymmetries between convergent and divergent responses have been demonstrated by Zuber and Stark,[8] inspection of their records shows that this asymmetry is not present in the early, constant-velocity part of the response to which this proposition applies. The second implication is that there is no dead-zone. Disparity, however small, evokes a responding vergence movement. Whence follows the next proposition.

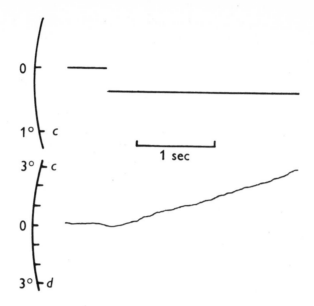

FIGURE 1. The open-loop response to a step change of disparity is a vergence movement that proceeds at constant velocity.[6]

D. Proposition 4
"In the steady state, when the target vergence is constant, disparity is zero."

This is a logical consequence of Proposition 3. It is at variance with a large body of observations that suggest that disparities of a degree or more can exist during steady binocular fixation. This issue has been extensively discussed by Alpern.[9] No clear resolution of this descrepancy has been proposed, but methodological and individual differences may be responsible. It is certainly the case that disparities that, by being contained within Panum's fusional area, are too small to cause diplopia, are sufficient to evoke vergence responses, just as they are able to give stereoscopic sensations. The vergence control system is thus a system working to reduce disparity to zero, and not to reduce diplopia to fusion. "Fusional" vergence is a confusing term used by some authors.

E. Proposition 5
"Disparity is monitored continuously."

Disparities as short-lived as 20 ms have been shown to evoke vergence movement. In this respect, vergence movements are again seen to resemble smooth-tracking version movements, and to contrast with saccadic movements.

F. Proposition 6
A period during which disparity is continuous, but not constant, evokes a vergence movement that is determined not simply by the moment-to-moment value of the disparity, but also, in a nonsimple way, by the time differential of the disparity.

This proposition embodies most of the complexities of the vergence control system, and owes its vagueness to the present inadequacy of our knowledge.

On the basis of Propositions 1 through 5, it is possible to suggest a model for the vergence control system. The simplest model, compatible with those propositions, is one in which the velocity of vergence movement at any time is a function of the instantaneous value that the disparity had some 160 ms previously. The function of disparity that specifies velocity of vergence movement is described under Proposition 3, and

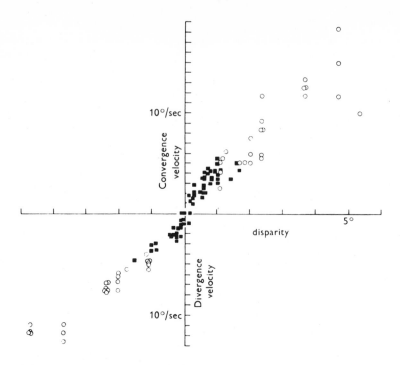

FIGURE 2.   The constant velocity of vergence movement as a function of the constant disparity that evokes it. Black squares are from open-loop observations, open circles from closed-loop observations.[6]

illustrated in Figure 2. This function is nonlinear, but the model just defined is not unduly complex, having just this one amplitude-dependent nonlinearity. For small disparities, the relation of vergence movement velocity and disparity seems from Figure 2 to be linear, and investigation of the system behavior under small-signal conditions is indicated. Of course, linearity can never be proved. At best, extensive investigation may fail to reveal nonlinearity.

Disparities that vary sinusoidally with time are a suitable input with which to begin such an investigation. If small-signal linearity holds, then a sinusoidally varying disparity will evoke a vergence movement that is a sinusoidal function of time, with the same frequency as the disparity, and, at any given frequency, has an amplitude proportional to the amplitude of the varying disparity. This is found to be the case, provided that the amplitude of the disparity variation does not greatly exceed the bounds set by the small-signal condition, about ±0,2°. Furthermore, the ratio of the amplitude of the sinusoidal vergence movement to the amplitude of the disparity variation, the gain of the open-loop, will be inversely proportional to the frequency of the variation, and have a value calculable from the slope of the velocity-of-vergence-movement vs. disparity curve (Figure 2) at its origin. This is also found to be the case. Another expectation of the small-signal model is that, at any frequency, the sinusoidal vergence movement will lag behind the disparity variations by a period of time equal to 160 ms added to one fourth of the sinusoidal period. This is found not to be the case. The measured phase lags are always much smaller than this, usually no more than half the expected value.

On the basis of this observation, it is not possible to maintain the small-signal model proposed above. However, the implications of this observation are deeper than that. Not only is that particular model untenable, but so also is the assumption of small-signal linearity. This is because, in any linear system, there exists a relationship between the gain as a function of frequency and the phase lag as a function of frequency. This relationship is such that if the gain is known for all frequencies, then a minimum value of the phase lag is calculable for all frequencies. In our case, the gain is known over a range of frequencies. Any reasonable extrapolation of the values of gain outside the measured range gives minimum values of phase lag in excess of those found. The rejection of the assumption of linearity is forced.

There is reason to believe that this nonlinearity is involved when the variation of disparity is continous and has a finite velocity less than some upper bound. Under these conditions, the output of the vergence control system is affected by the disparity velocity and not just by its moment-to-moment magnitude. When the disparity changes at a rate in excess of the limiting value, the vergence movement is determined in the way described in Propositions 2 through 5. Thus, if disparity is made to change according to a step-ramp waveform, the vergence-movement response shows that the velocity of the ramp produces a vergence movement that anticipates the course of the disparity change. This suggests one possible function for the processing of the velocity of disparity change in the generation of vergence movement. Clearly, knowing not only the instantaneous magnitude of the disparity, but also the way it is changing, allows the possibility of short-term anticipation.

It must be borne in mind that the velocity signal that is processed is the velocity of the disparity change, not the velocity of the target vergence movement. The magnitude of the target vergence and the velocity of its movement are quantities not entering directly via the retina, but they could be reconstructed by a combination of retinal information with information, internally generated, about where the eyes are directed. However, it is clear from the open-loop response to a step change or a square wave of disparity, where the target vergence movement has a prolonged and substantial continuous velocity component but the disparity change has none, that velocity of the target vergence movement evokes no velocity-generated component in the response. When target vergence is constant, and disparity nonzero, as is the case when gaze is transferred from one target to another having different vergence, the vergence movement that takes place in order to cancel the disparity, itself introduces a velocity into the disparity. The response to this velocity will be to slow the vergence movement and give greater stability to the control system.

Comparison with the control of versional movements suggests another possible function for the use of disparity velocity in the control of vergence. In the control of version, smooth-tracking movements are directed towards matching the velocity of the eye's version movement to that of the target's version movement, thus, aiming at achieving a stationary retinal image, even if it is not centrally fixated. Saccadic movements look after fixation. Similarly, in the case of vergence control, the reduction of the velocity of disparity change would carry the benefit of reducing any impairment of vision that might be caused by the movement of the images over retina.

III. THE PREDICTOR

There is another possible property that would have the effect of reducing the phase lags of the responses to sinusoidally varying disparity. It could be that the vergence control system has the ability to predict the future behavior of a target's vergence when that vergence moves in a repeating pattern. It is a remarkable characteristic of the version control system, whether producing saccades or smooth-tracking, that it shows predictive responses to repetitious inputs.[13,14] This appears as a reduction in the phase lag of the response after a few cycles of a periodic tracking task, be it sinusoidal or square wave. This adaptive behavior suggests a level of complexity in the control system beyond that usually found in manmade systems, particularly, as this ability to predict is achieved without any apparent sacrifice of performance in response to unpredictable tasks. It is of considerable interest, therefore, to know whether a similar ability exists in the vergence control system. However, the evidence is against this suggestion. The open-loop response to a square-wave change of disparity, where repetitiousness is present in the disparity, shows that phase advance is absent in the response. It is possible that prediction is based on repetitiousness in the velocity of the disparity change, but this has the ring of implausibility. It seems more plausible to reject the hypothesis that the vergence control system can predict on the basis of repetitiousness and attribute the phase advance of the open-loop sinusoid responses to a nonlinear process applied to the moment-to-moment value of disparity velocity. The crucial experiment involves examining the phase lags of the vergence movement response to the first few cycles of a sinusoidally changing disparity, but this has not been done. It is invalid to argue that such a predictor exists by comparing the phase lags of responses to sinusoidally varying disparities with the phase lags of the simple harmonic components of the responses to unpredictable mixtures of several different sinusoidal variations of disparity, because Fourier analysis cannot be legitimately or safely applied to a nonlinear system.

The observed open-loop response to sinusoids of disparity change remain puzzling. Part of this puzzle may derive from an unwarranted assumption made by Rashbass and Westheimer.[6] In their determination of the open-loop characteristics, they restricted their experiments to sinusoidal disparity changes, whose amplitudes at any given frequency were confined to a range in which they had shown that the output amplitude was proportional to the input amplitude. This is a necessary condition for linearity, but not a sufficient one. With hindsight, having seen the response characteristic to be inexplicable in linear terms, and finding that it is the phase observations that are difficult to explain, the question arises whether, within the range of input amplitudes for which output amplitude is proportional to input amplitude, phase lag is independent of input amplitude. If it is not, then the phase lags observed may be the result of the arbitrary selection of input amplitudes, and may, therefore, not show any meaningful relationship to frequency.

IV. WHY OPEN THE LOOP?

In the above discussion, the terms "open-loop" and "closed-loop" have been used freely. These terms should be familiar to anyone involved in eye-movement studies. The closed-loop condition is the normal viewing state, where the disparity is determined not only by the target vergence movement, but also by the vergence movement of the eyes themselves. The open-loop condition is achieved by moving the target in such a way that any eye vergence movement is accompanied by a target vergence movement that removes any change the eye movement may otherwise have imposed on the disparity.

The impression can sometimes be obtained from reading accounts of open-loop exeriments, that the system behaves differently in this condition from the way it behaves when the loop is closed. This is, of course, not so. Whether the loop is open or closed, the subject is doing his best to view a moving target, and it should be no concern of his whether the movements originate from his own eye or from an independent signal generator. Ideally, he should not be aware of which is the case. If the subject did behave differently in the two conditions, the whole purpose in opening the loop would be undermined.

The reason for opening the loop is to give the experimenter complete control of the input to the system, in this case, disparity. It is obvious that this is the only way in which the response to simple transient changes can be studied, because, with the loop closed, the response itself destroys the simplicity of the input. That is less obviously so in the study of the response to sinusoidal inputs, because, in a linear system, sinusoidal inputs evoke sinusoidal outputs, and disparity would then also be sinusoidal. Where nonlinearity is expected, opening the loop is again the only way to give the experimenter control of the signal entering the system.

The amplitude and phase of the sinusoidal vergence movements of the target can be represented by a vector. Where the system is essentially linear, the vergence movement will be sinusoidal and can be represented by another vector. The disparity change can then be obtained by vector subtraction. The vector of disparity change is commonly a small difference between two much larger vectors, and is susceptible to very large relative error. Opening the loop makes the disparity vector the controlled variable of the experiment. A good example of this use of the open-loop is provided by Zuber and Stark.[8] They illustrate a closed-loop response of the vergence system, at low-frequency, having a gain of about 1.3 and zero phase angle. These results would imply that the vergence movement is in antiphase with the disparity change, a phase angle of 180°. They, correctly, reject this implication in favor of the directly measured open-loop response, which is shown to be in phase with the disparity change. Inevitably, meticulous care is needed in the calibration of the recording system, whether the loop be open or closed.

V. CONCLUSION

It should be clear from this discussion that, in the present state of the art, theorizing has outstripped observation. The time is ripe for another careful look at the vergence control system. It is surely time for the Cinderella of eye movements to join her two versional sisters at the ball.

ACKNOWLEDGMENT

The author is deeply indebted to Dr. Frans Veringa for his keenly analytical reading of the original draft of this chapter. If the present version has any merit, much of it must be ascribed to his helpful suggestions.

REFERENCES

1. Kertesz, A. E. and Jones, R. W., Human cyclofusional response, *Vision Res.,* 10, 891, 1970.
2. Helmholtz, H. von, Handbuch der Physiologischen Optic, translated as *Treatise on Physiological Optics,* Vol. 3, Southall, J. P. C., Dover Publications, New York, 1962, 58.
3. Rashbass, C. and Westheimer, G., Independence of conjugate and disjunctive eye movements, *J. Physiol.,* 159, 361, 1961.
4. Westheimer, G. and Mitchell, A. M., Eye movement responses to convergence stimuli, *AMA Arch. Ophthalmol.,* 55, 848, 1956.
5. Riggs, L. A. and Niehl, E. W., Eye movements recorded during convergence and divergence, *J. Opt. Soc. Am.* 50, 913, 1960.
6. Rashbass, C. and Westheimer, G., Disjunctive eye movements, *J. Physiol.,* 159, 339, 1961.
7. Robinson, D. A., The mechanics of human vergence eye movement, *J. Pediatr. Ophthalmol.,* 3, 31, 1966.
8. Zuber, B. L., and Stark, L., Dynamical Characteristics of the fusional vergence eye movement system, *IEEE Trans. Syst. Sci. Cybern.,* SCC-4, 72, 1968.
9. Alpern, M., Vergence movements, in *The Eye,* Vol. 3, 2nd ed., Davson, H., Ed., Academic Press, New York, 1969.

10. Carpenter, R. H. S., *Movements of the Eyes,* Pion, London, 1977.
11. Clark, M. R. and Crane, H. D., Dynamic interactions in binocular vision, in *Eye Movements and the Higher Psychological Functions,* Senders, J. W., Fisher, D. F., and Monty, R. A., Eds., Lawrence Erlbaum Associates, New Jersey, 1978.
12. Westheimer, G. and Mitchell, D. E., The sensory stimulus for disjunctive eye movements, *Vision Res.,* 9, 749, 1969.
13. Westheimer, G., Eye movements responses to a horizontally moving visual stimulus, *Arch. Ophthalmol.,* 52, 932, 1954.
14. Stark, L., Vossius, G., and Young, L. R., Predictive control of eye tracking movements, *IEE Trans. Hum. Factors Electron.,* HFE-3, 52, 1962.

Chapter 8

DONDERS', LISTING'S, AND HERING'S LAWS AND THEIR IMPLICATIONS

Gerald Westheimer

TABLE OF CONTENTS

I. INTRODUCTION

To be taken seriously, a model must constitute an economically phrased description of a range of happenings. It facilitates learning and practical application, and to the curious it becomes an invitation to search for substrates.

On all these counts, the models proposed by Donders, Listing, and Hering have never been bettered. They all date back to the middle of the last century, but a book devoted to models of oculomotor behavior is not complete without giving thought to these modelling attempts of earlier generations.

All three laws imply yet another model which is taken so much for granted that its enormity is seldom realized: the behavior of the eyeball in the orbit as if there were a ball-and-socket joint. As is well-known in anatomy, the head of the femur and the acetabulum make up an actual ball-and-socket joint, constructed of bone. But the constraints on the globe in the orbit are exercised by soft and elastic tissues: fat, muscle, tendon, and the skin. That the overall effect so closely approximates a ball-and-socket joint is a minor miracle.

The term ball-and-socket joint is self-descriptive. Technically, it states the requirement that a point in the moving part (the eye) never shift its location within the fixed part (the orbit). That point is called the center of rotation, because the only movements possible in a ball-and-socket joint are rotations of the moving components. A single such rotational movement is characterized by the fact that whatever else changes position, one line in the moving body does not. The center of rotation is the one point which all possible axes of rotation have in common. The other class of motions, the translations, are excluded in a ball-and-socket joint; in a translation, all points of the moving part experience equal and parallel displacements.

The deviation of a given construction from a perfect ball-and-socket joint can, in fact, be nicely specified by the extent to which all translations have been excluded.

Accordingly, the questions asked of the eyeball and its movements are

1.   Where is the center of rotation?
2.   What translational movements, if any, are associated with the rotational movements of the eye in the orbit?

The measurements needed to answer these questions are exercises in ingenuity that have occupied many fine minds in physiological optics. The consensus now is that:

1.   The center of rotation is where one might expect to find it: near the center of curvature of the eyeball, i.e., approximately 13 mm behind the corneal apex.
2.   Stability of the center of rotation is good to perhaps 0.1mm, but it can be much less stable on occasions.

The practical consequences of the occurrence of translational eye movement are slight under most circumstances. They do not matter for visual purposes, if the viewing target is far from the eye. The eye rotation necessary to bring a peripheral target onto the fovea is, in fact, independent of translational eye shifts if the target is at infinity.

For the researcher, however, these lateral translational movements may mean trouble. If the eye acted as a perfect ball-and-socket joint and the head were kept still, the position of any single point in the eye (unless it lay on the axis of rotation) would be a unique indicator of the rotational stance of the eye. This is the basis of the methods of determining eye position which record the corneal reflection or the limbus position. It can be calculated that a pure translational movement of 0.1 mm, which does not displace the retinal image of a distant object at all, would be equivalent to, and hence be registered as, a one-half degree rotational movement. This problem has given impetus to the design and use of the more refined techniques of recording eye movements, such as the contact-lens or search-coil techniques which isolate the rotational movements by optical or electronic means through an attachment to the eyeball, or the technique described by Rashbass and Westheimer, which utilizes the difference signal between the locations of two identified landmarks on the eye, a signal which is substantially free from artifacts due to translational eye movements.

II. DISCUSSION OF LAWS

The laws to be discussed now, those of Donders, Listing, and Hering, all rest on the premise that the eyes execute only rotational movements. Such movements require, in the general case, three independent numbers for their unambiguous specification. The simplest approach is to begin with the eye looking straight ahead. (This itself is not an easy situation to define unambiguously, but there have been good attempts to do so.) Any other eye position can be defined by the rotation necessary to move the eye to that new position from the original straight-ahead position. This rotation is most readily characterized by the orientation of the axis and the extent of the rotation around the axis. There are, thus, three angles, two to define the inclination of the axis with respect to the basic coordinates (say the horizontal and the frontal planes of the head) and another one to define the angle through which the globe has rotated around this axis. A simple example will illustrate: the eye is looking up 30° in its median plane. In this case, the axis of rotation is horizontal and has remained in the frontal plane (zero inclination with respect to the frontal and horizontal planes), and the angle of rotation is 30°. Or another case: suppose the eye is looking just 20° to the right. The axis of rotation is in the frontal plane, but vertical, i.e., inclined by 90° with respect to the horizontal plane, and the extent of rotation around this axis is 20°. Now take the situation of an eye which starts off in the first position, viz. 30° up, and moves to occupy the second position, viz. 20° purely right. This change can be accomplished by a single rotation. It has an axis whose orientation is in the plane through the center of rotation that is normal to the eye's fixation line in its positions of origin and destination, an axis evidently inclined with respect to both the frontal and horizontal planes. To appreciate the problem to which Donders' and Listing's laws address themselves, one needs to consider two possible ways in which the transfer of gaze from the 30° up position to the 20° right position can be carried out: the single rotation just described and, alternatively, the sequence of first moving from 30° up to straight-ahead, and then moving from straight-ahead to 20° right. The inclination of the vertical meridian of the retina with respect to gravity, i.e., the cyclotorsion of the eye, will have a certain definite value when the eye arrives in its position of destination through the single rotation from the position of origin to the position of destination. However, this value of cyclotorsion will be different from its value had the eye arrived in its position of destination through the maneuver of first rotating down 30° to look straight ahead and then 20° right. Rotations of a rigid body in a ball-and-socket joint do not obey the laws of vector addition. As distinct from translations, which are simple vector operations and can be executed in arbitrary order, rotations are not commutative and the orientation of the retinal vertical meridian in one and the same position of destination will be different, depending on the orientation of the axis of rotation that brought it there.

A. Donders' Law

This is precisely where Donders' law comes in. It postulates the invariance of the orientation of the eye's vertical meridian with respect to gravity in any given eye position occupied by voluntary fixation, regardless of where the eye looked before. In other words, the simple conceptual scheme of establishing an *ad hoc* axis of rotation predicated by the prevailing pre- and post-movement positions is not applied. Instead, another simple conceptual scheme prevails: only the position of destination matters.

In practice, Donders' law is very well obeyed (to better than one half degree of cyclotorsion) provided one considers only eye positions reached after voluntary saccades, and not those reached *en passant* during a smooth movement, or after a convergence movement. There are some exceptions, but they involve either oculomotor pathology or deliberate training.

The eye, thus, follows one simple conceptual scheme (only the destination matters), rather than other equally good conceptual schemes. The recognition that there are other equally good schemes (i.e., that Donders' law is not obvious and inescapable) opens to us a search for a context which makes it obvious. The situation may be likened to a legal one when there is more than one precedent case. Only when we know the equally applicable alternatives can we estimate the bias inherent in a given juridical opinion.

The implication of Donders' law is that, at the peripheral level, neural coding is for eye position rather than movement. Coding that is strictly for movement would be organized as follows. Every time there is a need to bring the fovea onto an eccentric retinal stimulus of given radial orientation and angular distance from the fovea, one and the same eye rotation is called for; i.e., related to that stimulus is a particular axis of rotation and angle of movement around it. However, as we have seen, such a movement would produce a resultant cyclotorsional stance that depended on the eye position of origin from which the fixed movement started. Donders' law, however, states that the cyclotorsional stance associated with a given eye position is independent of the movement that brought the eye there.

A good visualization of this state of affairs is afforded by the operation of the type ball in a selectric typewriter. Regardless of how the ball gets there, it needs to have a fixed angle of orientation with respect to the vertical when it is poised to strike any letter. When I first studied the problem of coding of eye movements I came to the conclusion: "On the whole, the present findings are best explained by postulating the existence of a one-to-one relation between innervation sets to the extraocular muscles and positions of the eye in the orbit. A saccadic movement would then be no more than the practically instantaneous changeover from one innervation pattern to another, and this would occur as a unitary phenomenon, in which instructions for all necessary changes in muscle tension are issued and effected simultaneously, the eyeball coming to a stop in an equilibrium position dictated by the new forces applied to it.'''

When the first recordings of impulse rates to alert monkey eye muscles came in, it was indeed found that steady and often quite high impulse rates, graded for eye position, issue from the nuclei of the eye muscles in the brainstem continuously. They cease during sleep and anesthesia, but start up immediately on awakening, even in a monkey whose voluntary movements had previously been eliminated by brainstem lesion.

The story does not end here, however. Movement-coding is not only an interesting concept, but also one that has been observed in brain stimulation studies in monkeys. The strong inference of position-coding, which can be drawn from Donders' law, might have led one to expect that the representation in the brain which one addresses by electrical stimulation is in the form of a position-coded map. The result of stimulation of such a position-coded map would be what have been called goal-directed movements. It would be as if one could get at the wiring emerging from the keyboard of a selectric typewriter, and found that electrical pulses delivered to a given wire would always move the type ball to a fixed letter. In the monkey frontal eye fields and colliculus, however, the findings indicate not the position coding expected on the basis of Donders' law, but movement-coding: electrical stimulation of a given site yields a stereotyped movement, of a given direction and extent, bringing the eyes to a new position which depends on the position of origin and the site stimulated. Since such movements presumably bring the eyes into their new position according to Donders' law (this has, however, yet to be demonstrated experimentally), a recoding process must be at play which translates a retinotopic map into an orbital position-coded map.

The unraveling of the brainstem oculomotor networks is an important current undertaking (see the relevant chapters in this volume), but in the final picture there must be room for the recoding of signals implied by the simultaneous demands of Donders' law and the retinotopic stimulation maps. Perhaps a little-noticed irregularity will be of help here. Stimulation of any spot in the colliculus causes identical movements only when they originate near the middle of the field of fixation. A sequence of identical stimuli does not usually trigger movements of equal magnitude. The evoked movements tend to be larger when the eyes are pointing in the direction of origin of the movement, and get smaller as the eyes move into the opposite field. This invites the interpretation that the translation of movement-coding to position-coding is not perfectly unique, an interpretation which may actually be welcome. The mechanical forces acting on the eyeball (due to the layout of the muscles in the orbit) are so complex in their arrangement that too tight a coupling of the movement-coded neural instruction to the final muscular contraction could be disastrous. A glance at any of the schemes describing the tension set of each of the muscles for various orbital positions[2-5] makes it apparent just how unlikely it would be to get equal position changes for equal collicular signals, regardless of initial eye position.

B. Listing's Law

We now come to Listing's law. Donders' law may be rephrased to say that the eye ordinarily utilizes only two degrees of freedom of rotational movements. Once the line of sight has been rotated from the straight ahead position to fix another point, the eye occupies the new position with a fixed cyclotorsional stance, though Donders' law does not specify what that stance is. Listing, however, succeeded in deducing the applicable rule. Here again the recognition that there are many alternative arrangements makes us seek out the context within which Listing's law is an inevitable consequence.

Obviously, once we have a position-coded system, where the cyclotorsion associated with each position is independent of the movement that brought the eye to that position, the rules governing that cyclotorsion can be arbitrary. In clinical instruments for testing ocular muscle balance and giving orthoptic exercises, the torsional positions are determined by the constraint of the mechanical design, e.g., the way the axes of the moving parts are fixed to the frame and to each other. The simplest of these designs is to have a grid of great circles of longitude, and then small circles of latitude, like the ones used in geography. The vertical meridian then always stays vertical (with respect to a plumb bob) for all displacements. However, Listing found that when the eye has moved into a tertiary position, i.e., into oblique quadrants, the retinal meridian which was vertical in the straight-ahead position is no longer vertical (Figure 1). It occupies a cyclotorsional stance as if the eye had been brought into the tertiary position from the primary (i.e., ideally straight-ahead) position by a rotation around an axis which is situated wholly within a fronto-parallel plane through the eye's center of rotation. As we have seen, the eye does not actually rotate around a system of such axes; if it did, starting positions other than the primary positions would lead to a violation

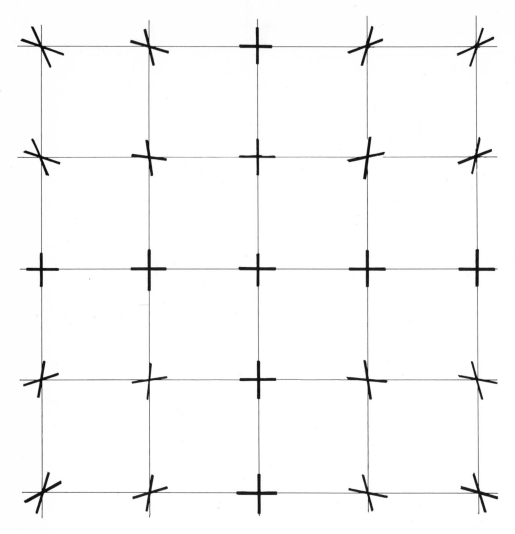

FIGURE 1.   Schematic diagram (not to scale) illustrating cyclotorsional consequences of Listing's law. Short horizontal foveal line after-images (heavy line segments) do not coincide with horizontal grid lines representing planes of constant elevation and depression. Such planes create great circles when they intersect a sphere centered on the eye and these, in turn, become horizontal straight lines when projected onto a fronto-parallel plane (shown here). The same holds for the relationship between short vertical foveal line after-images and vertical grid lines representing planes of constant longitude which have been projected onto a fronto-parallel plane. In either case, the eye exhibits a cyclotorsion in tertiary positions, i.e., positions which cannot be reached by rotations around a purely horizontal or vertical axis. Lines of constant elevation and lines of constant longitude are not orthogonal on the surface of a sphere, but become so when projected onto a fronto-parallel plane, whereas the real right angle between the eye's horizontal and vertical meridians becomes distorted due to foreshortening.

of Donders' law. Listing's law, thus, fills in the set of particular cyclotorsional numbers which Donders' law says are fixed; the two laws tell us that the eye occupies carefully defined positions, but do not address themselves to the mechanics of the movements. For example, in a mechanical system operating on a different system of axes than Listing's, a tertiary position would not exhibit the cyclotorsion demanded by Listing's law and a mechanism would have to be interfaced to supplement the cyclotorsion that the device displays in each tertiary position to accord with whatever torsion is needed by Listing's law. In a computer-operated display, we can provide this by a look-up table or by the requisite algorithm. In the actual operation of the oculomotor apparatus, neural circuitry has to be involved, and this opens the question of whether these laws are due to an open-loop, hard-wired circuit, or whether they constitute the command variable (*Sollwert*) of a feedback organization. Secure, broad-based studies of how well Listing's law is actually obeyed by a given eye have yet to be undertaken, but whenever good specification of an eye's cyclotorsion in a tertiary position is needed, the investigation usually shows that it is not exactly what Listing's law predicts. Unless detailed investigations give more solid support to the universality of Listing's law than is available now, it is more of a sketched-in ideal than a set of firm facts. The difference is important. Whenever behavioral measurements come up with extremely precise values, invariant with many conditions, this points to the existence of a stabilizing feedback system, complete with error detecting sensors. On the other hand, should it turn out that Listing's law is obeyed in a more haphazard, less rigid and less universal way, this might indicate a neural intent insufficiently important to warrant continuous monitoring and refining.

Also, indeed, the common justifications for Listing's law are sufficiently tentative and noncompelling to allow for this view. Helmholtz, for example, suggested that the cyclotorsional arrangement of Listing's law is to be expected if, during its gradual adaptation to day-to-day operating conditions, the oculomotor apparatus settles into a model of behavior where least effort is required to move from one position to the next. This view betrays Helmholtz's great prejudices: an excellent understanding of and feel for the physical realities of sense organs, and an unwillingness to posit much in the way of innate neural arrangements. On the other hand, Hering preferred to think of Listing's law as a meaningful expression of a specific neural intent. He had an extraordinary outlook in these matters, best expressed in his own words: "It is obvious that the motor apparatus of the visual organ has to fit the sensory apparatus as the shell does an egg. For, whether one assumes that they were set up according to a wise plan, or that they developed with each other and through each other in an inevitable way as the evolutionary series is traversed, in any case: the capabilities of the one have to correspond to the needs of the other.²'''

While Listing's law does not help in the detection of the vertical, nor of the horizontal, e.g., of the horizon when the head is tilted up or down, it does have an interesting effect that may possibly be of consequence in perception: there is self-congruence of the retinal image of line elements of all long straight lines passing through the primary position. It manifests itself in the following observations, which in fact constitute the specific test for the location of the primary position and the validity of Listing's law: an after-image is created in the fovea of a short segment of a long line, vertical, horizontal or oblique, passing through the primary position. Fixation of the line in other positions reveals coincidence of the after-image with the line. This kind of congruence of a foveal line segment is not displayed in other situations, which to us might intuitively seem more appropriate. Suppose we imagine ourselves surrounded by a grid on a sphere marking off lines of longitude and latitude. First, a short horizontal line after-image is generated in the fovea when the eye is looking straight ahead. The after-image will stay within the horizontal line marking the equator, but it will not do so when other horizontal lines, representing various upper or lower lines of latitude, are traced out. A similar observation will apply to a vertical line after-image in the fovea, and the tracing of the lines of longitude. This situation prevails even when the grid is projected from a sphere onto a fronto-parallel plane. Only lines generated by great circles through the primary position will exhibit self-congruence for the foveal line after-images of the appropriate direction. One can obviously make a lot of the possibility of this kind of invariance for perceptual processes; on the other hand one can sympathize with the nervous system for not bothering to build in an elaborate verification apparatus for ensuring that this "law" be obeyed, come what may.

C. Hering's Law

In contrast to Donders' and Listing's laws, which apply to each eye separately, the rule to which Hering's name is attached refers to the yoking of the two eyes; both eyes behave as a single unit under almost all circumstances. To emphasize how remarkable this performance is, and to offset his explanation from Helmholtz's, Hering enumerated a series of situations in which this parallelism of ocular movements of both eyes is manifested in spite of formidable counterindications:

1.   When one eye is covered, the nonseeing eye goes along with the seeing eye.
2.   The nonseeing eye goes along with the seeing eye when one eye is blind from birth on.
3.   The nonseeing eye goes along with the seeing eye in cases of strabismus when only one eye is utilized for vision.
4.   Both eyes move together in involuntary nystagmus.

Hering here is strongly sponsoring the view that coordination of the movement of the two eyes is an innate affair. How else can one explain its presence in individuals who have never used both eyes together?

To realize the full implications of Hering's law, one needs to visualize the layout of the muscles in the orbit. Although they exist in the appropriate number — six, to accommodate the three rotational degrees of freedom in push-pull fashion — the muscles do not follow any reasonable or appropriate geometrical pattern, except for the horizontally acting muscles, i.e., the medial and lateral rectus muscles. For vertical and oblique movements, there are no strictly agonistic-antagonistic pairs, nor is there accurate correspondence between the action of a particular muscle in the right orbit with that of any other muscle in the left orbit. Yet, activity of this complex of nonparallel muscles in mirror-symmetrical orbits still results in parallel movement. Also, this parallelism, or concomitancy as it is called, already exists at birth (certainly in the monkey, but also to a considerable extent in the human infant) and shows up, as Hering has pointed out, even under conditions of congenital uniocular blindness. The conclusion is inescapable that there is an innate apparatus which converts movement-coded signals issuing from, say, the cortex or the colliculus, into properly graded and appropriately distributed position-coded activity in the complex of the involved twelve muscles in the two orbits.

The task that falls to this apparatus is well illustrated by the numbers in Figure 2. Shown are estimates of the steady innervation levels of the twelve muscles which are required to hold the eyes in three positions of gaze. From the standpoint of mechanics, these three eye positions are separated by equal movements. So, presumably, the supranuclear signal that results in the movement of the eyes from occupying the position 20° down/20° right to looking straight ahead would, when applied for the second time, result in the movement of the eyes from the straight-ahead position to a position 20° up/20° left. The assumptions underlying the estimates of the innervation strength are as good as can be developed at this stage and included the appropriate cyclotorsion to bring the eyes to these tertiary positions according to Listing's law. One can begin to imagine the characteristics inherent in the distributing network. The same signal that changes the RIR from 31 to 7 and the LIR from 26 to 7, must, on a second application, change the values of both muscles from 7 to 0.8 g. This points to interesting properties relating to the relative strength of the synaptic signals. There are on the order of 4000 motoneurons in each of the twelve muscle nuclei. A motoneuron has a very extensive dendritic tree (Figure 3) with tens of thousands of synaptic sites, doubtless of both excitatory and inhibitory nature. There is no difficulty in envisaging that

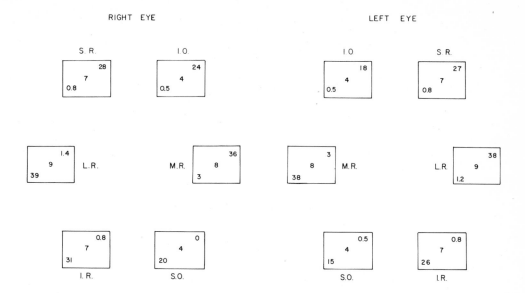

FIGURE 2. Innervation strengths (in grams) in the 12 extraocular muscles for steady binocular fixation in three eye positions: 20° down and 20° right; straight ahead; and 20° up and 20° left. Data from Robinson's calculations.[5] Change in fixation from down-and-right position to straight-ahead position represents the identical rotation as the change in fixation from straight-ahead position to up-and-left position.

differences in strength of synaptic connections, including quite complex nonlinear ones, can result from differences in the projection of the presynaptic signals onto the motoneurons. However, what is difficult to envisage is a state of affairs in which this is achieved with the preestablished harmony demanded by the observed exactness of Hering's law, for the error in parallelism of the two eyes under ordinary vision is only a fraction of a degree. Fortunately, we have a well-developed apparatus for fine-tuning of the positions of the eyes relative to each other. It has the character of a feedback system, with a delay of less than 200 msec (see Rashbass, this volume). In addition, as everyone who has been involved in orthoptics knows, there are long-time tonic changes which can produce variations of the open-loop binocular balance position by several degrees. Thus, while neural plasticity is undoubtedly a major factor in the excellence of Hering's law as a description of oculomotor behavior, its main implication is the existence of a sophisticated distribution pattern in the brainstem which partitions in a carefully regulated way the prenuclear movement-coded signals into portions appropriate to the mechanical action of the twelve individual muscles. The observed concomitancy of ocular excursion in the newborn, and in the functionally uniocular, makes it certain that this distribution pattern is primary and innate, with only a secondary overlay of fine-tuning.

III. CONCLUSION

We have seen that the three models of oculomotor behavior discussed here, the laws of Donders, Listing, and Hering, are as relevant to our understanding of the system as ever. The significant recent advances in neuroanatomical pathway tracing, and in electrical stimulation of and recording from the pertinent loci of the brain of the alert primate have given us information which allows us to view these laws in newer perspectives. The rigor and invariance with which they apply are clues to the basic innateness of the neural connection which underlies them, and as a corollary, to the parts

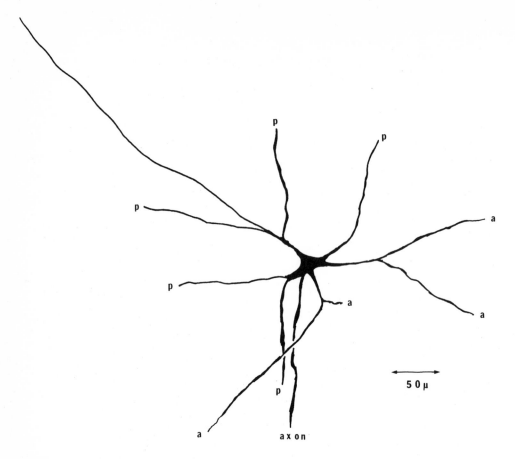

FIGURE 3.   Drawing of the dendritic tree of a single third-nerve motoneuron in a Golgi-Cox preparation from an infant macaque. The illustration shows, collapsed onto a single plane, all dendritic branches contained in a frontal section of 150μ thickness. Excluding the longest, which extends at least 600μ from the cell body, all branches probably spread much further than shown, because their observed end always coincided with either the posterior (p) or the anterior (a) limit of the section. Compared to a section cut normal to the axis of the brainstem, the dendrites seen here appear longer, though no less numerous. The dendritic pattern of these motoneurons must thus be interpreted as neither random in geometrical configuration nor, in view of the inordinate branch lengths, as functionally insignificant in spite of the difficulty of dendritic electrotonic conduction.

which long-term neural plasticity or short-term feedback circuitry play in their makeup.

BIBLIOGRAPHY

The monographs by Alpern[6] and Carpenter[7] contain good textbook treatments of the concepts here overviewed. The Chapter by Rashbass in this Volume contains a full description of the vergence system superimposed on the innate conjugacy of versional movements, which is the subject of Hering's law.

REFERENCES

1. **Westheimer, G.**, Mechanism of saccadic eye movements, *Arch. Ophthalmol.,* 52, 710, 1954.

2. **Hering, E.,** *Die Lehre vom binocularen Sehen,* Leipzig: Engelmann, 1868.

3. **Boeder, P.,** The cooperation of extraocular muscles, *Am. J. Ophthalmol.,* 51, 469, 1961.

4. **Krewson, W. E.,** The action of the extraocular muscles, *Trans. Am. Ophthalmol. Soc.,* 48, 443, 1950.

5. **Robinson, D. A.,** A quantitative analysis of extraocular muscle cooperation and squint, *Invest. Ophthalmol.,* 14, 801, 1975.

6. **Alpern, M.,** Movements of the Eyes, in *The Eye,* 2nd ed., Vol. 3, Davson, H., Ed. Academic Press, New York, 1969.

7. **Carpenter, R. H. S.,** *Movements of the Eyes,* Pion, London, 1977.

Chapter 9

OCULOMOTOR RESPONSES TO NEAR STIMULI: THE NEAR TRIAD

John L. Semmlow

TABLE OF CONTENTS

I. INTRODUCTION

A. Definitions

Changing gaze from a far to near object provokes activity in three oculomotor mechanisms: the eyes turn inward (converge), the lens increases dioptric power through a change in shape, and the iris sphincter muscle contracts, causing a decrease in pupil diameter (constriction). The general motive for these neuromuscular responses is, as in most oculomotor behavior, the production of "the clearest possible perception of an object".[1] Specifically, lens and pupil responses improve the quality of the retinal image, while ocular convergence moves the retinal images into topographically similar areas (retinal correspondence) permitting perceptual fusion. (Fusion is a cortical phenomenon wherein the two retinal images are perceived singly.)[2]

The three motor responses, collectively termed the oculomotor near triad, or simply near triad, are driven by stimuli associated with object distance. Retinal blur and retinal disparity (the lack of correspondence between retinal images) are related to object distance by basic geometrical and optical rules and are each sufficient to evoke all three motor responses. Additional features related to object distance which may modulate near triad response include perspective, apparent size, chromatic and spherical abberations, and subtle "psychic" clues.[2,3]

Both retinal blur and disparity drive neurological feedback control systems. As the lens changes its refractive power, blur and its analogous neural signal will change. Similarly, vergence eye movements alter retinal disparity. These feedback pathways are independent from one another and, as we shall see later, the regulatory control exercised by the two systems is quite different, the dispartity vergence response being very tightly regulated, while the accomodative system tolerates substantial blur.

Because of their effectiveness in evoking a motor response and the ease with which they can be manipulated in the laboratory, movements driven by blur and/or disparity have received the most attention. Lens and ocular vergence response to blur stimulation are termed accommodation and accommodative convergence, respectively, while similar motor responses driven by disparity are termed convergence accommodation and fusional, or disparity vergence (the latter term will be used here). Pupil near triad responses are not specifically named.

Lens response is quantified in terms of the distance, in diopters, of the object on which the lens is focused (i.e., one over the object distance in meters). Ocular vergence is measured as the angle of intersection of the lines of sight from the two eyes. This angle is expressed in either degrees, prism diopters, or meter angles (see Reference 26 for definitions). Iris response is usually quantified by the pupil diameter in millimeters.

Retinal disparity is the consequence of overlapping visual fields between the two eyes, and vergence movements are prominent in only the few species (primates and cats) which have forward facing eyes.[4] The phylogentically late development of the near triad has resulted in relatively underdeveloped control processes. Thus, it is diplopia (double vision) and other disorders caused by near triad malfunctions which "form the largest single group of oculomotor disturbances in clinical practice."[2]

B. Early History

While the synkinetic motor activity of the oculomotor near triad was accurately described by Porterfield in 1759,[5] it was not until the mid-nineteenth century that organized inquiry into the various component mechanisms began. The founding and rapid growth of the science of physiological optics was paralleled during this period by similar explosive activity in other areas of biology and physiology.

The early studies of ocular movement involved the center of rotation.[6] During these studies, Müller[7] described the relationship between blur and blur-driven vergence, the accommodative convergence response. Later, Herring[1] demonstrated that this relationship was the result of an inborn synergy between the medial recti muscles and the lens muscles. Herring is also attributed with the first control system approach to the near triad by defining vergence eye movements as a single response of the "double-eye" organ.[8] Further elaboration of this idea led to what is now known as Herring's Law, that corresponding muscles of each eye are equally innervated during vergence movements.[1]

Experiments on convergence accommodation were also performed by Herring and when these lens responses resulted in a defocused image, he described the compensatory action of the accommodative system.[1] Pupil size changes in response to disparity stimulation are also described by Herring. The fact that both disparity-driven lens and iris response are equal in the two eyes was reported and used as further evidence supporting a common neural origin for these near triad responses.

The limits of accommodative and vergence response during normal binocular viewing, the so-called relative responses, were investigated by Donders[9] and Volkmann.[10] These limits, which define the zone of clear single vision, (See Section IV-A) are particularly important in many clinical disorders. Through the work of Donders, Volkmann, Herring, and others of that period, a scientific basis for the treatment of oculomotor imbalances was firmly established.

By the late nineteenth century, all of the major near triad response behaviors had been qualitatively documented and a few, such as accommodative convergence, had been quantatively measured. In 1886, the first comprehensive theory to explain near triad synkinesis was proposed by Maddox.[11] This theory stood essentially unchallenged for nearly 50 years when objective measurements of lens response stimulated an alternative proposal.[12] As the mechanisms underlying near triad synkinesis constitute a major focus of this Chapter, these theories will be detailed in a later section (Section V).

II. STIMULUS AND RESPONSE MECHANISMS

As mentioned in the Introduction, the near triad involves three motor response mechanisms driven primarily by two quite different stimuli. Before describing the behavior of the various stimulus-response combinations, a description of the major individual elements will be given.

A. Stimulus Mechanisms
1. Accommodative Stimulation
While blurring of the retinal image provides an obvious stimulus to accommodation, chromatic and spherical aberrations, psychic proximal factors, and lens oscillations have been proposed as contributing to the monocular sensory signal. That the reflex can be driven by blur alone has been demonstrated through experiments by Allen,[13] Stark and Takahashi,[14] and others.[15] These experiments show that when such clues as changes in target size, color, brightness, lateral position, and binocular parallax were eliminated, initial accommodative movements were sometimes incorrect. Initial response errors are expected from a stimulus, such as blur, which does not contain direction information. While attempting to eliminate directional clues, Campbell and Westheimer[16] and Fincham[17] found that chromatic aberration or any of a variety of other complex stimuli could be used to provide this information. Additionally, Fincham[17] has determined that direction information is lost when small "scanning" eye movements are prevented, indicating image movement may be important in the detection process.

Recently, Phillips and Stark[18] showed that accommodation can be stimulated simply by defocusing a target image. Thus, it is probable that retinal blur alone supplies the primary drive in an accommodative response, while a combination of other sensory stimuli provide direction information. Accordingly, the terms blur stimulus and blur-driven components will be used synonymously with accommodative stimulus and components.

The neural process used to abstract blur information from the retinal image is not understood. The complexity of clues which may be involved in the accommodative response suggest the visual cortex must play a role. However, under normal viewing circumstances, Fincham[17] found that lenses can induce accommodative changes without subject awareness. This suggests that the accommodative response is a true reflex,[17] though a voluntary component may also be involved.[19] Assuming that the brain has at its disposal only two types of fundamental visual information (differences in light intensity and differences in color), Fincham[17] has proposed a process which provides for detection of converging and diverging retinal light rays. His proposal combines the directional sensitivity of foveal cones (the Stiles-Crawford effect) with the added information provided by scanning eye movements to obtain signals related to image blur.

Near triad responses influence the accommodative error signal. Clearly, the refractive state of the lens directly modifies blur providing a negative feedback pathway. Additionally, the pupil response can also influence the blur stimulus. Finally, the disparity stimulus may also act to modify the effective blur signal.

Pupil size influences accommodative stimulation by modifying the ocular depth-of-focus, the dead-space operator associated with the optical properties of the lens and iris. This fact is sometimes used to eliminate the feedback influence of lens refractive state on blur. By presenting the stimulus target through an optical pinhole, blur components can be eliminated from near triad responses. While classical optics predicts a hyperbolic relationship between pupil diameter and depth-of-focus, Ripps et al.[20] found that neither the steady accommodative or accommodative convergence response was influenced by pupil size if the diameter was larger than 1.5 mm. Similarly, the dynamic accommodative convergence response has been shown to be unaffected by variations in pupil size ranging between 3.0 and 7.0 mm.[21] Since the undrugged iris rarely constricts to diameters less than 2 to 3 mm,[22] modification of the blur stimulus by the normal iris can be ignored.

During a symmetrical vergence movement, as occurs when the stimulus target is moved along a midline between the two eyes, the target will be off the fovea until the movement is complete, and all disparity stimuli will produce a temporarily off-foveal image. As off-foveal images are less effective in generating accommodative responses,[23] disparity response does influence the blur signal. Whiteside[23] subjectively measured the accommodative response to peripheral stimuli and found that images "making an angle of four degrees or more with the fovea constituted but a weak stimulus for the accommodative reflex". Measuring the amplitude of dynamic accommodative convergence to increasingly off-foveal targets, Semmlow and Tinor[24] found the response rapidly diminished so that targets five degrees from the foveal fixation point evoked less than half the response of an equivalent foveal stimulus (Figure 1). Thus, during binocular stimulation when both disparity and blur are present, the accommodative component should be less than predicted by the same blur stimulus presented monocularly.

Accommodative stimuli may be generated in the laboratory using either variation in target distance or lenses. A Badel optometer, which employs a lens with secondary focal point optically conjurgate to the ocular entrance pupil, is sometimes used to vary accommodative stimulation while maintaining image size constant.

2. Disparity Stimulation

Retinal disparity, as defined in Section I-A, is the only stimulus required to drive

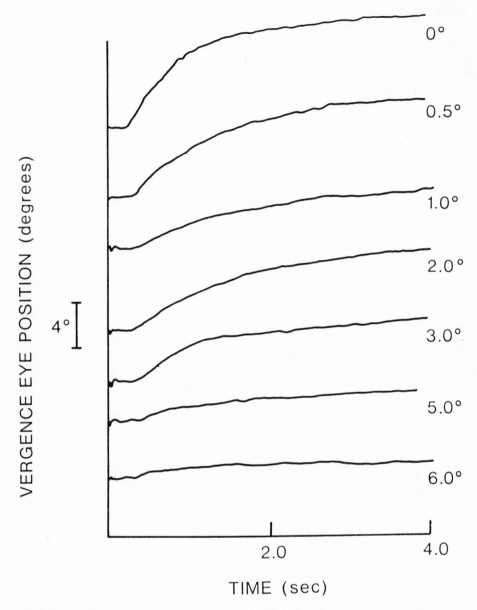

FIGURE 1. Accommodative convergence responses to a 3.0 diopter accommodative stimulus for various retinal image positions with respect to the fovea.[24](Note: Convergence is always plotted upward.)

the disparity vergence response.[25] Diplopia, the conscious awareness of double vision, is not a prerequisite for the generation of this reflex if the disparity stimulus is sufficiently small.[26] Clearly, binocular vision is required to produce a disparity stimulus, and the occlusion of one eye is a simple and frequently used technique to eliminate disparity-driven components from other near triad responses. With the exception of the obvious feedback effect of vergence eye position on disparity, stimulus effectiveness is independent of other near triad stimulus or response states.

As with blur, little is known about the neural processing used to detect disparity. Cells selectively sensitive to disparity have been found in the visual cortex[27] and striate cortex of cat,[28] and similar cells in humans may provide the basis for neural control of disparity vergence.[3] Based on the oculomotor response to combined disparity and version stimuli, Toates[29] has proposed a theory for the computation of the respective drive signals. His proposal uses the sum and difference of retinal image to fovea distance in the two eyes to calculate the appropriate version and vergence response for any binocular stimulus condition. Responses usually observed under combined vergence/version stimulation support the basic notions of Toates' theory.

Disparity vergence stimulation can be independently altered by inserting prisms in the visual pathway, or through the use of movable mirrors as in the haploscope and Dynamic Binocular Stimulator.[30] Alternatively, the distance can be varied between two identical images viewed stereoscopically. This latter technique is frequently used when time-varying stimuli are required.

3. Proximal Stimulation and Voluntary Responses

Both accommodative and vergence responses maybe influenced by proximity stimuli, a subconscious awareness of the target's actual distance. Itlelson and Ames[31] found that both accommodative and vergence response varied as the size of a monocular target was varied. Accommodation responses were also noted when the target was viewed binocularly. However, several subsequent experiments[32,33] including one by Morgan,[34] which used size, light intensity, and relative position to alter apparent distance, have shown no accommodative response to proximal stimuli.

The influence of proximal stimulation on vergence response, termed proximal vergence, has been documented in both monocular[32,33] and binocular viewing conditions.[35,36] While the influence of this stimulus varies widely among subjects and measuring techniques,[26,34,35] several investigators report the response is roughly linear with the stimulus (when apparent distance is expressed in diopters).[35,36] This has led to the use of a single response to stimulus ratio (PC/A) to quantatively describe steady state proximal vergence, though the appropriateness of this linear description is in question.[26,37] Typical reported values range between 0.5 to 1.0 deg/dio. Finally, it is possible that proximal convergence is simply a conditioned reflex associated with disparity vergence[38] having no separate neural processes.[29]

Both accommodation and vergence responses may also be subject to some voluntary control. In an extensive study, Fincham[39] reported that accommodation is entirely involuntary, at least in younger subjects. However, Marg[19] has found significant voluntary accommodation in similar subjects. It is possible that the difference depends on the blur magnitude, with accommodative errors of 2.5 diopters or less, evoking an involuntary reflex, while larger errors require some voluntary correction.[39]

Though voluntary accommodation is somewhat controversial, voluntary convergence is well-known and easily demonstrated. It can operate over greater disparities than the disparity reflex, but does require conscious identification of the double images (diplopia).[4]

While proximal and voluntary components may contribute to the day-to-day operation of the near triad, they are of little use in experimentation, as they are difficult to control in any quantative manner. Thus, most experimental studies presented in the following Sections use only disparity or accommodative stimulation, or both. In these experiments it is generally assumed, not always correctly, that proximal and voluntary responses have been eliminated.

B. Neural Processes

The synkinetic action of near triad motor responses is reflected in the structure of controlling neural processes. Both the lens and iris receive most of their neural control via the IIIrd Cranial nerve and the ciliary ganglion.[41] In addition, the iris dialator muscle receives sympathetic innervation via the superior cervical ganglion; however this muscle may not be involved in the near response.[4,41] The extraocular muscles which mediate vergence eye position are also innervated by the IIIrd, along with the IVth and VIth Cranial nerves.

In the brain stem, the final common pathway for most near triad responses begins in the Edinger-Westphal nucleus, a subdivision of the oculomotor nucleus. Electrical stimulation of cells in this center has resulted in pupillary constriction, accommodation, and lateral adduction.[41-43] However, the integrated vergence response does not appear to be represented at this level,[43,44] nor does the near triad synkineses.[44]

Searching for higher levels of near response control, Jampel[44] elicited all possible combinations of near triad responses (except accommodation alone and accommodation with pupillary constriction) by cortical stimulation of small portions of areas 19 and 22. These and other results led him to propose a three-tiered control structure: the cortex, which "integrates and synthesizes" the total synkinetic response, the midbrain, which "modifies the impulses on a more primitive level", and the oculomotor nuclear complex which "acts as a final common pathway".

Few additional neurological studies have been done which confirm or expand Jampel's original proposals. Bender and Shanzer[45] have located an integrating relay in the prerubal field which projects to the Edinger-Westphal nucleus. These cells which receive inputs from a variety of midbrain structures, as well as from the cortex, could form the basis of Jampel's second level of control.

C. Response Mechanisms

Neural signals evoked by near triad stimuli are distributed to three neuromuscular structures: the lens, iris, and extraocular muscles (EOM). Each of these motor processes has been extensively studied, both as an anatomical structure and as a dynamic mechanical process functioning as an output transducer.

1. The Lens

Accommodative responses are mediated by shape changes in the lens. These changes are produced by altering the tension on the lens and its highly elastic capsule.[46,47] The theory first proposed by Helemholtz in 1855[6] is now generally accepted as an explanation for lens shape changes. In this theory the unaccommodated (focused for infinity) lens is under maximum tension, stretched by its attachments (the zonule of Zinn) to the ciliary muscle. As the circular sphincter of the ciliary muscle contracts, tension in the suspensory ligaments is reduced and a redistribution of stress in the lens capsule produces a more spherical shape.[46-48] The initial tension is supplied by either the meridonal fibers of the ciliary muscle,[49] which would have to be innervated reciprocally with the sphincter fibers,[50] or the passive elastic properties of the suprachonoidal connective tissue.[51] The arguements supporting reciprocal innervation as opposed to a single muscle acting against a passive elastic element have been summarized by Toates.[3]

In senile presbyopia, a reduction occurs in maximum lens refractive power with age. While this reduction is definitely attributed to increased viscosity of the lens substance due to progressive sclerosis,[46,52,53] there is controversy regarding the specific relationship between ciliary muscle contraction and lens power[54] as the lens hardens. Nonetheless, it is agreed that neural innervation becomes less effective in producing refractive change as sclerosis advances.[54,55]

Several models of the lens mechanical structure have been developed.[3,56,58] Fisher[52,57] has made a thorough quantative analysis of the mechanical characteristics of the isolated lens. Using dynamic data obtained from ciliary nerve stimulation (in cat), O'Neill et al.[56] developed a nonlinear, first-order model for the lens neuromuscular apparatus. Their model indicated that the transport delay and primary dynamics of an accommodative response reside in the lens plant.

2. The Iris

The iris is a delicate, mobile diaphragm stretching across the anterior portion of the eye having, at its center or slightly to the nasal side, a generally circular opening, the pupil. Its size may vary from 1.3 mm to 10 mm in man, and in other species, even more.[59] The known functions of the iris include light regulation, increasing depth of focus, and the reduction of optical aberrations. The pupillary border rests upon and is supported by the lens and, being pushed forward by this curved body, has the shape of a truncated pyramid.

Iris mobility is provided by two smooth muscles: the spincter pupillae and the dilator pupillae. The sphincter pupillae lies in a concentric ring 0.7 mm to 1 mm wide near the inner edge of the iris. It is a powerful and unique muscle capable of contraction to less than one fourth its maximum length in seconds.[59] Both the existence and the function of the radial dilator muscle have been in doubt.[60] Currently, it is not certain whether the dilator merely sets a slowly varying tone against the swift moving sphincter[61,62] or plays a fully active role in the dynamic response,[60] though experimental evidence tends to favor the latter.[60,63]

A quantative model of the iris muscular apparatus has been developed by Stark, Hansman, and Semmlow.[64,65] Rather than stimulating the controlling nerve fibers to obtain information on the isolated iris, we used a comparative analysis between light-induced and near triad responses.[66] As with the lens, the iris motor apparatus was found to be dynamically limiting in the near response, but with second-order over-damped characteristics. Two distinct nonlinear behaviors were isolated[66] and attributed to specific muscle properties.[64,65] This iris model has been used successfully as a component in a larger model representing the entire pupil light reflex.[67]

3. The Vergence Plant

A vergence response consists of equal, but opposing horizontal movements of the two eyes; hence, vergence neural processes must share control of the horizontal rectus muscles with other eye movement systems. This shared control is effected without interference, so that complex vergence responses may take place simultaneously with other ocular responses.[68] Though it was once thought that vergence may employ a specific subset of motor neurons and muscle fibers,[69] it is now generally agreed that a given muscle fiber type is not reserved for a specific oculomotor task.[29,70]

The oculomotor apparatus mediating horizontal position control has been the focus of numerous quantative models[71-75] usually with regard to its role in saccadic eye movements. Though these movements are about ten times faster than vergence movements of the same magnitude,[73] much of this speed is attributed to a time optimal innervation pattern, not to the inherent dynamics of the motor apparatus.[73,76] These modeling studies also suggest that disparity vergence dynamics are the result of a step change in neural innervation.[73] Hence, even in the disparity vergence response, it is probably the plant which is dynamically limiting. However, vergence response latencies (transport delay) and accommodative convergence dynamics are probably of control origin.

III. RESPONSES IN ISOLATED SYSTEMS

As noted in the last section, two of the near triad responses, accommodation and vergence, are controlled by feedback systems. Through appropriate adjustment of the visual stimulus, it is possible to selectively disable one or the other system, permitting the remaining system to be studied in relative isolation. This section deals with experimental findings from such isolated systems: their static and dynamic behavior under closed-loop and, in some cases, open-loop conditions.

To isolate the accommodative system, the disparity vergence system is disabled by eliminating binocular stimuli. This is accomplished simply by blocking one eye (monocular vision). Under these circumstances, there can be no disparity, and disparity-driven components are assumed to be zero, or perhaps, some constant value. Changes in monocular target depth or insertion of lenses will produce blur-driven responses free of interference from disparity components.

The elimination of blur can be used to isolate the disparity vergence system. This is usually accomplished by having the subject view the stimulus through an optical pinhole. The large depth-of-field produced insures zero blur, irrespective of lens dioptric power. Often, "isolated" disparity vergence responses are obtained simply by maintaining accommodative stimulation constant, the assumption being that accommodative motor components will also be constant. While this assumption does not lead to significant errors in the dynamic vergence response,[77] it does lead to inaccuracies in the description of the steady state response (See Section VI-C).

The two techniques described above can also be used to obtain open-loop behavior. That is, pinhole viewing will disable accommodative feedback and monocular viewing disrupts the disparity vergence. Unfortunately, these techniques do not permit variation of the stimulus; it is always zero under these circumstances. To obtain open-loop responses with varying inputs, it is necessary to use an "error clamping" technique,[78] in which the resonse is monitored and the stimulus continuously varied to enforce constant error. Alternatively, with accommodation it is possible to open the loop by paralyzing the ciliary muscle of one eye, presenting blur stimulation to that eye, and monitoring the response of the unparalyzed eye.

A. Accommodative Responses
1. Static Behavior

Maintained changes in all three near triad motor responses are evoked by accommodative stimulation. The lens response, under feedback control, follows an increase in blur stimulation, but not without some error.[79,80] This error, sometimes termed a "lazy lag" because the response is less than the stimulus, is due in part to the accommodative dead-space[81] mentioned previously (Section II-A-1). Toates[3,82] argues that these steady state errors are the consequence of a proportional control system one with a simple gain term (and no integrator) in the forward path. Such control systems require a finite error to maintain the desired output. Krishnan and Stark[83] modelled the accommodative system with a "leaky integrator" (first order lag term) in the forward path, a representation which has the same steady state error characteristic as a proportional system .[84] Some of the error may be associated with sensory mechanisms, since the error tends to increase as visual accuracy decreases, as when the illumination level is reduced.[85,86] Finally, at high levels of accommodative stimulus, the error may increase substantially due to saturation of the lens plant (See Section II-C-1).

At very low levels of accommodative stimulus, the error usually changes sign with the response greater than the stimulus. This is due to the fact that the accommodative system has a nonzero output in the absence of blur stimulation. This physiological resting state, or tonic accommodation, ranges between 0.5 and 1.5 diopters[87,88] and occurs normally in darkness or when viewing an empty field.[89] The source of this tonic component is not known.

The lens response to constant blur stimulation is not itself constant, but fluctuates over a range as large as 0.4 diopters.[90] These fluctuations increase at higher accommodative responses and are eliminated when the ciliary muscle is paralyzed, suggesting they are of neural origin. Phillips and Stark[18] recently suggested these fluctuations are used in a "hunting" scheme to distinguish target blur from an out-of-focus image and to provide direction information.

The vergence response to a steady accommodative stimulus is easily measured during monocular fixation when the disparity system is disabled. In addition to a tonic vergence component, most subjects show a change in vergence response linearly related to accommodative stimulation.[34,91-93] Thus, steady state characteristics of this interactive process can be quantatively defined by a single number: the accommodative convergence to accommodative stimulus ratio (AC/A$_s$). This ratio describes the relative effectiveness of blur stimulation to produce a vergence movement. The value of this ratio varies widely between individuals with an average from one study of 3.39 prism diopter/diopter.[36] To adequately fixate a binocular target at any given depth requires an AC/A$_s$ ratio of around 6 prism diopter/diopter (based on the geometrical relationship between target distance and vergence angle required); thus, for most people accommodative convergence cannot provide the total required binocular vergence.

The iris also responds to changes in accommodative stimulation. The response is basically nonlinear, with the movement induced by a given stimulus decreasing, as mean pupil diameter varies either side of a midrange value.[21] This "range" type nonlinearity has been attributed to a property of the iris muscle.[65] If pupil size changes are restricted to a sufficiently limited range, a linear approximation may be made and a ratio similar to the AC/A$_s$ can be used to qualify the response-stimulus relationship. Common values lie between 0.35 and 0.75 mm (change in diameter) per diopter.[94]

2. Dynamic Behavior

Near triad responses to time varying blur stimulation have been documented for a number of stimulus patterns, notably sinusoids and step changes. Accommodative step changes were first measured by Kirchhof[95] using a high-speed photographic technique. He found considerable intersubject variation with an average movement time of around 0.5 sec (not including the latent period). Subsequent step response data show a generally exponential, overdamped response,[96] with a latent period around 0.3 to 0.4 seconds.[58,96,97] From step and impulse responses, Campbell and Westheimer[96] concluded that the accommodative system operates in a continuous manner (no sampled data behavior).

Sinusoidal responses have been recorded in a number of studies,[96,98-100] sometimes in conjunction with a servoanalytic treatment of the closed-loop accommodative system.[98,99] Frequency characteristics are dependent on stimulus amplitude demonstrating the presence of an amplitude dependent nonlinearity.[99] For larger inputs (greater than around 0.5 diopter), the frequency response resembles that of a second-order, overdamped system with a bandwidth of around 0.4 to 0.8 hz.[96,99,100]

The dynamics of an accommodative convergence step response closely resembles that found in accommodation; however, the response latency is from 100 to 200 msec shorter.[101] Pulse stimulation shows that this response, like accommodation, is the result of a continuously operating control system.[102] Open and closed-loop sinusoidal data also show a frequency characteristic similar to accommodation, provided the stimulus is presented in such a manner as to be unpredictable.[100] The similarity in dynamic features, along with the consistency of the of the AC/A$_s$ ratio (within a given subject),[34] has been cited as evidence that these two responses share a common neural center.[92,101,103]

The pupil response to step on sinusoidal changes in accommodative stimulation has been documented by Stark, Hansmann, and Semmlow.[65,66] Step responses show roughly second-order dynamics and two nonlinear behaviors: the range type nonlinearity mentioned earlier and a direction dependence in which constrictive movements were faster than dilation. Both the dynamics and nonlinearities have been attributed to elements in the neuromuscle apparatus.[64,65]

B. Disparity Driven Responses
1. Static Behavior
The steady state response of vergence to disparity is quite accurate with positional errors of the order of minutes of arc. These errors, termed fixation disparity, are usually measured subjectively with a fully functional accommodative system. Thus, these measurements do not represent the behavior of the isolated disparity vergence system and will be covered in the section on binocular responses.

When the lens is isolated from blur components and driven by disparity, a significant response is generally observed. Though this reponse is not very linear with the stimulus, it has often been approximated by a ratio similar to the AC/A_s ratio. This approximation, termed the convergence accommodation to convergence ratio, CA/C, can be as large as 1.2 DIO/MA in younger subjects, but decreases with age[12,104] probably due to decreasing responsiveness of the presbyopic lens. The CA/C value cited above represents more lens drive than would be required under binocular viewing conditions and indicates that convergence accommodation is a stronger interactive process than accommodative convergence.

The iris also responds to changes in disparity stimulation at least for most subjects. Though the relationship between stimulus and response is subject to the same nonlinear motor process as blur-driven signals[105] and the relationship in basically nonlinear,[106] a single ratio valid over a limited range of pupil diameters is often used to define the response. Reported values for this ratio, defined as change in pupil diameter with disparity stimulation, range between 0.0 to 0.127 mm/prism diopter.[93,107] Sharkhnovich[108] observed that changes in pupil diameter are directly related to convergence response, irrespective of whether accommodation or disparity stimuli generated the response. Thus, it is likely that both near triad pupil responses are mediated by a single neural center which receives input from the vergence motor center.

2. Dynamic Behavior
Most disparity-driven dynamic components have been studied without isolating the vergence system from accommodation. However, Semmlow and Venkiteswaran[77] have observed that disparity vergence dynamics are the same when the accommodative system is fully functioning, as when accommodation is open-loop. Thus, the results described below will be assumed to represent disparity components responding in isolation.

Both sinusoidal and step responses show that disparity vergence has faster dynamics and occurs after a shorter latent period than the blur-driven movement.[100,109] In general, the step response is exponential, overdamped (or slightly underdamped), and sometimes faster during convergent movements.[109,110] While direction dependence indicates the presence of nonlinearity, Rashbass and Westheimer[25] have found no indication of nonlinearity in response to open-loop step stimulation. Responses to pulse stimuli indicate that the controlling system operates continuously, and both open and closed-loop sinusoidal and step responses suggest the presence of a linear integral controller.[25,110] A further description of disparity vergence control characteristics is found in Toates[29] and elsewhere in this book.

Dynamic responses of the lens to disparity stimulation are difficult to record, since lens movement must be continuously monitored while the eye is moving (in response to the disparity stimulation). Recently, Krishman et al.[111] simultaneously measured the step response of convergence accommodation and disparity vergence. They noted that the lens response was similar in form, but slower in dynamics than the vergence movement. It is likely that plant dynamics are responsible for response differences; however, their experimental conditions did not eliminate accommodative feedback, and it is possible that regulatory action from the accommodative control system influenced the lens response.

IV. BINOCULAR RESPONSES

A. Steady State Behavior

1. Relative Responses and the Zone of Clear Single Vision

Responses of the visual motor triad during maintained binocular fixation have been extensively studied. In general, such static experiments measure the change in one or more motor outputs, as one stimulus is varied and the other held constant. The response of a motor component to changes in its analogous stimulus component is termed the relative response.[10,112] Thus, relative accommodation is the change in lens power due to blur stimulation, while vergence stimulation is held constant. Similarly, relative vergence is the vergence response to disparity stimulation while accommodative stimulation is fixed. Since the two relative responses are mediated by feedback systems, the relative response should track the stimulus within reasonable error limits. The degree to which this is true provides a measure of both the control effectiveness of the feedback system and its independence from other near triad components.

The maximum and minimum values of relative accommodation and relative vergence are of particular interest, since they define the range of stimulus combinations over which clear and single vision can be maintained. A plot of the boundaries imposed by these limits (in the accommodative/vergence response plane) is termed the zone of clear single vision[10,112-114] and is shown in somewhat idealized form in Figure 2. Such plots are obtained simply by increasing or decreasing one stimulus component while the other is held fixed until either blur or diplopia occurs. Most subjects experience blur before diplopia, irrespective of which component is varied.[26,114] A possible explanation for this phenomenon is offered in the next section.

Blur occurring at the top and bottom horizontal boundaries of the zone (Figure 2) is attributed to range limitations of the accommodative plant. That is, the crystalline lens is simply incapable of further change in dioptric power at these boundries. Evidence for the mechanical nature of this limitation is seen in the lowering of the upper boundary with advanced age, a decrease which correlates with the decrease in lens capsule flexibility due to progressive sclerosis (see Section II-C-1).

The negative (left-hand) side of the zone represents the limits of both negative relative vergence and positive relative accommodation, while the positive (right-hand) boundary represents the limits of positive relative convergence and negative relative accommodation.[34,114] The mechanism which produces the diagonal boundaries of the zone is not well defined, but is definitely of neural origin, since both lens and eye positional mechanisms are capable of greater range. A curious feature of the zone is the extension of positive relative vergence often found along the upper boundary where lens response is in saturation (line AB in Figure 2). The mechanism underlying this feature is discussed in the next section.

2. Response Error During Relative Accommodation

As mentioned, relative response errors and the dependency of such error on the status of other triad components provides important information on the autonomy of the underlying feedback control system. Large sustained errors between stimulus and

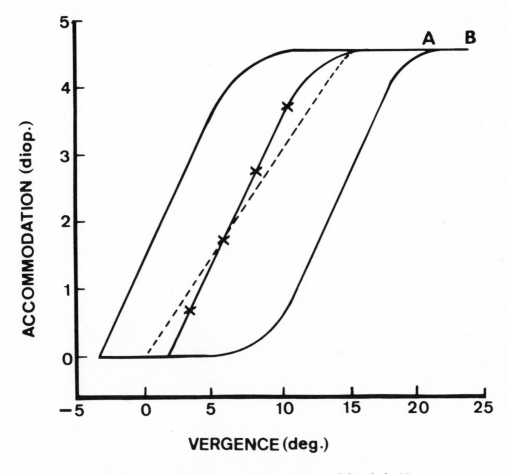

FIGURE 2.   The idealized representation of the zone of clear single vision.

relative response indicate ineffectiveness in the mediating control system. Further, a large variation in such errors produced by interactive stimulus components indicates a strong influence from these components. Conversely, small relative response errors suggest good regulatory control and errors independent of the other stimulus or response states indicate comparative isolation of the mediating control processes.

An example of the former situation is seen in the response characteristics of relative accommodation. As shown in Figure 3A, relative accommodation only approximates blur stimulation values. This indication of poor regulation is also seen in the "lazy lag" during isolated accommodative responses as described earlier (Section III-A-1). Figure 3 also shows that the error in relative accommodation is quite sensitive to disparity stimulation. Thus, as disparity stimulation increases, the accommodative response also increases even though blur stimulation is held constant. Decreasing accommodation is seen when disparity stimulation is decreased. Eventually, accommodative error becomes so large that the target image becomes noticeably blurred and the boundary of the zone of clear single vision is reached.

Two somewhat different explanations have been suggested for the strong influence of disparity stimulation on relative accommodation. The occurence of blur at the zone boundary is most often explained as a recruitment of accommodative drive and associated accommodative convergence to help forestall diplopia.[26,113,115] The mechanism for this recruitment is unexplained, though a semivoluntary process is usually implied.

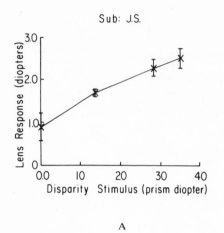

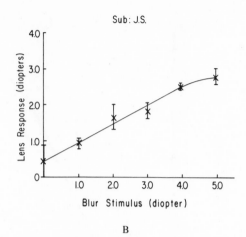

A

B

FIGURE 3.   Lens responses to steady state blur and disparity stimulation under binocular viewing conditions.

(A) Lens response to blur stimulation when disparity stimulation is held constant at 0.0 prism diopters.

(B) Lens response to various levels of disparity stimulus while blur stimulus is held fixed at 0.5 diopters.

An alternative explanation, originally suggested by Fincham and Walton[12] and later by Morgan[34] is that the blur is produced by excessive convergence accommodation associated with a strong fusional effort. Given a significant convergence accommodation to convergence (CA/C) ratio (as suggested by the findings of Fincham and Walton[12] and Kent[104]) the convergence accommodation expected at high (or low) disparity stimulus levels could simply overwhelm the feedback regulation provided by the accommodative control system.

Both of these hypotheses are consistent with the data of Figure 3B as both predict a similar change in lens power with increased disparity stimulation. However, the two hypotheses imply opposite roles for accommodative convergence near fusional limits. Under the "recruitment" hypothesis, accommodative convergence provides positive convergence in support of the fusional effort. The "lens overdrive" hypothesis requires active compensation from the accommodative controller in an effort to negate the disparity-induced lens drive; hence, the associated accommodative convergence must necessarily be in opposition to the vergence response. As these alternate hypotheses have important theoretical implications (presented in Section VI), the author has devised an experiment to distinguish between them.[116]

Since the two hypotheses imply opposite roles for accommodative convergence at the zone boundary, the most direct test would be simply to measure the accommodative convergence component under limit conditions. Normally, it is impossible to measure accommodative convergence during forced vergences, since disparity stimulation requires binocular vision and accommodative convergence is measured monocularly. An experimental paradigm was designed to indirectly measure the direction (divergent or convergent with respect to monocular value) of accommodative convergence under strong fusional effort. Essentially, advantage is taken of the faster response dynamics of disparity vergence. Initially, a binocular stimulus was presented requiring either a strong overconvergence or undercovergence. The disparity stimulus was then quickly reduced to near the monocular accommodative convergence value. The disparity system rapidly responds with a vergence movement to the new vergence position; however, as the accommodative convergence response is somewhat slower, it will require more time to return to its phoria value. If immediately after the disparity vergence movement one eye is blocked, the ongoing readjustment of the accommodative con-

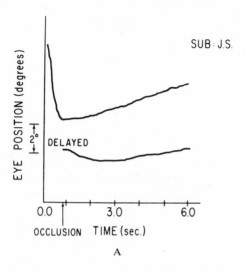
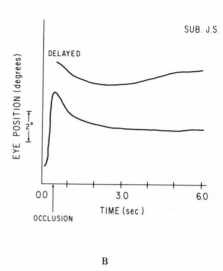

FIGURE 4. Response of one eye to occlusion (at the time indicated by the arrow) immediately following the reduction of a strong disparity stimulus. The response marked "delayed" occurs when occlusion is delayed ten or more seconds after disparity stimulus reduction and provides a control.
(A) Responses when the initial disparity stimulus is convergent.
(B) Responses when the initial disparity stimulus is divergent.[116]

vergence component should be exposed as a monocular vergence movement. A control experiment was also included to compensate for monocular movements not related to accommodative convergence.[116]

Results showed that an initially overconverged position produced a converging monocular response while, initial divergence produced a diverging response after occlusion, Figure 4. A converging monocular response indicates that accommodative convergence was divergent (with respect to the phoria position) and vice versa. All subjects showed monocular movements which indicated that accommodative convergence is divergent during forced convergence and convergent during forced divergence.

Accordingly, the increase in relative accommodation with increased disparity stimulation must be due to convergence accommodation, since the accommodative drive and the associated accommodative convergence is actually decreasing under these circumstances. Hence, the blur experienced at the diagonal boundaries of the zone is due to the inability of the poorly regulated accommodative feedback control system to compensate for the "overdrive" produced by convergence accommodation.

The "lens overdrive" hypothesis also provides a straightforward explanation of the additional vergence response seen at maximum accommodative response (Region A-B of Figure 2). In this region, lens responsiveness to neural stimulation is severely diminished; thus, disparity vergence can continue to increase to its "theoretical limit"[114] without inducing blur through convergence accommodation. Those subjects who do not experience blur at the limits of relative vergence[114] may have either a low CA/C ratio or a better regulated accommodative system providing more effective compensation.[116]

3. Response Error During Relative Vergence: Fixation Disparity

Regulation in the disparity vergence system is much more precise than in accommodation; hence, response errors for relative vergence are quite small. Nonetheless, small errors of the order of minutes of arc do exist as first reported by Hofmann and Bielchowsky.[117] Since these errors result in a sustained disparity between retinal images

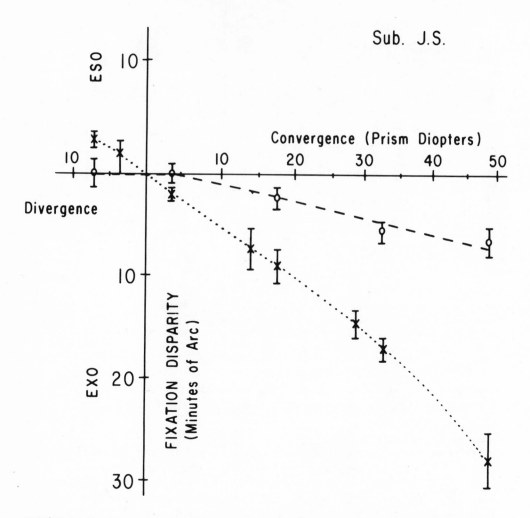

FIGURE 5.   Fixation disparity as a function of disparity stimulation (dotted line). The dashed line shows the vergence response error when accommodation is open-loop and is discussed in Section VI-C.[137]

(which is still fused by central processes), the term "fixation disparity" is often used to label relative vergence error. Later work has confirmed the existence of these errors,[118-120] and more recently Ogle and his collegues[36,121-123] have studied this phenomenon extensively.

Figure 5 shows a typical fixation disparity curve as a function of disparity stimulation. Though individual curves show considerable intersubject variation,[121] there is a general trend of increasing fixation disparity as the disparity-driven component approaches greater output levels. Further, since fixation disparity is generally measured subjectively,[122] there is some controversy regarding the absolute magnitude of vergence positional errors,[29] and it is clear that fixation disparity values are somewhat dependent on stimulus conditions.[124] Though small, a finite error has important implications regarding the disparity vergence central controller,[29] as is discussed elsewhere in this book.

As with accommodation, relative vergence error is also influenced by the other near triad stimulus, in this case, blur. Relating blur-induced fixation disparity to the disparity vergence stimulus required to produce an equivalent fixation disparity, Ogle and Martens[36] found a linear relationship was generated with a slope related to the AC/A, ratio. This indicates that changes in fixation disparity brought about by blur stimulation are the direct result of accommodative convergence. More importantly, this finding indicates that accommodative convergence, though only observed directly under monocular vision, plays an active role in binocular vergence.

The relationship between binocular AC/A_s, as measured using fixation disparity, and monocular AC/A_s, as measured using traditional methods (such as the Maddox rod), is not exact. In a comparative study, Ogle et al.[121] found monocular and binocular values differing by a factor of 2 or more. Differences were attributed, in part, to a more effective accommodative stimulus under binocular stimulation. Similarly, comparing the vergence response which gives zero fixation disparity (termed the "associated phoria") with the monocular vergence response (the "disassociated phoria") under the same accommodative stimulus, Ogle[122] found little correlation. Thus, while accommodative convergence is active during binocular fixation and it does influence the vergence system, its binocular role cannot necessarily be predicted from monocular measurements.

Measurements of fixation disparity have been used to demonstrate the existence of long-term adaptation in disparity vergence control processes.[125,126] Unlike the control processes mediating transient responses, the slow disparity vergence processes show considerable direction dependence, indicating separate adaptive mechanisms for divergence and convergence.[126]

B. Dynamic Behavior

1. Binocular Accommodative Convergence

Considerably less experimental data are available on the dynamic characteristics of near triad components during binocular vision. A few recent experiments have brought light to the role of accommodative convergence during binocular vergence movements.

While the fixation disparity experiments just described show that accommodative convergence may be active during maintained fixations, until recently there was no evidence that this component contributed to the dynamics of a binocular vergence response. If disparity stimulation is present, as it would be during a normal binocular response, the target image will be off the fovea, at least through part of the movement. As mentioned previously (Section II-A), the effectiveness of blur stimulation in producing accommodative convergence is substantially reduced when the stimulus image is more than a few degrees off-fovea.

More significantly, Alpern[127] was unable to find blur-induced vergence movements during steady binocular fixation. In these experiments, disparity stimulation was held constant and the confounding problem of an off-foveal target image was not present. However, as previously noted, disparity vergence is a very tightly controlled system and, with a constant stimulus, any externally manifested accommodative vergence is likely to be small and transient in nature. For example, if a subject is binocularly viewing a target and a blur stimulus is generated, say, through the interposition of lenses, an induced accommodative convergence movement would create a disparity which would be rapidly compensated by the feedback control of the disparity vergence system.

Accordingly, Semmlow and Venkiteswaran devised an experiment to carefully monitor eye movements in response to a step change in binocular blur stimulation under constant disparity stimulation.[30] The averaged movements to a number of stimulus presentations showed a small transient movement followed by a return to approximately the initial position, Figure 6. The direction of the initial movement was related to the accommodative stimulus in the same manner as a monocularly induced accommodative vergence movement. The return movement occurred around 200 to 300 msec after the initial movement and was completed in another 500 to 800 msec. These dy-

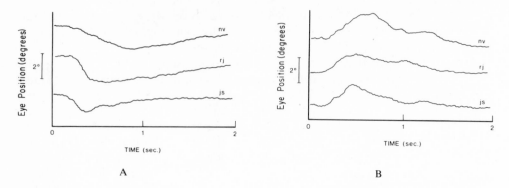

FIGURE 6.   Averaged responses of the right eye in three subjects to a 3 diopter step change in blur stimu-
lation with disparity held constant.
(A) Movements due to increasing accommodative stimulation (1-4 dio.).
(B) Movements produced by decreasing stimulation (4-1 dio.).
The final position will not be exactly the same as the initial position due to a blur-induced change in fixation
disparity.[30]

namical features are consistent with the assumption that the net response was made
up of an initial accommodative vergence movement followed, after the appropriate
delay, by a corrective disparity vergence movement. Thus, binocular blur stimulation
is capable of producing a vergence movement, at least when the target image is initially
on the fovea.

2. Dynamic Component Addition

The question remains as to whether the blur-driven component participates in a normal binocular vergence response when both blur and disparity stimulation are present.
The isolated component dynamics presented in Section III show that vergence response
to a step change in disparity stimulation is faster and has a shorter latent period than
the blur-driven response. Given a simultaneous change in both blur and disparity stimulation, as occurs when binocular fixation is switched between targets at different dis-
tances, disparity vergence would be expected to dominate the early portion of the dynamic response. Any contribution from the slower responding accommodative
convergence component would be expected during the latter portion of the movement.

To confirm this prediction, Semmlow and Wetzel did a comparative study of vergence movements generated by coordinated binocular stimulation (simultaneous blur
and disparity) and those produced by disparity stimulation alone.[109] A special stimulus
apparatus was used which permitted both stimulus conditions to be generated under
identical viewing conditions and eliminated cues to proximal vergence.[30] The average
vergence responses produced by coordinated binocular step stimulation are shown for
one subject in Figure 7 A and B (upper curves), along with the responses to disparity-
only stimulation (middle curves).

Qualitative comparison of the response pairs shows that the initial portion of the
movements are similar with differences occurring in the final portion of the dynamic
response. The contribution of the accommodative convergence components is more
clearly demonstrated in the lower curves in Figure 7 A and B which show the computed
difference between the vergence movements produced by coordinated and disparity-
only stimulation. From these curves, we see that the maximum difference between
responses occurs near the completion of the dynamic response. Little or no accommodative convergence contribution is seen during the first third of the movement, nor is
the contribution of accommodative convergence detectable at the end of the movement.

In an effort to quantify the accommodative convergence contribution to binocular vergence movement, we measured the difference between the responses with and without accommodative stimulation at two selected time points during the dynamic movement (t(τ) and t(max) in Figure 7). We then compared this measured difference with values predicted by the addition of isolated components. Calculation of the predicted values took into account the relative differences between accommodative and disparity vergence latencies and dynamics, as well as the subject's AC/A, ratio. Results of this calculation done on five subjects showed that the combined stimulus movement could be modelled as a linear addition of blur and disparity-driven components up to time t(τ). At the later time, t(max), the accommodative convergence contribution, though noticeable, was less than predicted by a simple addition of the two isolated responses. The final position was roughly the same for both responses; hence, any accommodative convergence contribution was not externally visible at the end of the response. (This is intuitively satisfying, since an externally manifested accommodative vergence contribution would cause diplopia under the experimental conditions.)

An important question generated by this study concerns the behavior of accommodative vergence during the late and posttransient period of the response. At the final position, the combined component response is less than the sum of isolated component responses to the same stimulus. Explanations for this lack of component addition are intimately related to theories of near triad synkinses and will be discussed in detail in the following section.

V. THEORIES OF NEAR TRIAD SYNKINESIS

During normal binocular viewing, both blur-driven and disparity-driven components are active and must combine in some manner to produce a coordinated near triad response. Since each stimulus operates through a feedback control system which, in turn, may interact with the other system, the two systems may operate jointly in a way quite unlike their independent behavior. Mutual interactions, while probably advantageous to near triad neurological control, hinder research efforts to define the controlling processes, since binocular operation cannot be directly inferred from isolated behavior. Thus, despite extensive research, fundamental questions regarding the specifics of binocular synkinesis and the relative importance of disparity and blur stimuli remain unresolved.

Theories of near triad interaction divide into two general categories depending on the form of interactive mechanism postulated. Specifically, the synkinetic interaction between accommodative and vergence feedback control systems could be the result of two separate central mechanisms or a single interactive process. Theories in the latter category usually assume that one component is not involved under normal stimulus conditions, or that the two components are manifestations, of a single bilateral linkage. That is, the two interactive components, accommodative convergence and convergence accommodation, may be that aspect of a single interactive process which is observed when one, or the other feedback control system is open-loop.

A. Single Interaction Theories

The earliest theory for the interaction of these components during binocular fixation was proposed by Maddox in 1886.[11] This theory, which will be referred to here as the Maddox Hierarchy, holds that the primary support for maintained binocular vergence is supplied by accommodative convergence along with a tonic component (and, presumably, proximal effects), while the disparity-driven component provides a "fusion supplement". The function of disparity vergence then is to compensate for error be-

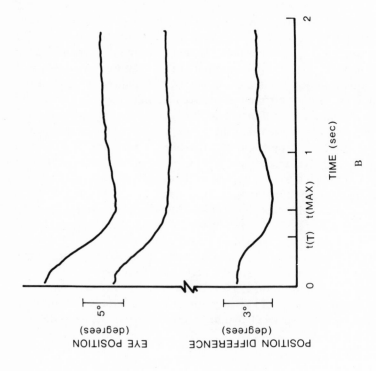

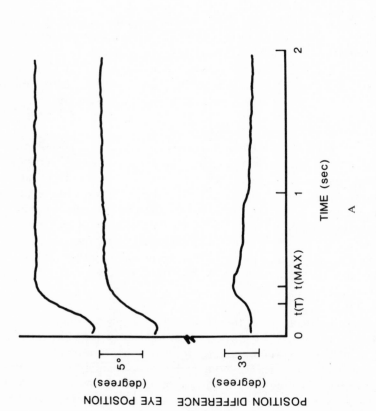

FIGURE 7.   Vergence movements produced by disparity step stimulation with (upper curve) and without (middle curve) accompanying blur step stimulation. The computed difference between the two responses is shown in the lower curve. (A) Responses due to increasing stimulation (0-3 meter angles and 0-3 diopters). (B) Responses due to decreasing stimulation (3-0 meter angles and 0-3 diopters).[90]

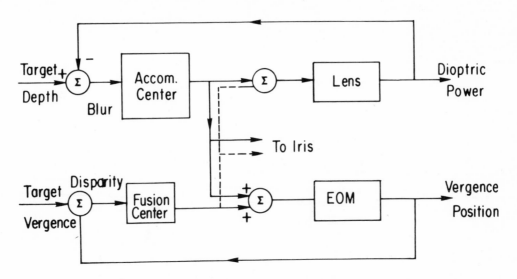

FIGURE 8. Organizational structure of major near triad processes consistant with the Maddox/Alpern theory of binocular synkinesis. Dashed lines indicate functionally unimportant pathways.

tween the position caused by the combination of components mentioned above and the required vergence position. This theory falls into the category of single interactive process, since no provision is made for the influence of a separate convergence accommodation link. Many current clinical and research concepts such as "fusional demand" and "fusional reserve" are directly related to the Maddox structuring of vergence components.[26]

Theories supporting a single functional linkage may be subdivided into two additional categories depending on which stimulus, blur or disparity, is considered dominate. In the Maddox Hierarchy and its refinements, blur-driven components play the major role.

Expanding on the basic assumption of blur dominance, Alpern et al.[92] propose a specific neural mechanism for near triad synkinesis. They suggest the motor innervations to both the lens and vergence plants "have a common point of origin in the central nervous system, that these innervations are linearly related to each other, and that they are evoked simultaneously by a change in accommodative stimulation". Based on this proposal, Zuber[103] constructed a schematic organizational block diagram showing the functional relationship between near triad components. This general structure, expanded to include the vergence system and feedback pathways, is shown in Figure 8. In the Maddox/Alpern theory, the existence of a separate convergence accommodation link is not excluded, but its role under normal circumstances is considered "small and relatively unimportant for the basic process of near-seeing".[54] Alpern[54] cites evidence, including the neurophysiological findings of Jampel[44] (Section II-B), to support the fundamental role of blur-driven components in near triad responses.

In an alternative theory, Fincham[128] and Fincham and Walton[12] maintain that disparity-driven components dominate the near triad. Here, only a single interactive process is presumed to exist: a process linking the lens to the vergence system termed "convergenced-induced accommodation". Accommodative convergence is described as "the evidence [i.e., open-loop manifestation] of the convergence effort which is called into play to induce the necessary amount of accommodation".[128] In other words, when the vergence system is open-loop, as in monocular vision, blur stimulation acts through the vergence system generating a convergence with an associated convergence accom-

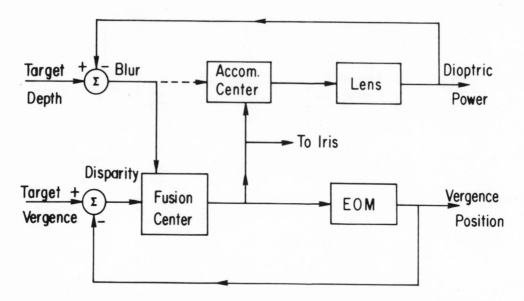

FIGURE 9.   Organizational structure of near triad processes based on the Fincham theory of synkinesis. Dashed line indicates functionally unimportant pathway.

modation of sufficient magnitude to produce the desired lens response. During binocular fixation, Fincham predicts that most of the required accommodative response results from convergence accommodation. The accommodative system is only required to "act as a fine adjustment of accommodation . . ."[12] A neural center for accommodation is presumed to receive both blur and convergence signals and "from the integration of this knowledge determines the necessary innervation to the ciliary muscle".[128] The general arrangement of near triad processes implied by Fincham's theory is shown in Figure 9.

Arguments supporting the concept that disparity-driven components dominate near triad motor responses have been summarized by Crone.[4] In addition to the fact that CA/C ratios generally exceed AC/A ratios, the response latency of disparity-driven movements is less than blur-driven movements. Finally, the disparity stimulus is more accurate and without the direction ambiguity of blur. Unfortunately, the Fincham theory of near triad synkinesis has not been as extensively developed as the Maddox/Alpern theory.

B. Dual Interaction Theory

A theory of near triad synkinesis which includes two separate functional interactive processes and provides a partial resolution of the question of stimulus dominance has recently been proposed and developed by Semmlow, Jaeger, and Hung.[129-131] As mentioned in the preceeding section (IV-B-2), a quantitative comparison of blur and disparity components in the binocular response showed a linear addition of the two components during much of the movement.[109] However, during the late and posttransient period, the combined response was less than the sum of the two isolated components (Figure 7). The Maddox/Alpern theory, in assigning the primary maintenance of steady fixation to accommodative convergence, requires a posttransient readjustment of disparity vergence, since this component clearly dominates the initial dynamic response. Fincham's theory is compatible with the initial and final values of the response, but cannot explain the blur contribution during midresponse.

The implications of this experiment led us to conjecture that both blur and disparity

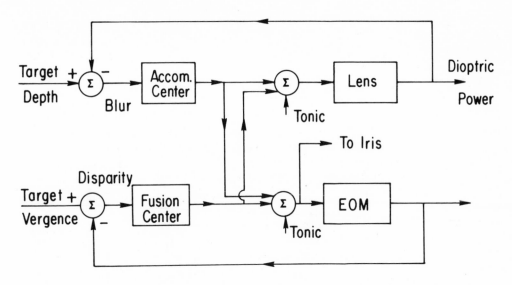

FIGURE 10. Organizational structure of near triad components featuring two separate interactive processes. Modified after Semmlow and Venkiteswaran.[30]

components are significant in near triad responses. Such conjecture leads directly to the structural arrangement shown in Figure 10, in which separate neural centers receiving blur and disparity stimuli each interact with the other system through separate neural pathways. This arrangement evolved from a basic scheme originally proposed by Westheimer[132] and is similar to a more detailed model constructed by Toates.[133] Note that innervation to the iris is in accordance with the findings of Sharkhnovich[108] described in Section III-B-1.

While none of the three theories of binocular synkinesis presented above has been extensively developed, they do provide experimentally verifiable predictions. The next section examines these theories with respect to relevant experimental findings.

VI. EXPERIMENTAL EVIDENCE ON THEORIES OF NEAR TRIAD SYNKINESIS

A. Maddox/Alpern Theory

The Maddox/Alpern theory of near triad synkinesis requires two basic assumptions: (1) accommodative convergence adds algebraically to other vergence components to produce a binocular response; (2) the value of accommodative convergence during binocular fixation is the same as that observed monocularly for the same accommodative stimulus. The most direct support for the first assumption is provided by the shape of the zone of clear single vision. In its usual representation, the horizontal boundaries of the zone depicting maximum and minimum vergence response are assumed to be parallel to the phoria line[26,113] (Figure 2); that is, these vergence limits are related to the phoria position by a positive and negative constant. Assuming that the maximum and minimum attainable magnitude of the disparity component is a constant, or at least independent of accommodative stimulation,[134] then the vergence limits are easily explained as the sum of this component (positive and negative) and the monocular accommodative convergence.[30]

Additional support for the first assumption of the Maddox theory is seen in the fixation disparity experiments (Section IV-A-3) which indicate that the AC/A_s ratio under binocular viewing conditions is similar to that measured monocularly.[36,121] These results indicate that accommodative convergence is an active, additive component of binocular vergence. Finally, the summation of accommodative convergence with other components during dynamic binocular responses is demonstrated in two experiments previously described: the binocular accommodative convergence experiments[30] and the experiments comparing vergence dynamics with and without blur stimulation.[109]

While there exists evidence that the first assumption is correct, there is little support for the second necessary assumption. In fact, evidence reflecting a difference in monocular and binocular accommodative convergence values is indicated by the lack of correspondence between disassociated (monocular) phoria and associated phoria mentioned earlier (Section IV-A-3). These results, coupled with their clinical experience, led Ogle, Martens, and Dryer[121] to conclude that monocular phoria measurements "cannot be presumed to be a measure of the oculomotor imbalance when fusion is maintained".

Further evidence for a difference in monocular and binocular accommodative convergence is seen in recent experiments by Semmlow and Heerema[135] which examined the disparity component during binocular fixation of an orthophoric stimulus (that is, a binocular stimulus in which the vergence requirement was carefully adjusted to exactly equal the monocular response produced by accommodative convergence and tonic components). Under this stimulus condition, the Maddox/Alpern theory predicts the disparity component will be zero since no "supplemental vergence" is necessary. Interruption of binocular fixation produced a slow transient divergence movement followed by an eventual return to the initial position (Figure 11, upper curves). The time characteristic of the slow divergence was identical to a normal fusional decay movement produced by blocking one eye while the subject was strongly over-converged (Figure 11, lower curve of each pair). This led us to conclude that the slow divergence was due to the decay of a nonzero disparity component followed by the even slower return of accommodative convergence to its monocular level. The presence of this fusional component violates a crucial prediction of the Maddox/Alpern theory. We concluded that during binocular fixation, the fusional component is always greater than, and the accommodative convergence component correspondingly less than, indicated by the Maddox/Alpern theory and traditional measurements of monocular accommodative convergence. This finding explains the difference between associated and disassociated phorias mentioned previously.

B. Fincham Theory

Fincham's theory differs from that of Maddox/Alpern theory in that disparity is considered the dominant stimulus and only a single interactive process exists. This latter feature implies some behavioral characteristics which can be experimentally verified. Specifically, AC/A_s and CA/C ratios should be reciprocally related in any given subject. Also, it should be impossible for accommodative convergence and convergence accommodation to maintain different values at the same time, since they are two manifestations of the same interactive process.

Most available data suggests that the first prediction is not true. Fincham himself reports CA/C ratios of around 1 dio/meter angle for younger people[12] as opposed to AC/A_s ratios around 0.7MA/dio.[136] However, experimental errors in measuring the two ratios (particularly the CA/C) make it impractical to use existing data as a conclusive test of Fincham's theory.

An experiment described previously, originally designed to investigate the blur at high-disparity stimulus levels, provides a formal test of the second prediction of Fincham's theory,[116] that accommodative convergence and convergence accommodation are the result of a single process. The basic approach consists simply of measuring the accommodative convergence component when a subject is strongly overconverged. Un-

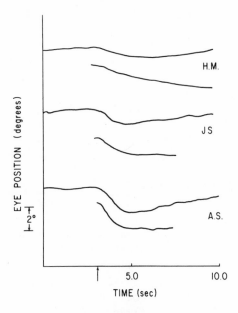

FIGURE 11. Averaged response of the right eye in three subjects to the interruption of binocular vision. In the upper curves of each pair, the initial binocular stimulus was identical to the monocular phoria (accommodative convergence and tonic components). The lower responses are produced when the initial stimulus required strong overconvergence.[135] (Lower curves scaled down.)

der these circumstances, convergence accommodation will increase and, as described in Section IV-A-2, will lend to an increase in the dioptric power of the lens. If only a single interactive process exists, accommodative convergence must necessarily follow the increase in convergence accommodation. Yet, the results of Figure 4 were interpreted as demonstrating a decreased accomodative convergence component under these conditions. Accordingly, accommodative vergence and convergence accommodation must be mediated by separate interactive processes supported by distinct neural mechanisms, and a fundamental prediction of Fincham's theory has been experimentally disproven.

C. Dual Interaction Theory

The experimental evidence used to refute the Maddox/Alpern and Fincham theory can be used in support of the Dual Interaction theory outlined in Figure 10. In fact, the configuration shown in Figure 10 is the simplest arrangement of near triad elements which is consistant with the evidence cited above.

Additional support for the Dual Interaction Theory comes from experiments which simultaneously measure both accommodation and vergence responses to isolated blur or disparity stimulation. Measuring lens and accommodative vergence dynamic response to step changes in blur stimulation, Wilson[101] found "close coupling" between the two, indicating that much of the central neural control is shared by the two motor responses. When these same responses are evoked by disparity stimulation, Krishman et al.[111] also found a similarity in the dynamic response features, implying these near triad responses were mediated by a common neural center. These were done on isolated systems. Taken together, they imply common central mechanisms for both blur-driven responses and disparity-driven responses.

The Dual Interaction Theory predicts certain behavioral features which may be experimentally verified. In particular, since separate neural centers and interactive pathways are assumed, the errors seen in relative responses (Section IV-A) should be due, in part, to an inhibiting interaction between the two systems. For example, the fixation disparity observed in relative vergence responses should be enhanced by effort on the part of the accommodative system to maintain a constant output in the face of increasing convergence accommodation. That is, as relative vergence response increases, so does the associated convergence accommodation. Since accommodative stimulation is traditionally held constant during this measurement, blur-driven components, including accommodative convergence, should decrease to compensate for the increased disparity lens drive. A decrease in accommodative convergence will oppose the ongoing fusional effort causing larger relative response errors. Thus, the Dual Interaction Theory predicts that relative response error will be reduced if interaction with the other system is eliminated. In the case of fixation disparity (relative disparity vergence error), lower values should be observed if the accommodative system is made open-loop.

Semmlow and Hung have recently completed an experiment comparing fixation disparity curves with the accommodation system open and closed-loop.[137] The open-loop accommodation values were obtained simply by having subjects view a standard fixation disparity target through an optical pinhole. Results presented in Figure 5 show a substantial reduction in fixation disparity when accommodation is open-loop (dashed curve). Hence, normal fixation disparity measurements contain components related to the accommodative feedback system as predicted by the Dual Interaction Theory. This may explain the observation by Shor[126] that fixation disparities are influenced by factors unrelated to disparity adaptation (Section IV-A-3), factors which are external to the isolated disparity vergence control system.

By similar arguments, errors in the accommodation response should be less when interaction with the disparity system is eliminated as in monocular vision. However, experiments have not been done to specifically test this prediction of the Dual Interaction Theory.

VII. SUMMARY

All motor responses of the near triad are composed of reflexive components driven by blur and disparity stimulation. Additionally, vergence responses are influenced by proximal stimuli (a subconscious estimate of target distance) and may be elicited by voluntary effort. The effectiveness of these latter inputs on lens responses is controversial.

The behavior of isolated near triad motor responses to blur and disparity has been quantitively documented for both fixed and transient stimuli. Systems models have been developed for disparity vergence, blur accommodation, and blur vergence, many of them evaluated by computer simulation.

Under binocular viewing conditions, the static responses of vergence and accommodation have been studied with emphasis on response range (the zone of clear single vision) and response error (relative response) under various stimulus combinations. Since binocular responses are the result of multiple components, these studies provide little information on the principles underlying near triad control. Mutual interactions between the major feedback control systems make it difficult to infer binocular roles from studies on isolated systems, and the inability to measure internal states during a binocular response has resulted in continued confusion and conjecture on questions regarding basic control strategy and general organization.

A few recent experiments shed some light on the internal states of triad components. These experiments essentially utilize the difference in dynamics between blur-driven and disparity-driven components to expose the binocular activity of these internal components. Experimental results indicate that both blur and disparity components share in the maintenance of steady state lens and vergence responses though the disparity component dominates the transient response. These results support a basic organizational structure of near triad components termed the "Dual Interaction Theory" in which the control is mediated by two distinct feedback systems. Though each is capable of independent operation, they mutually interact during a binocular response through two separate neural linkages.

Though primative and undeveloped, the Dual Interactive Theory does provide predictions which may be experimentally verified. One prediction, that relative response errors are dependent on components in both feedback systems, has been demonstrated experimentally, at least for vergence responses. Other predictions await experimental testing. Finally, the Dual Interaction Theory provides an organizational framework for the vast amount of experimental evidence cited in this Chapter. This framework should serve as a stimulus for renewed efforts in modeling near triad responses. In fact, this overview of a rich observational and experimental history suggests a comprehensive quantative model capable of computer simulation as an essential next step to furthering our understanding of this complex oculomotor response.

REFERENCES

1. Herring, E., On the Motives of Eye Movement, in *The Theory of Binocular Vision,* (transl.), Bridgeman, B. and Stark, L., Eds., Plenum Press, N.Y., 1977.
2. Carpenter, R. H. S., *Movement of the Eyes,* Pion Ltd., London, 1977.
3. Toates, F. M., Accommodation function of the human eye, *Physiol. Rev.,* 52, 828, 1972.
4. Crone, R. A., *Diplopia,* American Elsevier, New York, 1973.
5. Potterfield, W. A., *A Treatise on the Eye,* Vol. 1, Edinburgh, 1759, 410.
6. Helmholtz, H., Movements of the Eye, in *Physiological Optics,* Vol. 3, (transl.), Dover Press, New York, 1962.
7. Müller, J., *Elements of Physiology,* Vol. 2, (transl.), Taylor, W. and Walton, J., London, 207, 1842.
8. Bridgeman, B., Introduction, in *The Theory of Binocular Vision,* by E. Herring, Plenum Press, New York, 1977.
9. Donders, F. C., *On the Amomalies of Accommodation and Refraction of the Eye: With a Preliminary Essay on Physiological Dioptrics,* (transl.), New Syderham Soc., London, 1864.
10. Volkmann, A. W., Neue Beiträge zeu Physiologie des Gesichtsinnes, 1836.
11. Maddox, E., Investigations on the relationship between convergence and accommodation of the eyes, *J. Anat.,* 20, 475, 1886.
12. Fincham, E. F. and Walton, J., The reciprocal actions of accommodation and convergence, *J. Physiol. (London),* 137, 488, 1957.
13. Allen, M. J., The stimulus to accommodation, *Am. J. Optom,* 32, 422, 1955.
14. Stark, L. and Takahashi, Y., Absence of an odd-error signal mechanism in human accommodation, *IEEE Trans. Biomed. Eng.,* BME-12, 138, 1965.
15. Troelstra, A., Zuber, B. L., Miller, D., and Stark, L., Accommodative tracking: a trial-and-error function, *Vision Res.,* 4, 585, 1964.
16. Campbell, F. W. and Westheimer, G., Factors influencing accommodation responses of the human eye, *J. Optom. Soc. Am.,* 49, 568, 1959.
17. Fincham, E. F., The accommodation reflex and its stimulus, *Br. J. Ophthalmol.,* 35, 381, 1951.
18. Phillips, S. and Stark, L., Blur: a sufficient accommodative stimulus, *Doc. Ophthalmol.,* 43, 65, 1977.
19. Marg, E., An investigation of voluntary as distinguished from reflex accommodation, *Am. J. Optom. Arch. Am. Acad. Optom.,* 28, 347, 1951.

20. Ripps, H., Chin, N. B., Siegel, I. M., and Breinen, G. M., Effect of pupil size on accommodation, convergence, and the AC/A ratio, *Invest. Ophthalmol.*, 1, 127, 1962.
21. Semmlow, J., Hansmann, D., and Stark, L., Variation in pupillomotor responsiveness with mean pupil size, *Vision Res.*, 15, 85, 1975.
22. Lowenstein, O. and Loewenfeld, I. E. The Pupil, in *The Eye,* Vol. 3, Davson, H., Ed., Academic Press, New York, 1962, 231.
23. Whiteside, T. D. C., The Relation of the Effectiveness of a Stimulus at the Fair Point to its Angular Distance from the Fovea, in *The Problem of Vision in Flight at High Altitude,* Butterworths, London, 1957.
24. Semmlow, J. and Tinor, T., Accommodative convergence response to off-foveal retinal images, *J. Opt. Soc. Am.*, 68, 1497, 1978.
25. Rashbass, C. and Westheimer, G., Disjunctive eye movements, *J. Physiol. (London),* 339, 1961.
26. Alpern, M., Types of Movement, in *The Eye,* Vol. 3, 2nd ed., Davson, H., Ed., 65, Academic Press, New York, 1969.
27. Barlow, H., Blakemore, C., and Pettigrew, J., The neural mechanism of binocular depth discrimination, *J. Physiol. (London),* 193, 327, 1967.
28. Bishop, P. O., Henry, G. H., and Smith, C. J., Binocular interaction fields of single units in the cat striate cortex, *J. Physiol. (London),* 216, 39, 1971.
29. Toates, F. M., Vergence Eye Movements, *Doc. Ophthalmol.,* 37, 153, 1974.
30. Semmlow, J. L. and Venkiteswaran, N., Dynamic accommodative vergence in binocular vision, *Vision Res.,* 16, 403, 1976.
31. Itlelson, W. H. and Ames, A., Accommodation, convergence and their relation to apparent distance, *J. Psychol.,* 30, 43, 1950.
32. Hoffstetter, H. W., Proximal factor in accommodation and convergence, *Am. J. Optom. Arch. Am. Acad. Optom.,* 19, 67, 1942.
33. Alpern, M., Vergence and accommodation. I. Can change in size induce vergence movements, *AMA Arch. Ophthalmol.,* 60, 355, 1958.
34. Morgan, M., Accommodation and vergence, *Am. J. Optom. Arch. Am. Acad. Optom.,* 45, 417, 1968.
35. Knoll, H. A., Proximal factors in convergence, *Am. J. Optom. Arch. Am. Acad. Optom.,* 36, 378, 1959.
36. Ogle, K. N. and Martens, T. G., On the accommodative convergence and the proximal vergence, *AMA Arch. Ophthalmol.,* 51, 702, 1957.
37. Alpern, M., Testing distance effect on phoria measurement at various accommodation levels, *AMA Arch. Ophthalmol.,* 54, 906, 1955.
38. Morgan, M., A comparison of clinical methods of measuring accommodative convergence, *Am. J. Optom.,* 27, 385, 1950.
39. Fincham, E. F., Factors controlling ocular accommodation, *Br. Med. Bull.,* 9, 18, 1953.
40. Lowenstein, O., The Argyll Robertson Pupillary Syndrome: mechanism and localization, *Am. J. Ophthalmol.,* 42, 105, 1956.
41. Bender, M. B. and Weinstein, E. A., Functional representation in the oculomotor and trochlear nuclei, *Arch. Neurol. Psychiatr.,* 49, 98, 1953.
42. Crosby, F. C. and Woodburne, R. T., The nuclear pattern of the nontectal portions of the midbrain and the isthmus in primates, *J. Comp. Neurol.,* 78, 441, 1943.
43. Warwick, R., The so-called nucleus of convergence, *Brain,* 78, 92, 1955.
44. Jampel, R. S., Representation of the near-response on the cerebral cortex of the macaque, *Am. J. Ophthalmol.,* 48, 573, 1959.
45. Bender, M. B. and Shanzer, S., Oculomotor Pathways Defined by Electric Stimulation and Lesions in the Brain Stem of Monkey, in *The Oculomotor System,* Bender, M., Ed., Harper & Row, New York, 1964, 81.
46. Fincham, E. F., The function of the lens capsule in the accommodation of the eye, *Trans. Optom. Soc. London,* 30, 101, 1928.
47. Fisher, R. F., Elastic constants of the human lens capsule, *J. Physiol. (London),* 201, 1969.
48. O'Neill, W. and Doyle, J. M,. A thin shell deformation analysis of the human lens, *Vision Res.,* 8, 193, 1968.
49. Henderson, T., The anatomy and physiology of accommodation in mammolia, *Trans. Ophthalmol. Soc. U. K.* 46, 280, 1926.
50. Cogen, D. G., Accommodation and the autonomic nervous system, *Arch. Ophthalmol.,* 18, 739, 1937.
51. Wolff, E., Discussion of a paper by T. Henderson, *Trans. Ophthalmol. Soc. U.K.,* 72, 538, 1952.
52. Fisher, R. F., The significance of the shape of the lens and capsular energy changes in accommodation, *J. Physiol. (London),* 201, 21, 1969.

53. Duane, A., Are the current theories of accommodation correct?, *Am. J. Ophthalmol.*, 8, 196, 1925.
54. Alpern, M., Accommodation: Evaluation of Theories of Presbyopia, in *The Eye*, Vol. 3, 1st ed. Davson, H., Ed., Academic Press, New York, 1962.
55. Morgan, M. W., The ciliary body in accommodation and accommodative convergence, *Am. J. Optom. Arch. Am. Acad. Optom.*, 31, 219, 1954.
56. O'Neill, W. D., Sanathanan, C. K., and Bradkey, J. S., A minimum varience time optimal, control system model of human lens accommodation, *IEEE Trans. Syst. Sci. Cybern.*, SSC-5, 290, 1969.
57. Fischer, R. F., Elastic constants of the human lens capsule, *J. Physiol. (London)*, 201, 1, 1969.
58. Tompson, H., The Dynamics of Accommodation in Primates, Ph.D. thesis, University of Illinois Medical Center, 1975.
59. Lowenstein, O. and Loewenfeld, I., Influence of retinal adaptation upon pupillary reflex to light in normal man, I, *Am. J. Ophthalmol.*, 48, 536, 1958.
60. Loewenfeld, I., Mechanisms of reflex dilation of the pupil. Historical review and experimental analysis, *Doc. Ophthalmol.*, 12, 185, 1958.
61. Seybold, W. D. and Moore, R. M., Oculormotor nerve and reflex dialation of pupil, *J. Neurophysiol.*, 3, 463, 1940.
62. Apter, J. T., Studies on the autonomic innervations of iris, *Am. J. Ophthalmol.*, 42, 122, 1956.
63. Lowenstein, O. and Loewenfeld, I., Role of sympathetic and parasympathetic systems in reflex dilation of the pupil, *Arch. Neurol. Psychiatr.*, 64, 313, 1950.
64. Semmlow, J. and Stark, L., Simulation of a biomedical model of the human pupil, *Math. Biosci.*, 11, 109, 1971.
65. Hansmann, D., Semmlow, J., and Stark, L., A Physiologial Basis of Pupillary Dynamics, in *Pupillary Dynamics and Behavior*, Janisse, M., Ed., Plenum Press, New York, 1974, 39.
66. Semmlow, J. and Stark, L., Pupil movements to light and accommodative stimulation: a comparative study, *Vision Res.*, 13, 1087, 1973.
67. Semmlow, J. and Chen, D., A simulation model of the human pupil light reflex, *Math. Biosci.*, 33, 5, 1977.
68. Rashbass, C. and Westheimer, G., Independence of conjurgate and disjunctive eye movements, *J. Physiol. (London)*, 159, 361, 1961.
69. Alpern, M. and Wolter, J. R., The relation of horizontal saccadic and vergence movements, *Arch. Ophthalmol.*, 56, 658, 1956.
70. Breinin, G. M., The structure and function of extraocular muscle. An appraisal of the duality concept, *Am. J. Ophthalmol.*, 72, 1, 1971.
71. Thomas, J. G., The torque-angle transfer function of the human eye, *Kybernetik*, 3, 254, 1967.
72. Cook, G. and Stark, L., Derivation of a model for the human eye-positioning mechanism, *Bull. Math. Biophys.*, 29, 153, 1967.
73. Bahill, A. T. and Stark, L., The trajectories of saccadic eye movements, *Sci. Am.*, 240, 108, 1979.
74. Robinson, D. A., Models of the saccadic eye movement control system, *Kybernetik,*, 14, 71, 1973.
75. Collins, C., Orbital Mechanics, in *Control of Eye Movements*, Bach-y-Rita, P., Collins, C., and Hyde, J., Eds., Academic Press, New York, 283, 1971.
76. Clark, M. and Stark, L., Time optimal behavior of human saccadic eye movement, *IEEE Trans. Auto. Cnt.*, AC-20, 345, 1975.
77. Semmlow, J. and Venkiteswaran, N., Comparison of disparity vergence dynamics with accommodation open and closed loop, unpublished experiments.
78. Stark, L., Environmental damping of biological systems: pupil servomechanism, *J. Optom. Soc. Am.*, 52, 925, 1962.
79. Morgan, M. and Olmstead, J. H. D., Quantative measurements of relative accommodation and relative convergence, *Proc. Soc. Exp. Biol. Med.*, 41, 303, 1939.
80. Heath, G. G., The influence of visual activity on accommodative responses of the eye, *Am. J. Optom. Arch. Am. Acad. Optom.*, 33, 513, 1956.
81. Westheimer, G., Focusing responses of the human eye, *Am. J. Optom. Arch. Am. Acad. Optom.*, 43, 221, 1966.
82. Toates, F. M., A model of accommodation, *Vision Res.*, 10, 1069, 1970.
83. Krishnan, V. V. and Stark, L., Integral control in accommodation, *Comp. Pro. Biomed.*, 4, 237, 1975.
84. Hung, G. and Semmlow, J., Static behavior of Accommodation and Vergence: Computer Simulation of an Interactive Dual Feedback System, *IIEE Trans. Biomed. Eng.*, BME-27, 439, 1980.
85. Heath, G. The influence of visual acuity on accommodative responses of the eye, *Am. J. Optom. Arch. Am. Acad. Optom.*, 33, 513, 1956.
86. Alpern, M., Variability of accommodation during steady fixation at various levels of illuminance, *J. Optom. Soc. Am.*, 48, 193, 1958.

87. **Morgan, M.,** The resting state of accommodation, *Am. J. Optom. Arch. Am. Acad. Optom.,* 34, 347, 1957.

88. **Heath, G.,** Components of accommodation, *Am. J. Optom. Arch Am. Acad. Optom.,* 33, 569, 1956.

89. **Campbell, F. W. and Primrose, J. A. C.,** The state of accommodation of the human eye in darkness, *Trans. Ophthalmol. Soc. U.K.,* 73, 353, 1953.

90. **Campbell, F. W., Robson, J. G., and Westheimer, G.,** Fluctuations of accommodation under steady viewing conditions, *J. Physiol. (London),* 145, 579, 1959.

91. **Morgan, M.,** Accommodation and its relationship to convergence, *Am. J. Optom. Arch. Am. Acad. Optom.,* 21, 183, 1944.

92. **Alpern, M., Kincaid, W., and Lubeck, M.,** Vergence and accommodation. III. Preposed definitions of the AC/A ratios, *Am. J. Ophthalmol.,* 48, 143, 1959.

93. **Flom, M. C.,** On the relationship between accommodation and accommodative convergence, *Am. J. Optom. Arch. Am. Acad. Optom.,* 37, 517, 1960.

94. **Marg, E. and Morgan, M.,** The pupillary near reflex: the relation of pupillary diameter to accommodation and the various elements of convergence, *Am. J. Optom. Arch. Am. Acad. Optom,.* 26, 183, 1949.

95. **Kirchhof, H.,** A Method for the Objective Measurement of Accommodation Speed of the Human Eye, (transl.), *Am. J. Optom. Arch. Am. Acad. Optom.,* 27, 163, 1950.

96. **Campbell, F. W. and Westheimer, G.,** Dynamics of accommodation responses of the human eye, *J. Physiol. (London),* 151, 285, 1960.

97. **Phillips, S., Shirachi, D., and Stark, L.,** Analysis of accommodation response times using histogram information, *Am. J. Optom. Arch. Am. Acad. Optom.,* 49, 389, 1972.

98. **Carter, J. H.,** A servoanalysis of the human accommodative mechanism,. *Arch. Soc. Am. Ophthalmol. Optom.,* 4, 137, 1962.

99. **Stark, L. Takohoshi, Y., and Zmes, G.,** Nonlinear servoanalysis of human lens accommodation, *IEEE Trans. Syst. Sci. Cybern.,* SSC-1, 75, 1965.

100. **Krishnan, V. Y., Phillips, S., and Stark, L.,** Frequency analysis of accommodation, accomodive vergence and disparity vergence, *Vision Res.,* 13, 1545, 1973.

101. **Wilson, D.,** A centre for accommodative vergence motor control, *Vision Res.,* 13, 2491, 1973.

102. **Brodkey, J. and Stark, L.,** Accommodative Convergence -- an adaptive nonlinear control system, *IEEE Trans. Syst. Sci. Cybern.,* SSC-3r, 121, 1967.

103. **Zuber, B.,** Control of Vergence Eye Movements, in *The Control of Eye Movements,* Bach-y-Rita, P., Collins, C., and Hyde, J., Eds., Academic Press, New York, 1971, 447.

104. **Kent, P. R.,** Convergence-accommodation, *Am. J. Optom. Arch. Am. Acad. Optom.,* 35, 393, 1958.

105. **Hansmann, D.** Human Pupillary Mechanics: Physiology and Control, Ph.D. thesis, University of California, Berkeley, 1972.

106. **Backer, W. D. and Ogle, K. N.,** Pupillary response to fusional eye movements, *Am. J. Ophtholmol.,* 58, 743, 1964.

107. **Knoll, H. A.,** Pupillary changes associated with accommodation and convergence, *Am. J. Optom. Arch. Am. Acad. Optom.,* 26, 346, 1949.

108. **Sharkhnovich, A. R.,** Convergent Eye Movements, in *The Brain and Regulation of Eye Movements,* (Transl.), Plenum Press, New York, 1977.

109. **Semmlow, J. L. and Wetzel, F.,** Dynamic contributions of binocular vergence components, *J. Optom. Soc. Am.,* 69, 639, 1979.

110. **Zuber, B. and Stark, L.,** Dynamical characteristics of the fusional vergence eye-movement system, *IEEE Trans. Syst. Sci. Cybern.,* SSC-4, 72, 1968.

111. **Krishnan, V. V., Shirachi, D., and Stark, L.,** Dynamic measures of vergence accommodation, *Am. J. Optom. Physiol. Optom.,* 54, 470, 1977.

112. **Landolt, E.** Refractions and Accommodations of the Eye, (Transl.), Edinburgh, 1886.

113. **Balsam, M. H. and Fry, G. A.,** Convergence-accommodation, *Am. J. Optom. Arch. Am. Acad. Optom.,* 36, 567, 1959.

114. **Holfstetter, H. W.,** The zone of clear single binocular vision, *Am. J. Optom. Arch. Am. Acad. Optom.,* 22, 301, 1945.

115. **Alpern, M.,** The zone of clear single vision at the upper limits of accommodation and convergence, *Am. J. Optom. Arch. Am. Acad. of Optom.,* 27, 491, 1950.

116. **Semmlow, J. L. and Heerema, D.,** The role of accommodative convergence at the limits of fusional vergence, *Invest. Ophthalmol.,* 18, 970, 1979.

117. **Hofman, F. B. and Bielschowsky, A.,** Über die der Willkür Entzogenen Fusions-bewegungen der Augen, *Pflüg Arch. Physiol.,* 80, 1, 1900.

118. **Lau, E.,** Neue Untersuchungen über des Tiefen-und Ebenensehen, *Z. Psychol. Physiol. Sinnesorg. Abt. II,* 53, 1, 1921.

119. Lewin, K. and Sakuma, K., Die Sehrichtung Monokularer und Binokularer Objekte bei Bewegung und das Zustandekommen des Tiefeneffektes, *Physiol. Forsch.*, 6, 298, 1924-1925.

120. Ames, A. and Gliddon, G. H., Ocular Measurements, *Trans. Sec. Ophthalmol., A. M. A.*, 102, 1928.

121. Ogle, K. N., Martens, T. G., and Dyer, J. A., *Oculomotor Imbalance in Binocular Vision and Fixation Disparity,* Lear and Febigier, Philadelphia, 1967.

122. Ogle, K. N., *Binocular Vision,* Hafner, New York, 1964.

123. Ogle, K. N. and Prangen, A. de H., Further considerations of fixation disparity and the binocular fusion process, *Am. J. Ophthalmol.,* 34, 57, 1951.

124. Riggs, L. A., Discussion on the paper by K. N. Ogle, in *The Oculomotor System,* Bender, M., Ed., Hoeber Medical Div., Harper and Row, N.Y., 1964, 351.

125. Mitchell, A. M. and Ellerbrock, V. J., Fixation disparity and the maintenance of fusion in the horizontal meridian, *Am. J. Optom. Arch. Am. Acad. Optom.,* 32, 520, 1955.

126. Schor, C., Influence of rapid prism adaptation upon fixation disparity, *Vision Res.,* 19, 757, 1979.

127. Alpern, M., Does relative accommodation exist?, *Am. J. Optom,,* 43, 1957.

128. Fincham, E., Accommodation and convergence in the absense of retinal images, *Vision Res.,* 1, 425, 1962.

129. Semmlow, J. and Jaeger, R., Modelling the visual motor triad: an example of a multiple input-output biocontrol system, Proc. 25th ACEMB, Bal Harbor, Florida, 1972, 23.

130. Semmlow, J., and Hung, G., Binocular interactions of vergence components, *Am. J. Optom. Physiol. Optom.,* 57, 559, 1980.

131. Semmlow, J. and Hung, G., Experimental evidence for the independence of accommodative convergence and convergence accommodation, submitted.

132. Westheimer, G., Amphetamine barbituates and accommodative convergence, *Arch. Ophthalmol.,* 70, 830, 1963.

133. Toates, F. M., Accommodation and convergence in the human eye, *Trans. Inst. Meas. Contl.,* 2, 29, 1969.

134. Fry, G., Further experiments on the accommodative convergence relationship , *Am. J. Optom. Arch. Am. Acad. Optom.,* 16, 325, 1939.

135. Semmlow, J. and Heerema, D., The synkinetic interaction of convergence accommodation and accommodative convergence, *Vision Res.,* 19, 1237, 1979.

136. Morgan, M. and Peters, H., Accommodative convergence in presbyopia, *Am. J. Optom.,* 28, 3, 1951.

137. Semmlow, J. and Hung, G., Accommodative and fusional components of fixation disparity, *Invest. Ophthalmol.,* 18, 1082, 1979.

Chapter 10

EYE MOVEMENT DETERMINANTS OF READING RATE

B. L. Zuber and Paul A. Wetzel

TABLE OF CONTENTS

I. INTRODUCTION

The observation of eye movements during reading, and the utilization of these observations as a quantitative tool in reading research, have a long and distinguished history. Since the nineteenth century, Javal[1], Huey[2], Tinker,[3] and Taylor[4] are but a few of the researchers who have produced significant contributions to our understanding of this component of the reading process. A recent renewed interest in reading eye movements has taken place within the context of progress along a number of fronts. Eye movement monitoring techniques have improved in accuracy, ease of use, and general level of sophistication. Digital computers can be used to analyze data and control experiments, and, finally, our understanding of oculomotor behavior and control has made giant strides at all levels. This is crucial if we are to ultimately separate purely motor-based phenomena from the cognitive-based aspects of the reading process.

Eye movements are the only immediately available, objective, physiological manifestation of reading. It is clear that the parameters of these movements reflect, to an extent as yet not fully understood, the underlying information processing that occurs during reading. To approach an understanding of reading, we must begin to understand the nature of this information processing.

A. The Reading Eye Movement Pattern

The interesting "stop-and-go" or "staircase" pattern of eye movement utilized in reading was first observed nearly 100 years ago. A typical pattern of eye movements recorded during reading is shown in Figure 1. This pattern is deceptively simple. A series of "forward" or left-to-right eye movements (rapid saccadic eye movements) carries the eye across the line. Between each pair of forward movements the eye pauses, nominally for about 0.25 sec. Evidence at hand overwhelmingly indicates that it is during these fixation pauses that information processing occurs (Abrams and Zuber).[5] Occasionally, the eye makes a small regressive or right-to-left movement as indicated in the pattern. Although the information-processing implications of these regressions are not entirely clear, it has historically been assumed that the eye returns, by means of regression, for a "better look" at some segment of the line. Notice that regressions, like forward movements, are preceded and followed by fixation pauses. At the end of the line, a large right-to-left saccadic movement (return sweep) carries the point of fixation back to the beginning of the next line. At this point the process begins all over again.

When the pattern in Figure 1 is considered from an information processing point of view, the simplicity disappears very quickly. The pattern exhibits interesting spatial and temporal characteristics which, in fact, form the basis of our analysis. Although we can delineate clear spatial and temporal parameters, it is unquestionably true that these parameters are interrelated.

In a superficial sense, at least, the *temporal* processing of information during reading seems to be discrete, as indicated by a series of sequential fixation pauses. The duration of the fixation pause is a temporal parameter of prime importance for our analysis. Since about 90% of the time spent reading is spent fixating, it is clear that fixation pause duration plays a crucial role in determining such performance measures as reading speed (or rate). For some time, however, it has been less clear that performance improvements are directly attributable to systematic decreases in fixation pause durations. Change in this parameter elicited by experiment, or even conventional reading improvement training, tend to be less dramatic than changes in other parameters associated with the reading pattern (Ahlen, et al.).[6] Still, it seems clear that the duration of the fixation pause is related to the amount of text information processed during a fixation. During the fixation pause, both position information (i.e., where to move next) and text information are processed. If the area surrounding the point of fixation contains a reduced amount of text information (such as a deliberately placed blank area in the text), the duration of the fixation pause is significantly reduced (Abrams and Zuber).[5]

The nature of the pattern in Figure 1 provides us with some preliminary notions regarding the spatial aspects of information processing during reading. Given the normal decrease in acuity with distance from the fovea, it follows that, in any given fixation, the spatial extent of information processing will be limited. In other words, there will be a limited area (or span) surrounding the point of fixation over which text information will be processed. It is tempting to speculate that the size, and thus the number, of forward saccades will be related to the size of the span utilized in reading. Hence, in an attempt to understand the spatial aspects of information processing during reading, a variable of primary interest has been the size and number of forward saccadic movements. Of course, the occurrence of regressions also has important implications for the nature of spatial processing. It is interesting that these spatial variables appear to provide the plasticity required for changes in performance measures. In conventional reading improvement instruction, attempts are typically made to increase the size of the span used by the reader. The reasoning behind this is roughly as follows: increasing the size of the span increases the size of forward eye movements and decreases the number of such movements. Any saccadic movement in reading, whether forward or regressive, may be thought of as having a fixation pause associated with it. (Note that herein lies a crucial interaction between spatial and temporal parameters.) If the number of movements can be decreased, e.g., by increasing span size, reading time can be significantly shortened due to a decrease in the number of fixation pauses. The significance of this strategy becomes apparent when one considers that a typical line of print may be read with, say, six forward movements. The elimination of one of these movements — with its associated fixation pause — would reduce the processing time for the line by about 17%.

It is clear from the above that reading proceeds by means of information processing occurring simultaneously both in space and time. Both spatial and temporal aspects of this processing are reflected in the pattern of eye movements accompanying reading. Our research strategy, then, involves the careful quantitative measurement of spatial and temporal parameters of the reading eye movement pattern (output). In defining an input or independent variable for our experiments, we typically attempt to manipulate or control text characteristics, again either in terms of space, time, or information content.

B. Definition of the Input

One of the serious problems in reading research arises from the general unavailability of well-defined, canonical inputs. This situation can be attributed to the complexity of the language and from our inability to quantify the information content of language samples. The result is in some cases a lack of reproducibility, and in many cases, at least the suspicion that the conclusions of experimental studies are based on the specific language samples selected by the experimenter. Coleman,[7] among others, has emphasized that the results of studies on reading or verbal behavior are often of limited generality because they are specific to the language materials used in the study. In response, Miller and Coleman[8] developed a set of 36 prose passages ranging in difficulty from first-grade material to the most difficult technical prose. These were ranked on a scale of difficulty using three different cloze techniques and measurements from 479 subjects. The result of their study was a series of 36 texts, of graded difficulty,

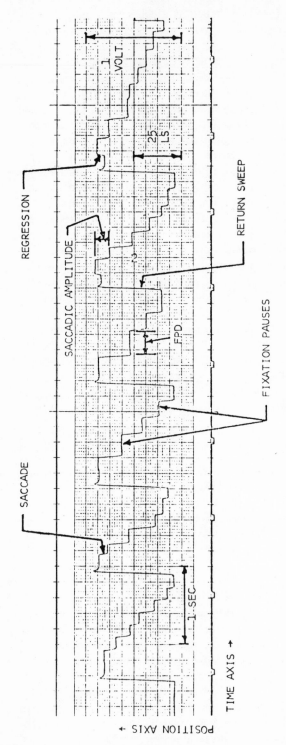

FIGURE 1.   The eye movement pattern recorded during the reading of six lines of text. The left margin of the text corresponds to the top of the trace. FPD - fixation pause duration, the amount of time the eye pauses during a fixation.

each containing 150 words, where the position of each text along the scale of difficulty was based on 2400 responses.

The validity of the original ranking by Miller and Coleman[8] was subsequently tested using different criteria for determining difficulty (Coleman and Miller[9] two additional criteria; Aquino[10] two additional criteria; Sticht[11] one additional criterion). The result of all of this testing has been to leave the original ranking essentially unchanged. Carver[12] did not challenge the difficulty ranking of the Miller-Coleman texts, but did question whether the texts had been ordered for readability. The difficulty/readability controversy is irrelevant for our purposes here, but in the process of answering Carver's objections, Miller and Coleman[13] did make a crucial observation. They found that ". . . reading speed, if measured in . . . letters per second . . . is constant across a range (of difficulty) that extends from first-grade texts to technical prose" (Miller and Coleman[13].) This is a truly compelling observation for it has extremely interesting implications for the nature of information processing in reading. The implication is that there is, somewhere in the information processing network, a rate-setting mechanism with a relatively simple relationship to the printed input medium. An elucidation of this constant-rate mechanism, intriguing in its own right, could well lead us to an understanding of other more complex information processing mechanisms underlying reading.

C. Definition and Statement of the Problem

A firmly entrenched observation in the field of reading is that reading rate in words per minute decreases as the difficulty of material read increases. Not only can this observation be objectively demonstrated, but it also has considerable intuitive appeal.

How does one reconcile the apparent contradiction that arises from one observation indicating a decrease in words per minute with difficulty, and another indicating a rate constancy when rate is measured in units smaller than the word? Consider the hypothetical experiment in which we have a series of texts of graded and quantified difficulty. All of the texts are the same physical length (same number of letters spaces). We ask a subject to read the texts and we measure the time required for reading. Reading rate is then calculated by dividing the number of words in the text by the total reading time. According to the observation of Miller and Coleman,[13] all texts will be read with a constant rate of letter spaces per second, and therefore, total reading time for all texts will be the same. In virtually all techniques for measuring text difficulty, there is a strong positive correlation between difficulty and word length — the more difficult a text, the greater the average word length. This is true of the Miller-Coleman texts, for example. Thus, when the constant reading times measured in this experiment are divided into the number of words, rate will decrease with difficulty because the number of words decreases with difficulty. Although all the texts have the same number of characters, as difficulty increases the words tend to become longer, and therefore fewer in number. The observed decrease in rate can be related exclusively to a physical text characteristic. Another hypothetical example will illustrate the point in a slightly different way. A text of 100 letter spaces (20 words) is read in 5 seconds. We add 100 letter spaces to the text, but the 100 letter spaces consist of 10 words in Case I and 20 words in Case II. The addition of 100 letter spaces adds an increment of 5 seconds to the reading time in both cases, and the rate remains at 20 letter spaces/second. Measured in words/second, the rate increases from 3 in Case I, to 4 in Case II, a 33% increase.

In summary, it is possible to explain contradictory results of rate dependence on difficulty by appealing to an analysis of physical text characteristics. When rate is measured in words per unit time, more difficult texts are read more "slowly" simply because there are fewer words per unit of physical space. As Miller and Coleman[13] and others have pointed out, much of the research on reading speed (where rate is typically measured in words per minute) could profitably bear reexamination, especially research where text difficulty is a variable.

None of the research following up on the observation of rate constancy by Miller and Coleman[13] has led to any contradiction of that original observation. Coke[14] used 90 passages (including 29 of the Miller-Coleman texts) in a study of oral and silent reading rate involving over one hundred subjects. In all of her experiments, subjects read at a constant rate in syllables per minute. When reading rate was measured in words per minute, there was linear decrease with difficulty level. This rate decrease was statistically associated with the average word length in syllables. Using several different tests, including correlation between comprehensability and readability, Coke demonstrated that the constancy of syllable rate was not due to superficial processing, i.e., reading without regard for comprehension.

With the phenomenon of rate constancy reasonably well established, the question we asked was "How are the parameters of the reading eye movement pattern related to rate constancy?" To answer this question, we must first explore the relationship between the eye movement parameters and difficulty level. Once this is done, we may begin to determine the role of reading eye movement parameters in the establishment of reading rate.

II. METHODS

A. Eye Movement Recording

To monitor eye position, we utilize the method of direct reflection of infrared light from the iris-sclera border on both sides of the pupil. An early use of this technique, described by Stark, Vossius, and Young[15] has been modified and improved for use in our laboratory. The basic technique involves collection of infrared light reflected from the front of the eye by two semiconductor light sensors. Each sensor is placed in one arm of a bridge circuit to increase sensitivity to changes in eye position and to decrease sensitivity to noise and thermal effects. In our apparatus, a high-output infrared source emits in the invisible part of the spectrum, and is driven by a high-frequency power source. The light-detecting part of the system incorporates demodulation circuitry to remove the high-frequency carrier. The result is a highly stable and very sensitive eye position monitor which can be utilized in a wide variety of ambient conditions. Normally, only the position of the left eye is monitored.

Major specifications for the system are a sensitivity of 0.1 to 0.4 volts per degree of eye rotation and a response time on the order of a fraction of a millisecond. In a typical recording situation, our resolution is on the order of 0.5 to 1.0 letterspace of text (0.4 degree/letterspace, typical).

The eye movement monitor is mounted on one end of the experimental table and is used in conjunction with a bite board and head rest for head stabilization. The vision of both eyes is totally unobstructed at all times. Calibration is accomplished by asking the subject to fixate a series of targets separated by a predetermined angular (or letterspace) distance.

B. Selection and Presentation of Texts

We used the first 35 Miller-Coleman texts. Each text was truncated to 100 words for use in our experiments, and then analyzed for physical characteristics (e.g., number of words, syllables, characters, and letterspaces).

Texts were typed on translucent white paper (no water mark) using an IBM Selectric element (Prestige Elite, 12 characters per inch). A typical text was typed within a field 45 character spaces wide by 10 single-spaced lines. Texts were left-margin justified only. After typing, the text occupied an area 3.75 (horizontal) × 1.67 (vertical) inches in the center of a 4 × 6 inch piece of paper. These were mounted on the front surface of what is essentially a light box. Texts were uniformly back-illuminated by means of a high-intensity lamp. Calibration patterns were produced, mounted, and illuminated in the same manner, and consist of crosses placed (horizontally) at the left margin, center and right margin, and (vertically) at the top, center, and bottom of the field. A typical calibration pattern, then, consists of nine fixation points.

When mounted for display, the text was 12 inches from the eyes, centered at eye level. The 45 character by 10-line field delineates an area 17.8 × 7.7 degrees of visual angle. Since the number of characters per horizontal inch is constant, we end up with 2.5 letter spaces per degree of visual angle.

The 35 texts, arranged from least difficult (Text 1) to most difficult (Text 35), were divided into five groups of seven texts each. Each subject read two texts randomly selected from each group. Order of text presentation was also randomized.

C. Subjects

Since most of our experiments are aimed at understanding the normal, mature reading process, our subjects are typically drawn from the college student population. Most of these subjects have normal, uncorrected vision, and all are naive subjects for the purpose of the experiment.

D. Data Analysis

Using a PDP 8/I digital computer, we have developed a computer program, RE-MAP (Reading Eye Movement Analysis Program), to analyze eye movement patterns on-line. The analog-to-digital capability of the computer is used to sample the output of our eye movement monitor (a voltage proportional to eye position). As sampling proceeds, the computer then detects eye movements and abstracts and stores the details of the eye movement pattern.

When REMAP is initialized, it enters an interactive mode and requests information from the user. Responding at a video terminal or teletype, the user supplies (and RE-MAP echoes) subject and text identification codes and the letter space distance between extreme points of the calibration pattern. The user then activates the calibration mode. The subject, at this point already in the apparatus, has been instructed to sequentially fixate a series of calibration points. REMAP measures and stores the eye position levels corresponding to each calibration point. Upon termination of calibration, RE-MAP computes an average calibration characteristic, and from this a measure of calibration linearity. The calibration characteristics in volts and letter spaces, along with the quantitative measure of linearity, are then printed on the line printer. With calibration completed, the user displays the text, places REMAP in a "run" mode and instructs the subject to begin reading. In this mode, REMAP searches for eye movements in the incoming data. When it detects a movement it stores the direction (forward saccade or regression) and size (saccadic amplitide) of the movement, and the elapsed time since the last movement (fixation pause duration). By using the return sweep as an end-of-line indicator, REMAP can keep track of the detailed sequence of pauses and movements corresponding to the reading of each line of text. Finally, when RE-MAP senses an end-of-text indicator it terminates data input and enters an analyze-and-print mode.

In this mode, REMAP prints out a line-by-line tabulation of all saccadic amplitudes (forward and regressive) and fixation pause durations. These are printed in the sequence of occurrence, and separated to correspond to each line of text read. Output proceeds with mean saccadic amplitude (forward saccades), mean fixation pause duration, number of fixations, and number of regressions for each line. The last part of the printout is descriptive of the entire text and includes mean and standard deviation for saccadic amplitude and fixation pause duration, number of fixations, number of regressions, total reading time, and the percentage of total reading time spent fixating. When the printout is finished, REMAP returns control to the user, who may recalibrate, proceed with the next text, or terminate.

We have tested REMAP in two ways. Accuracy was tested by comparing machine analysis against analysis by an experienced human, both operating on real data. In our tests, the difference between human and machine analysis was always less than ±5%. Repeatability was tested by having REMAP repeatedly analyze an electronically simulated reading pattern which was recorded on magnetic tape for analysis by REMAP on playback. In this test situation, the variability of results was never greater than ±1.5%.

III. RESULTS

Experimental analysis is designed to measure both reading rate and eye movement parameters as a function of diffculty level. Rate is measured in words per minute (WPM), syllables per minute (SPM), characters per minute (CPM), and letterspaces per minute (LSPM). This latter measure differs from CPM in that it takes into account spaces between words and punctuation, which presumably provide information to the reader. The eye movement parameters measured were (refer to Figure 1)

1. Mean fixation time (MFT) — the average time the eye is stationary between saccadic movements, i.e., the average value for FPD in Figure 1
2. Number of fixations (F) — the average number of pauses
3. Number of regressions (R) — the average number of regressive (right-to-left) saccades
4. Saccadic amplitude (SA) — the average size in letterspaces, of forward (left-to-right) saccades
5. Total reading time (TRT) — the total time required to read the text
6. Percent time (%T) — the percentage of TRT spent fixating

This last parameter (%T) is calculated by dividing the sum of all fixation pause durations (FPD) by TRT and multiplying by 100. This parameter clearly interacts with both MFT and TRT. In several other cases, there are clear interactions between parameters, and these interactions will have to be considered in drawing conclusions from trends in the data.

Measures of rate and eye movement parameters are computed from the reading of a single text at a given difficulty level by an individual subject. We, thus, generate individual data (ten values for each measure of rate and ten values for each eye movement parameter) for each subject across the range of difficulty. When the data are lumped together, we can look at relationships between rate and eye movement parameters as a function of difficulty for the entire population (100 points for each rate measure and a like number of points for each eye movement parameter).

A note is in order here about the scale of difficulty level. In our analysis, this scale is represented as linear, implying a proportionality in the measure of difficulty. In the determination of difficulty by Miller and Coleman and others, no such proportionality is implied or justified. That is, it is clear that text number ten is consistently judged more difficult than text number nine. One may not conclude, however, that text ten is *twice* as difficult as text five. This is a potential problem that will be important only if there are significant and widespread correlations between our dependent variables (rate

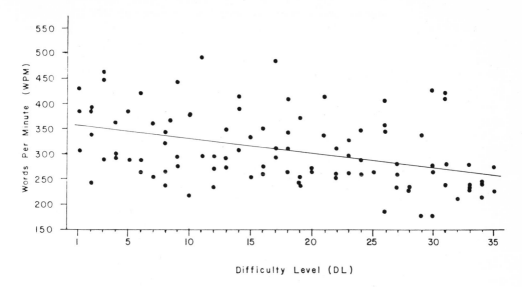

FIGURE 2. The decrease in reading rate (WPM) shows a statistically significant decrease as text difficulty level increases.

and eye movement parameters) and difficulty level, and if one wants to discover the detailed nature of such correlations.

Let us proceed with the results themselves. We will first consider population results and then individual results.

A. Population Results
1. Rate of Reading

Figure 2 is a plot of rate in words per minute vs. difficulty level. The straight line in the field of data is the calculated least squares regression line, and this type of statistic indicates that the relationship between WPM and difficulty level is significant at the 0.05 level. A similar analysis of the data where rate is expressed in LSPM, CPM, and SPM indicates no significant correlation (0.05 level) between any of these measures of rate and difficulty level. Figure 3 represents the population data for LSPM vs. difficulty. Note that although there is considerable spread in the data, the spread is accentuated by use of an expanded scale. The results shown in Figures 2 and 3 are essentially the same as those reported by Coke[14] and Streicher and Zuber.[16] Nine of the ten subjects comprising the population showed significant (0.05 level) decreases in WPM with difficulty level. For the population as a whole, the average decrease in WPM from difficulty level 1 to difficulty level 35 is 91 words per minute. This represents an average decrease of 30% of the overall mean WPM for the population across all difficulty levels. Sixty-five percent of this decrease can be attributed to the decrease in the number of words per text as difficulty level increases. Thus, the majority of the observed decrease in WPM can be attributed to a physical text characteristic, rather than to reading behavior.

2. Eye Movement Parameters

Of the six eye movement parameters we measured, only two showed any significant correlation with difficulty level. F, R, SA, and TRT were uncorrelated with difficulty level. MFT (mean fixation time) and %T (percent time fixation) both showed a slight increase with difficulty which was significant at the 0.05 level. Since %T is derived from MFT, the observed change in %T is no doubt related to the increase in MFT.

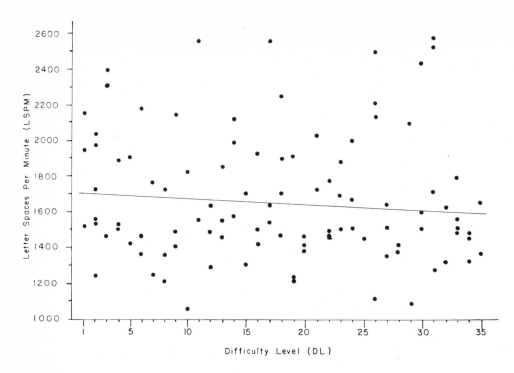

FIGURE 3.   The significant correlation between reading rate and difficulty level is not observed when rate is computed using units smaller than the word. In this case, rate is expressed in letterspaces per minute.

Over the entire range of difficulty, the average increase in MFT was 8% (0.018 sec) of the overall mean MFT for the population. Only three of the ten subjects showed a significant change in MFT with difficulty level. Any change in MFT will have an effect on WPM which can be calculated (Ahlen, et al.[6]) The observed 8% increase in MFT would cause a decrease in WPM of 24 words per minute. Since this is less than one third of the observed change in WPM, it does not significantly influence the observation that the major factor determining WPM is a physical text characteristic, namely, the number of words in the text. A plot of MFT vs. difficulty level appears in Figure 4. The straight line in the figure is the least squares regression line. Again, note that the vertical scale is expanded, with the entire vertical axis representing only 0.130 seconds.

B. Individual Results

In analyzing population results, individual subject data are lumped together in order to determine the influence of difficulty level as an independent variable. The only clear and strong correlation to emerge is that between WPM and difficulty. All other measures of rate and eye movement parameters remain essentially constant over the entire range of difficulty. In approaching the data for individual subjects, we wish to determine to what extent the subjects demonstrate independence from one another. Put another way, to what extent are the constant rate measures and eye movement parameters for a given subject unique to that subject? To test for independence among subjects, we used analysis of variance and t test statistics, again using the 0.05 level of significance as a criterion.

Independence — Reading Rate and Eye Movement Parameters — In this analysis, each subject's measures of rate and eye movement parameters are statistically tested for significant differences from those of all other subjects. For each rate and eye move-

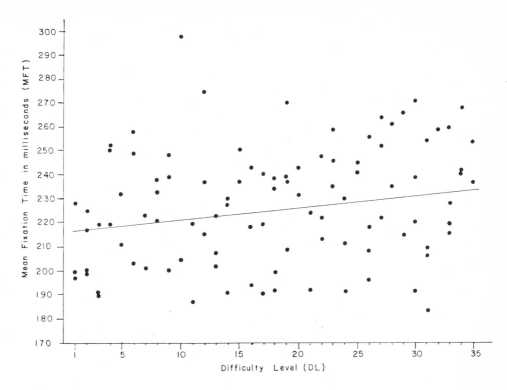

FIGURE 4. Mean fixation time is the only reading eye movement parameter statistically correlated with text difficulty. The overall change in MFT is not large enough to explain the change in WPM with difficulty level.

ment parameter, there are 45 possible comparisons. Figure 5 represents the independence matrix showing the results of all comparisons. Each box in the matrix is subdivided into ten positions. Each position represents either a rate measure or an eye movement parameter. An entry into a given position indicates independence which is statistically significant at the 0.05 level. Thus, when subject one was compared to subject four, only MFT for these two subjects was statistically different. On the other hand, subjects one and seven had statistically different rates and eye movement parameters across the board. A more compact way of looking at independence is to count the total number of cases of independence for each rate and eye movement parameter. These counts are tabulated in Table 1. The highest degree of independence appears in measures rate using units smaller than the word. Of the eye movement paremeters TRT, MFT, F and R show the highest degree of "uniqueness" among subjects. The lowest degree of independence is seen in WPM, SA, and %T, where independence appears only in 44 to 60% of the comparisons.

C. Rate-Determining Eye Movement Parameters

We return to the population results for a final exploration of the relationship between reading rate and eye movement parameters. We have reason to believe that two eye movement parameters — MFT and F — are of primary importance in determining rate of reading (Ahlen, et al.)[6] In order to carry out this analysis, we must first make some modification in our rate measures and eye movement parameters. First, we have converted LSPM to letter spaces per second (LSPS). This is purely for the convenience of dealing with smaller numbers. Second, certain eye movement parameter values are numerically related to text characteristics. F, R, and TRT are proportional to the phys-

SUBJECT NUMBER	1	2	3	4	5	6	7	8	9
2	WPM SPM CPM LSPM TRT F SA R								
3	WPM SPM CPM LSPM MFT TRT F R	SPM LSPM MFT SA							
4	MFT	WPM SPM CPM LSPM TRT F SA R	WPM SPM CPM LSPM MFT TFT F R						
5	MFT F	WPM SPM CPM LSPM %T TRT F SA R	WPM SPM CPM LSPM MFT %T TRT F R						
6	WPM SPM CPM LSPM MFT TRT F SA R	WPM SPM CPM LSPM MFT TRT F SA R		WPM SPM CPM LSPM MFT TRT F SA R	WPM SPM CPM LSPM MFT %T TRT F SA R				
7	WPM SPM CPM LSPM MFT %T TRT F SA R	WPM SPM CPM LSPM MFT TRT	WPM SPM CPM LSPM MFT %T TRT F SA R	WPM SPM CPM LSPM MFT %T TRT F SA R	WPM SPM CPM LSPM MFT %T TRT F SA R	MFT %T			
8	SPM CPM LSPM MFT %T TRT SA R	MFT %T F SA R	WPM SPM CPM LSPM %T TRT F SA R	SPM CPM LSPM MFT %T TRT SA R	SPM CPM LSPM MFT %T TRT F SA R	WPM SPM CPM LSPM %T TRT F SA R	WPM SPM CPM LSPM MFT TRT F SA R		
9		F SA R	WPM SPM CPM LSPM MFT TRT F R	SPM CPM LSPM MFT TRT	SPM LSPM MFT %T TRT	WPM SPM CPM LSPM TRT F SA R	WPM SPM CPM LSPM %T TRT F SA R	LSPM MFT %T SA R	
10	WPM SPM CPM LSPM TRT F	SA	WPM SPM CPM LSPM MFT TRT	WPM SPM CPM LSPM MFT TRT F R	WPM SPM CPM LSPM MFT %T TRT F R	WPM SPM CPM LSPM TRT F	WPM SPM CPM LSPM MFT %T TRT F	MFT %T F SA R	SPM CPM LSPM TRT R

SUBJECT NUMBER

FIGURE 5.   The independence matrix. The reading rates and eye movement parameters for each subject were statistically compared against those for all other subjects. When analysis indicated independence, an entry of the rate or parameter is made in the appropriate box. For example, when subject 4 is compared to subject 1 only values for MFT are statistically different; comparing subjects 5 and 7 indicates all rates and parameters are different.

Table 1
THE NUMBER OF CASES OF STATISTICAL INDEPENDENCE FOR READING RATES AND EYE MOVEMENT PARAMETERS ABSTRACTED FROM FIGURE 5.

Variable	Frequency of independence out of 45 possible subject comparisons	Variable rank
LSPM	35	1
SPM	34	2
CPM TRT	32	3
MFT	31	4
F R	30	5
WPM	27	6
SA	24	7
% Time	20	8

Note: Rates are parameters are listed in descending order of the number of cases of observed independence.

ical length of the text. A text which is physically twice as long will be read with twice the number of fixations (F) and regressions (R) and will be read in twice the total

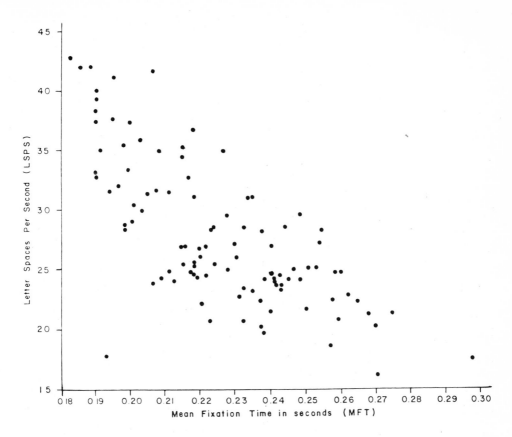

FIGURE 6.. Reading rate in letterspaces per second shows a clear inverse relationship with mean fixation time.

reading time (TRT). In the present case, the effect is very small, if not negligible, because our texts are designed to have about the same physical length, i.e., same number of letterspaces. We can get rid of this small effect by normalizing these parameters by dividing their values by the number of letterspaces in the particular text that was read. We, thus, end up with normalized variables F/LS, R/LS, and TRT/LS. In order to establish which of our eye movement parameters are crucial for determination of reading rate, we plot rate vs. each parameter. All measures of rate are clearly related to MFT, F/LS, and TRT/LS. Rate is not related to SA, R/LS, or %T. Figures 6 and 7 show LSPS vs. MFT and F/LS, respectively. Clearly, rate is a decreasing function of either of these parameters. If WPM is plotted on the vertical axis instead of LSPS, the spread in the vertical direction is greater due to the confounding influence of difficulty level. Finally, Figure 8 is a plot of F/LS vs. MFT. In this plot, the points for each subject are represented by different symbols. If there were no statistical scatter in the data, each subject would be represented by a single point such as the point representing the population mean for these two parameters. Notice that the points for each subject show different degrees of clustering, where the tightness of each cluster is determined by the amount of scatter present in the data points for a given subject. The numbers in the data field indicate the position of subject mean values for the two parameters.

IV. DISCUSSION AND CONCLUSIONS

The widely held and intuitively appealing notion that reading speed is inversely re-

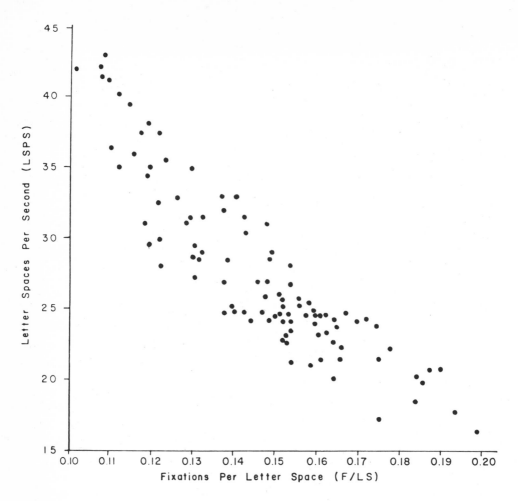

FIGURE 7.   The inverse relationship between letterspaces per second and the number of fixations per letterspace. The independent variable has been normalized to the number of letterspaces in the text.

lated to text difficulty appears open to very serious question. The results of the present study confirm earlier investigations (Miller and Coleman,[13] Coke,[14] and Steicher and Zuber[16]). and support the conclusion that reading rate when measured in units smaller than the word, is independent of difficulty level. Although reading rate measured in words per minute does significantly decrease with difficulty, the decrease can be related to a change in physical text characteristics. Thus, for texts of the same physical length, a more difficult text will contain fewer words than an easier one. The observed decrease in word rate is not related to reading behavior or information processing. When the effect of physical text characteristics correlated with difficulty is removed, dependence of reading rate on text difficulty disappears. The implication of this observation is that at some point in the information processing mechanism a constant rate of information flow is utilized.

As to the parameters of reading eye movements, none shows strong correlation with difficulty level. Of the primary parameters, only the mean fixation time (MFT) is correlated with difficulty. While the nature of this correlation is such as to reinforce a decrease in word rate with increasing difficulty, the magnitude of the overall change in MFT is insufficient to account for the observed decrease in word rate. Further, diminishing the importance of changes in MFT is the observation that only 30% of

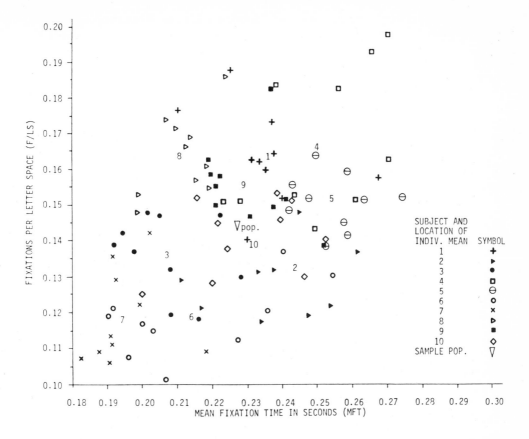

FIGURE 8. The one hundred data points for the entire population shown as a plot of fixations/letterspace vs. mean fixation time. The points for each subject form an operational cluster reflecting reading rate. In general, rate is higher as the cluster gets closer to either axis. Numbers in the data field represent the mean values for each subject. The mean values for the entire population is shown as a large open triangle designated "pop".

our subjects had statistically significant increases in MFT with difficulty. We feel that the present results justify the conclusion that virtually all eye movement parameters are essentially constant over the entire range of text difficulty studied. This conclusion is entirely consistent with the observation of rate constancy.

Rate constancy implies that a given reader approaches a wide range of textual material in essentially the same way. However, among readers in any population there will obviously be a distribution of reading rates. We expect that each reader will have a characteristic constant rate. The results of our statistical test of independence suggest that our subjects each utilized a unique constant rate in reading all of the texts presented to them. This uniqueness is evidenced not only by letterspace rate (LSPM), but also by a variety of eye movement parameters, most notably by mean fixation time (MFT) and the number of fixations utilized in reading a text (F). The least amount of uniqueness appears in word rate, saccadic amplitude (somewhat surprisingly), and percent time fixating.

Reading rate can be calculated with rather good accuracy by resorting to a simple equation in which two eye movement parameters (MFT and F) figure prominently (Ahlen, et al.[6]). In this equation, rate is inversely proportional to both parameters. This relationship is strongly suggested in Figures 6 and 7, where letterspace rate is plotted vs. MFT and F/LS, respectively. The clarity of the trends in these two plots may be partially attributed to the use of letterspace rate as the dependent variable, thus, removing the confounding effect of the relationship between word rate and difficulty.

The data in Figures 6 and 7 were used to construct Figure 8, a plot of F/LS vs. MFT. A point in this space defines a reading rate. In general, rate will increase as the point approaches the origin or either axis. Subjects are not represented by a point due to statistical spread. Rather, the data for each subject fall into an operational cluster defining the area of operation for that particular subject. The general location of the operational cluster defines a subject's reading rate.

Variability resulting in the kind of cluster dispersion seen in Figure 8 is one of the most unfailing characteristics of all reading studies. The present study is certainly no exception. The reasons for the consistent presence of statistical variability are unclear. Is it possible that we are dealing with information processing mechanisms that are inherently "sloppy", or is there some crucial variable yet to be discovered?

REFERENCES

1. Javal, E., Essai sur la physiologie de la lecture, *Ann. Oculist,* 82, 242, 1879.
2. Huey, E. B., *The Psychology and Pedagogy of Reading,* Massachusetts Institute of Technology Press, Cambridge, 1968.
3. Tinker, M. A., Recent studies of eye movements in reading, *Psychol. Bull.,* 55, 213, 1958.
4. Taylor, E. A., *The Fundamental Reading Skill,* Charles C Thomas, Springfield, Ill., 1966.
5. Abrams, S. G. and Zuber, B. L., Some temporal characteristics of information processing during reading, *Reading Res. Q.,* Vol. 8, 40, 1972.
6. Ahlen, J. W., Zuber, B. L., Carsello, C. J., and Ahlen, S. P., Reading improvement optimality reflected by eye movements, *Proc. 26th Ann. Conf. Engin. Med. Biol.,* 15, 148, 1973.
7. Coleman, E. B., Generalizing to a language population, *Psychol. Rep.,* 16, 219, 1964.
8. Miller, G. R. and Coleman, E. B., A set of thirty-six prose passages calibrated for complexity, *J. Verb. Learn. Verb. Behav.,* 6, 851, 1967.
9. Coleman, E. B. and Miller, G. R., A measure of information gained during prose learning, *Reading Res. Q.,* 3, 369, 1968.
10. Aquino, M., The validity of the Miller-Coleman readability scale, *Reading Res. Q.,* 4, 342, 1969.
11. Sticht, T. G., Learning by Listening in Relation to Aptitude, Reading and Rate Controlled Speech: Additional Studies. Technical Report 71-5, Hum. Resour. Res. Org., Alexandria, VA., 1972.
12. Carver, R. P., Evidence for the invalidity of the Miller-Coleman readability scale, *J. Rdg. Behav.,* 4, 42, 1971.
13. Miller, G. R. and Coleman, E. B., The measurement of reading speed and the obligation to generalize to a population of reading materials, *J. Rdg. Behav.,* 4, 48, 1971.
14. Coke, E. U., The effects of readability on oral and silent reading rates, *J. Ed. Psychol.,* 66, 406, 1974.
15. Stark, L., Vossius, G., and Young, L. R., Predictive Control of Eye Tracking Movments, *IRE Trans. Hum. Fac. Elecr.,* HFE-3, 52, 1962.
16. Streicher, T. W. and Zuber, B. L., Effect of text difficulty on reading speed and the parameters of reading eye movements, *Fed. Proc.,* 36, 561, 1977.

Chapter 11

CONTROL OF EYE MOVEMENTS DURING READING

Keith Rayner and Werner Inhoff

TABLE OF CONTENTS

I. INTRODUCTION

Interest in using eye movements as a means to study the reading process started with a surprising observation: our eye behavior during reading is opposite to our subjective impressions. Until 1878, it was assumed that our eyes travel smoothly along the line, make a "big jump" to the next line, and then continue with this smooth kind of movement. Javal[1] was apparently the first person to report that our eyes show a startling irregular movement pattern. They do not move continuously, but either make a pause or jump (saccade) with high velocity to a different location. This movement towards a new fixation location need not be in a forward direction (left-to-right for English readers), but the eye may jump to a part of the text which has already been read (regression). These observations were the impetus for a large scale research effort dealing with eye movements during reading. Huey[2] and Woodworth[3] each published a synopsis of early experimental data in the area of reading and specified our eye behavior at a descriptive level: the range of fixation duration in reading is between 100 to over 500 msec, saccade length covers 1 to 20 character spaces, and between 3 to 30% of our eye movements are regressions. Averaged over a number of readers, the mean fixation duration is generally 200 to 250 msec, the mean saccade length is 6 to 9 characters (2 to 3 deg. of visual angle), the mean frequency of regression is about 15 to 20%. Figure 1 shows a frequency distribution for saccade length and fixation duration for eight college-age readers. For these subjects, the mean fixation duration is 235 msec, the mean saccade length is nine characters, and the mean frequency of regression is 12.5%. The characteristics of the text were such that four character spaces equaled one degree of visual angle. The variance in the eye movement behavior is obvious in the figure. Our interest in this paper is focused on the source of this variance. That is, the question may be asked whether systematic factors underlie the observed variation and, if so, how can we account for their respective interpretations.

In this chapter, we will consider various views or models of how eye movement behavior in reading can be explained. Before describing different models of eye movements in reading, we would like to stress a point that is alluded to above. While there is a considerable amount of variability between readers in terms of eye movement behavior, there is also a fair amount of variability within subjects. While early workers were well aware of both sources of variability, later writers of books dealing with reading and perception often seem to have assumed that these mean indices of eye movement behavior during reading were relatively stable and invariant. In fact, this basic misunderstanding or oversimplification seems to be the primary motivation behind many remedial reading techniques. That is, it is often assumed that people who read poorly do so because they make inefficient eye movements. According to this assumption, good readers make smooth, efficient eye movements as each saccade covers about the same distance and each pause is approximately the same duration. As should be obvious from the basic facts about eye movements we presented above, it is a myth that good readers make smooth, regular eye movements; good readers are highly variable in terms of saccade length and fixation duration. Thus, it is not surprising that numerous attempts to train people to be better readers by making their eye movements more regular have led to failure.[4] Eye movements are a symptom of reading problems, not the cause.[4,5]

In the next section of the chapter, we will briefly review early research on eye movements in reading so as to put the remainder of the paper in historical perspective. Then we will describe a number of alternative models of how the eye movements during reading might be determined. We will conclude by reporting the characteristics of the data that are available and relate these data to the nature of the perceptual span in reading.

II. EARLY RESEARCH ON EYE MOVEMENTS IN READING

As we indicated previously, Javal's observation that the eyes make saccadic movements during reading was followed by a great deal of research on the topic. Pioneering researchers such as Dodge, Dearborn, Huey, Landolt, and Buswell vigorously carried out active research programs on reading using eye movements as the means to study the complex task. Most of the basic facts that we know about eye movements were obtained by these early researchers using rather crude recording techniques. Their research dealt with saccadic latency, suppressed vision during the saccade, perceptual span in reading, and other topics vitally related to an understanding of eye movements during reading. There was also considerable interest in the control of eye movements during reading. These early researchers found that the number of words per line seems to be more important than the visual angle subtended and that about 80% of the line is actually traversed in reading. That is, the first fixation on the line is indented four or five characters on the line and the last fixation is six or seven characters from the last letter on the line. Huey also went to considerable pain to point out the variability in fixation duration and saccade length that existed in the reading records. It was also emphasized that the reading material clearly had an effect on average fixation duration, saccade length, and frequency of regression with more difficult passages increasing fixation duration, decreasing saccade length, and increasing the probability of a regression.

A number of these early researchers speculated on how parafoveal and peripheral information may be important in reading. Dodge and Dearborn[6] both argued that peripheral retinal stimulation affords premonitions of coming words and phrases, as well as a consciousness of the relationship of the centrally fixated symbols to the larger groups of the phrase and the sentence. Gray[7] indicated that the successful strategy for obtaining meaning from written material occurs when a reader thinks ahead and tries to anticipate what is coming. He suggested that these anticipations are possible because of (1) grammatical relations that organize each sentence; (2) the context or knowledge of the subject matter; and (3) marginal impressions on the retina which help initiate the process of anticipation. Schmidt[8] on the other hand, argued that the anticipations and premonitions were not due to peripheral vision, but to the fact that the reader was immersed in the meaning of what was being read. In suggesting that anticipations (or hypotheses about what is coming next) were important in reading, these early researchers were laying the groundwork for a notion about reading that has become rather popular today. The idea suggested by Gray that anticipations and peripheral vision interact in reading is very close to the position taken more recently by Hochberg.[9]

Research dealing with eye movements in reading that led to theoretical advancement and understanding of basic underlying processes in reading probably reached its peak shortly after the publication of Huey's book. Thereafter, interest in the topic began to wane somewhat. There are probably a number of reasons for this decline in interest, but two possibilities seem to stand out. First, there were problems with apparatus. During these early years of eye movement recording, apparatus available for work on reading advanced from rather cumbersome crude techniques to the use of photographic methods. However, photographic corneal reflection techniques have certain problems of their own and given the vast amount of data collected on eye movements in reading between 1880 and 1925, researchers may have had the feeling that everything about reading eye movements that could be discovered with the methodology had been discovered. The second reason for the decline in interest in eye movements as a means to study basic processes in reading was the popularity of the behaviorist position in psychology which made questions dealing with the cognitive and perceptual aspects of

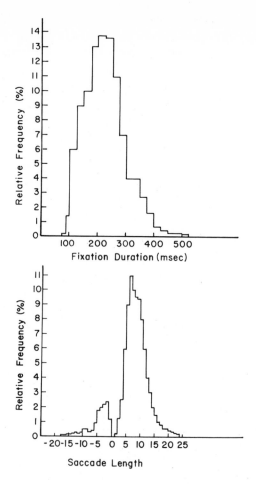

FIGURE 1.   Frequency distribution of fixation duration (upper graph) and saccade length (lower graph) for eight college-age readers. Return sweeps of the eye have been excluded from the distribution. Short fixations following the return sweep which are followed by corrective saccades have also been excluded.

reading taboo for experimental psychologists. A great deal of research on eye movements in reading did continue during this time, but it was largely confined to education where the emphasis was on applied issues. As a result, very little basic research or theory-building research was undertaken during this second era of eye movement research on reading. Tinker[4,10,11] has provided excellent reviews of the research on eye movements that was conducted between 1925 and 1958. With the advent of cognitive psychology in the mid 1960s, reading has once again become a popular area of investigation for experimental psychologists, and a number of researchers have once again been conducting studies dealing with basic questions about reading that lead to theory development. Foremost among these questions is how are a reader's eye movements controlled? That is, before we make use of the measurement of eye movements in the study of reading we have to know what mechanisms we are measuring. Each of the eye movement models we will describe offers a different answer to this basic issue of validation. However, once validated, eye movements bear a strong advantage over competing methods used in reading research: they yield objective data that are immune to systematic bias by the subject and the experimenter. The subject is unaware of eye movement behavior and, hence, would not be inclined to bias. If the data are collected on-line by a computer, there is no chance for experimenter dependent evaluation errors.

III. MODELS OF EYE MOVEMENT BEHAVIOR

There are many possible models which might be adopted to account for eye movements in reading. The task of these models is to account for the three sources of variability in eye behavior (fixation duration, saccade length, and regression) which we have described. In the present chapter, we will attempt to partition these possible models into classes of models and then to consider which of these classes are consistent with available data concerning the characteristics of eye movement behavior in reading. We will not attempt to deal with eye behavior differences between people.

We will describe five classes of possible models of eye movement control: minimal control models, low-level control models, high-level control models, process-monitoring models, and mixed models. Previously, Rayner[5] has referred to minimal control models as constant pattern models, low-level control models as stimulus control models, and high-level control and process-monitoring models as internal control models. However, here, we will adopt the more comprehensive categorization proposed by Rayner and McConkie[12] and discuss the five classes of models which they originally described.

We will make three distinctions which we believe are useful in classifying models of eye movements in reading. The first two distinctions are borrowed from Rayner and McConkie.[12] First, we will assume that processing activities involved in understanding text can exist at different levels. These levels reflect the characteristics of the code produced by the processing activities. Low-level processing activities are those in which the code produced is a rather direct representation of visual characteristics of the stimulus pattern, and higher-level processing activities are those in which the code represents information which is less directly tied to visual characteristics and more the result of previously stored information; for instance, codes which reflect syntactic parsings, meaning, etc.

The second distinction is between language processing itself (the activities directly involved in converting visual information to meaning) and process monitoring (processes which monitor some aspect of the language processing activities and produce events based on the state of those activities). Thus, eye guidance might be based either on some aspect of the language processing itself, or on some mechanism monitoring some aspect of that processing.

The third distinction we will make is between eye guidance in reading and fixation control in reading. These two components of eye behavior may not be under the control of a single mechanism; that is, the determination of where to look next may be made independently of how long to look there. The fact that there is no correlation between the length of a saccade and the preceding or following fixation duration[12,13] is consistent with this view and suggests that these two aspects of eye behavior must be accounted for separately. In this chapter, we will be primarily concerned with eye guidance, although for each of the models we describe we will also discuss fixation duration. Two basic positions can be taken with regard to the control of fixation duration. The first position suggests that the processing of the text must necessarily lag behind the perceptual input of the stimulus. This position, as will be seen in our later discussion, is basically that taken by theorists who adopt the minimal control and low-level control models. The assumption is that semantic comprehension of the text takes place independently of our eye behavior. The second position suggests that fixation durations are affected by the cognitive processes occurring during the time period of the fixation. This position is most closely identified with theorists taking the high-level control and process-monitoring positions. This distinction between control of fixation duration and control of eye guidance leads us to propose a general class of models referred to as mixed models.

Before discussing each of the models in depth, it should be noted that a certain degree of low-level control will probably be assumed by all theories of eye movement behavior in accounting for the fact that the reader typically tracks a particular line with successive fixations and detects the point at which the line no longer continues and, hence, successfully makes a return sweep to the beginning of the next line. A minimal amount of high-level control is also required to account for the reader's ability to move the eye backward in a regression when difficulty in understanding the text is encountered. Some models, however, require little guidance beyond these two characteristics and will be called minimal control models.

A. Minimal Control Models

Minimal control models are those which assume that the specific location or durations of fixations are of little importance, and that eye movements are based neither upon the visual patterns of the text, nor on the syntactic or semantic information being acquired from it. Rather, the eye is advanced in some regular pattern, habitual for the reader, simply under physiological and oculomotor control. The variance in eye movement behavior is assumed to be caused by internal motor irregularities or due to external distraction.

The minimal control model makes the least number of theoretical assumptions and may come closest to our intuition. In favor of this model is the fact that we cannot give account of our eye movement behavior, i.e., we cannot distinguish between relatively long or short fixations, and given the autokinetic effect, we may not even register regressive eye movements, but see our reading as a rather uniformly ongoing process. It also seems that certain known facts about timing constraints lend themselves most readily to this position.[14] That is, since the mean oculomotor latency period is in the range of 150 to 200 msec, many researchers have assumed that there is simply not enough time during the 200 to 250 msec of a normal fixation for the reader to process the material in foveal vision to a semantic level and at the same time determine where to look next. Thus, it seems to be the case that some researchers have adopted the minimal control model by default. It should also be noted that it may be incorrect to assume that timing factors are additive and serial, as it may well be that (as we have suggested above) the decision about where to send the eye next is made in parallel (and independently) with foveal processing. The major difficulty with a pure minimal control model is that it cannot incorporate experimental evidence that support the other conceptions. Furthermore, to assume that the variance in eye behavior is due to internal motor irregularities or due to external distraction does not seem reasonable in accounting for all of the variance observed. There seems to be too much variability in terms of saccade length and fixation duration within an individual reader for a pure version of the minimal control model to adequately explain important eye movement data.

A variation of the minimal control model does, however, have some credibility. According to this model,[15-17] eye movements are under oculomotor control, but there is a gain control that can be adjusted to account for the difficulty of the text; with difficult text the gain control is adjusted so that the eye does not move as far and remains fixated longer. In addition, some type of feedback to the oculomotor system from the higher processing centers could occur so that longer fixations and refixations occur. Hence, eye movements could be affected by syntactic and semantic variables according to this variation of the minimal control model. An experiment by Bouma and deVoogd[17] is often cited as evidence for this modified version of the minimal control model. In this experiment, subjects were asked to maintain fixation as text moved in front of the eye from right to left in a manner simulating an eye movement of about eight character spaces. Bouma and deVoogd found that subjects could read in this situation with good comprehension and argued that programming of eye movements is rather lax and that this lax control only insures that the proceeding of the eyes over the text keep pace with the proceeding of text recognition. Hochberg[18] has argued against their conclusion because of his objection to the task. He pointed out that finding that people can read when they have little control over visual exposure does not stand as evidence that they do not exercise such control when they have the opportunity to do so in normal reading. Finally, it should be noted that the modification of the minimal control model via a gain control that operates for textual difficulty can indeed account for much of the data that elludes the pure version of the model. However, if the modified version of the model is pushed to an extreme (as it might be forced to do to account for the data) so that the gain control works on a moment-to-moment basis, the model becomes indistinguishable from models which postulate that eye movements in reading are made on a nonrandom basis.

B. Low-Level Control Models

Low-level models assume that eye guidance is based on the visual characteristics of the text. It is commonly assumed that information acquired in parafoveal and peripheral vision is critical in this guidance, causing the eye to be sent to certain locations having visual characteristics of certain types. The low-level model does not make the efficiency of eccentric cues contingent upon the result of foveal processes. Foveal and eccentric vision may be affected by independent factors and this may be responsible for the lack of correlation between fixation duration and saccade length.

This model has gained plausibility as the result of research on the perception of pictures[19-21] and on visual search[22,23] in which it has been shown that peripheral visual information is critical in determining the location of fixations. Thus, there is the possibility that such visual characteristics of text as word length patterns to the right of the fixation point might influence where the eye is directed. It is important to note here that the type of information from eccentric vision that is useful in guiding the eye according to the low-level model is strictly visual in nature (such as word length) and semantic variables are not involved. This class of models would then predict that the locations and lengths of saccades vary in a nonrandom manner which reflects certain visual characteristics of the text pattern. The most common suggestion of this type has been that the eye is typically sent to regions containing longer words, since shorter words are frequently function words which are thought to contain less useful information.

According to the low-level model, fixation duration is affected by lateral inhibition and/or forward and backward masking effects.[14] Bouma demonstrated that adjacent contours affect each other; since there is less lateral interference for beginning letters of words or for one or two letter words these targets should yield shorter fixation durations than those registered for fixations in the middle of a multiletter word. Further, forward and backward masking occurs if two successive stimuli are presented in the same retinal location in close temporal proximity. Average fixation durations in reading approximate the upper temporal limit of backward masking effects. Backward masking exerts differential effects dependent on visual similarity[24,25] and semantic relatedness[26,27] in the stimulus material available across successive fixations. Thus, fixation duration and backward masking may be related: the stronger the backward masking effects over successive fixations, the longer the following fixation duration.

To summarize the low-level model, fixation duration guarantees encoding of visual information and saccade length is determined by eccentric cues (word length) which guide the eye through the text. The cognitive processes like lexical decision, semantic evaluation, or sentence comprehension take place independently of our eye behavior, or at least, find no direct expression in it.

C. High-Level Control Models

High-level control models assume that eye control is based on higher level processing, for instance on syntactic or semantic information from the text. The hypothesis testing models of reading[9,28-30] are examples of high-level control models. Central to Hochberg's theory[9] are the notions that the reader fixates on important cues in the text and decides where the next important cues reside so that the eyes can be moved to that area. He suggests that two control mechanisms are involved in reading, cognitive search guidance (CSG) and peripheral search guidance (PSG), both of which would be classified as high-level control. Hochberg argues that due to the redundancy of the language, the reader need not see every word in order to understand the text. Because of knowledge of the spelling, grammar, and idiom of the text, the reader can anticipate the message and strategically move the eyes to sample only certain visual features from the text needed to confirm anticipations. This process is CSG. In addition, peripheral visual input can be the basis for informed guesses about where the important words can be found and, hence, used to guide the eyes to those regions which will be most informative in testing expectations. This process is PSG. Hochberg suggests that the main parafoveal and peripheral cue used in guiding eye movements is word length, because shorter words are usually functors like "on, in, to, the", and so on. The reader is, thus, able to detect that a functor lies at some distance along the line of text, and then decide either to look at the word, or if it is likely to be redundant, to ensure that it is skipped. Although PSG involves low-level information, in fact, the reader is assumed to be also employing high-level information about the text, as well as knowledge of language constraints to decide whether to fixate given words or not. Thus, we, like Rayner and McConkie,[12] classify this theory as an instance of high-level control. An eye guidance mechanism would be considered to be of a low-level type only if guidance is based strictly on low-level information, and higher levels of information are not brought to bear on the decision. Although Hochberg does not discuss control of fixation duration, presumably if visual information acquired in the fovea (information used by CSG to confirm the hypothesis) is not in agreement with the generated hypothesis, further processing would be required, which would seem to result in longer fixations or regressions. However, it also seems that an implicit assumption of Hochberg's theory is that the reader is correct in his hypothesis or anticipation far more than he is wrong. Hence, the major source of variability for fixation duration according to this model might not be incorrect anticipations or hypotheses, but higher level processes of integrating semantic information.

Another possibility of high-level control is that some form of semantic preprocessing of text in the visual periphery occurs, and this incomplete analysis of the text provides enough information to send the eye judiciously to the place which will be the most informative about the meaning of the text. This kind of processing seems to operate in the auditory system. For example, Lewis[31] and Lackner and Garrett[32] have shown that unattended information which could not be reported by the listener, nevertheless influenced the attended information. In audition, both ears are functionally and physiologically equivalent. However, this symmetry does not hold for foveal vs. the parafoveal (plus peripheral) system in vision. Both systems differ physiologically and current data also support the notion of a functional difference. Further, if the semantic processing of the parafoveal or peripheral information were complete, it would make no sense for the reader to fixate an area that he had already identified. On the other hand, it has not been spelled out how semantic preprocessing could be partially completed to the extent that the reader knew whether or not to fixate a given area because he knew whether or not the area contained important information. Kolers and Lewis[33] have argued against this position on the basis of their demonstration that subjects are unable to obtain semantic information from two physically separate locations at the same time.

In summary then, the high-level model encompasses certain low-level processes. That is, visual processes precede cognitive evaluation, but the former are assumed to be constant and the variance in fixation duration and saccade length is due solely to higher order processes. How the model would account for the lack of a correlation between saccade length and fixation duration is uncertain. However, it might be quite possible for the high-level models to account for this lack of relationship, since the factors upon which predictions and hypotheses are made is very vague and unspecified. As McConkie and Rayner[34] and Gibson and Levin[35] have pointed out, it is unclear from the hypothesis testing models just what kinds of hypotheses the reader is generating (specific words, syntactic expectancies, semantic expectancies?), how the predictions are verified or confirmed, and what information is specifically sampled.

D. Process-Monitoring Models

There are several potential models of eye guidance in reading which assume that the eyes are not directly controlled by information in low-level or high-level codes, but rather they are controlled by a mechanism which monitors some aspect of the processes involved in generating these codes. We will describe two examples of such models here, visual buffer models and unbuffered process-monitoring models.

Visual buffer models assume that visual information acquired during fixations is held in a buffer until needed for further processing. The processing load of this buffer is monitored and the eye is sent ahead when further visual input can be accommodated. The goal of the eye movement mechanism is to ensure that visual input is acquired at the proper rate; fast enough that visual information is available when needed for further processing, but not so fast that the buffer overflows and information is lost. Once visual information is stored in the buffer, cognitive evaluation takes place in an independent system. Presumably, if reading was going quite smoothly and the text was of equal difficulty throughout, there would be little variability in saccade length and fixation duration as each new saccade brought exactly the same amount into the buffer as was transferred on to higher levels during the prior fixation. However, as the difficulty of text changed, presumably fixation durations and saccade lengths would be adjusted to meet the goal that the visual information be acquired at the proper rate.[16,17]

As Rayner and McConkie[12] pointed out, this simple model can take many forms depending upon the assumptions made about the size of the buffer and the nature of the eye control which can be exerted by the buffer monitoring process. In the simplest case, it reduces to a single gain control and becomes indistinguishable from the modified minimal control model we described previously. If the buffer is large, and the mechanism simply makes adjustments in fixation duration and saccade length which generally increase or decrease reading rate, no further specific control is required. On the other hand, if the buffer is small and capable of containing only slightly more information than is acquired on a single fixation, then the durations of fixations would reflect quite directly the type of processing taking place during the individual fixations. In this case, high-level processes (or semantic processing) would be very much involved, and to make predictions of eye movement behavior one would need a specific model of the types of cognitive processes required at specific locations in the text. This version of the process-monitoring model becomes indistinguishable from a high-level model in explaining fixation duration.

Unbuffered process-monitoring models assume that a visual buffer is not required in reading, since on each fixation a visual pattern is directly available. According to these models[36], during each fixation the reader processes the visually available information as far to the right as possible, at some criterion level of certainty. Thus, the eye remains fixated until the semantic processing has been achieved and is then sent to the next location. Since the duration of a fixation is determined by the time required to process visual information (including the syntactic and semantic processing made possible by the visual information), the duration of the fixation would be quite variable. When the eye is advanced, the length of the saccade reflects the distance to the right that words have already been identified. That is, saccade length depends on the size of the perceptual span for semantic identification. If it is supposed that word identification is based on some combination of contextual information and visual information, then the lengths of saccades would be quite variable depending on the characteristics of the text at each point. McConkie[36] has explicitly related this type of model of eye guidance to attention shifts of the eye. That is, the reader processes the text as far to the right for meaning as possible given the limited visual acuity (and lateral masking), and when semantic identification is no longer available, the reader shifts attention by making an eye movement. It should be noted that this model of eye guidance faces a potential difficulty since according to this model the eye movement is programmed dependent upon the output of a semantic evaluation, the proper saccade length can only be programmed at the end of the individual fixation duration. However, an average saccade latency of 150 to 175 msec[37], given an average fixation duration of 200 to 250 msec, argues in favor of a relatively early decision concerning the initiation of the saccade.

E. Mixed Models

As we indicated previously, it is quite possible to construct models of eye control in reading which are a mixture of certain of the previously described models. Thus, it would be quite possible to assume that fixation durations are determined by high-level or process-monitoring control, but that where the eye is sent is not under specific control (minimal control), or that it is determined by visual characteristics of the text (low-level control). Another possibility is that where the eye is sent is under some form of high-level control, but that fixation duration is not under momentary control.

The rate of reading is the result of both fixation duration and saccade length, as well as the frequency of regression.[5] It is possible that a single mechanism, such as a gain control or buffer monitor, might adjust both of these aspects of eye behavior together in order to increase or decrease the reading rate. If so, one would expect a negative correlation between the durations of fixations and the lengths of the saccades prior to or following them. However, as we have pointed out, Rayner and McConkie[12] and others found no correlation between these two aspects of eye movement behavior. In addition, they found no correlation between successive saccade lengths nor between successive fixation durations. These results seem to place important restrictions on acceptable models of eye movement control. If some form of control is assumed, it cannot be of a type which adjusts (via a linear relationship) fixation duration and saccade length together as simple gain control or buffer monitoring positions would suggest. Also, it appears that we cannot account for fixation duration or saccade length alone on the basis of such mechanisms. Rather, the determination of the length of the saccade and the duration of the fixation seems to be made on the basis of some momentary state existing at that time, rather than on some more slowly changing state that exists over more than one fixation, i.e., each fixation and each following eye movement seem to represent a processing cycle of their own. Still, momentary control of this sort might result either from a random variability component of a model assuming minimum control, or it may result from some specific form of control, whether low-level, high-level, or process-monitoring in nature. This conclusion indicates that gain control models are unlikely to be useful in accounting for eye movement behavior during reading. It also leads to the same conclusion about buffer monitoring models. In order to predict momentary control, the type of buffer that would be required would be a small one, with control of eye movements very directly reflecting cognitive processes which are occurring (and removing information from the buffer), rather than a large buffer which mediates over several fixations. If the buffer is not capable of mediating across fixations, it would not seem to hold a very interesting place in the theory; that is, eye movements must be assumed to reflect some aspect of the reading process rather directly, and the properties of the buffer add little to the theory.

In this section, we have attempted to describe the characteristics of a number of potential models of eye movement control in reading. The mixed models of eye movement control are logically quite possible and gain added credibility from the fact that there is no relationship between fixation duration and saccade length. This finding, we suggest, implies that separate control mechanisms may be responsible for these two aspects of reading behavior. However, we should also point out that the lack of a correlation between these two aspects of eye behavior can be accommodated by the low-level, high-level, and process-monitoring models. This can be done by assuming, for example, that although fixation duration and saccade length are controlled by high-level processes, a different mechanism (controlled by different high-level activities) accounts for each aspect.

It should be obvious that we did not discuss regressive eye movements in our characterizations of eye movement control models. Although there has been very little empirical research on regressive eye movements during reading, it appears that regressions occur when the reader has difficulty understanding the text, when the reader misinterprets the text, and when the reader overshoots the target word. Generally speaking, then, it would appear that either high-level control or process-monitoring control is involved in the decision to send the eyes backward in order to get more useful information. However, this need not bear implications for the eve guidance models outlined earlier, since the reader regresses to a section of text which he has already stored and identified, while there is no corresponding storage and identification for the to-be-encountered text when the reader makes a forward (left-to-right) saccade.

In summary, we have argued that the minimal control model cannot account for the variability that exists in a single reader's eye movement behavior. Furthermore, we have argued that a minimal control model with a gain control and a buffered process-monitoring model may not be useful in characterizing eye movement control, because in order to account for the variation that exists in eye movements, the gain control would have to be operating on a moment-to-moment basis and the buffer would have to be very small also operating on a moment-to-moment basis. In both cases, the models become indistinguishable from other models that do directly posit cognitive involvement in eye movement control and, hence, not very useful. In the next section, we will discuss the empirical evidence that exists concerning eye movement control in reading.

IV. EMPIRICAL EVIDENCE RELATED TO EYE MOVEMENT CONTROL

In this section, we will describe the results of descriptive and empirical studies dealing with eye movement control. The section will be divided into three main parts. First, we will discuss research dealing with the perceptual span in reading, and then we will discuss other data that are relevant to the question of whether or not eye movements in reading are made on a nonrandom basis. In particular, we will discuss research relevant to control of fixation duration and then discuss eye guidance.

A. The Perceptual Span in Reading

Once the discovery was made that the observable reading behavior consists of a series of discrete behavioral events, the interest turned to finding a psychological equivalent of these processes. The term "perceptual span" was agreed upon to describe the information available to the reader during an individual fixation; less agreement was attained in determining the effective information available to the reader during this temporal frame. Huey[2] and Woodworth[3] both devoted a considerable amount of space to discussing the effective stimulus in reading and more recent research has also focused on the size of the perceptual span.[38]

In normal reading, the horizontal line of text that is projected on the reader's retina can be divided into three major anatomical regions: foveal, parafoveal, and peripheral. The fovea is the area of clear visual acuity and extends 2 deg. across the fixation point. Beyond the fovea, the parafoveal region spreads 5 deg. to the left and 5 deg. to the right of the fixation point and the remainder is peripheral region. One topic of interest was whether this anatomical structure bears a functional relationship to the information available to the reader.

It is obvious that any estimate of the size of the perceptual span one obtains is very much dependent upon the technique used. Many different techniques have been used in the past, but the most precise, and at the same time most ecologically valid technique used to determine the size of the perceptual span is one that enables the experimenter to control the amount of information available to the reader at a given moment, yet the reader controls the variables governing timing and sequence of information extraction. This is obtained by making the visual stimulus display contingent upon the reader's eye movements.[39-42] In the first experiment of this type,[39] passages of text were mutilated in systematic ways so that various types of information from the original text were maintained or altered. For example, in one condition, every letter in the original text was replaced by an *x*, thus, preserving word length and punctuation information, but altering word shape information. Initially, a passage of mutilated text appeared on a Cathode Ray Tube (CRT). However, as soon as the reader fixated on the first line of text, the display changed so that within a certain area (eight character spaces to the left and right of the fixation point, for example) the *xs* were replaced by corresponding letters from the original text. This area within which the normal text appeared was called the *window*. When the reader made a saccade, those letters became *xs* once again, and the *xs* within the window area around the new fixation point were replaced by the corresponding letters from the original text. Thus, wherever the reader fixated, there was readable text, while the mutilated text appeared outside of the window area. The experimenters varied the size of the window area and the characteristics of the mutilated text and found evidence which indicated that readers do not obtain useful information more than 12 to 15 characters to the right of the fixation point. However, it was also clear from the experiment that useful information is obtained further to the right than would be represented by the average saccade length. That is, the average saccade length was eight characters, but useful information was obtained from an area extending at least 12 to 15 characters away from fixation. If the effective information which is available to the reader depends on the anatomical structure of the eye, then the incoming information should be symmetrically evaluated and semantic information should be restricted to the area of clear vision (fovea). To test this, the window was varied so that a symmetrical window (20 letters displayed to the right, as well as to the left of the point of fixation), a right shifted window (4 letters to the left, 4 to the right), and a left shifted window (20 characters to the left, 4 to the right) were displayed.[43] For each subject, there was no difference in reading performance between the symmetrical and right shifted condition, while the left shifted window resulted in reading impairment. Thus, although anatomical symmetry might suggest a psychological symmetry in information extraction, the readers made more efficient use of information displayed to the right of fixation.[43,44] Other recent experiments[41,42] have also found evidence to suggest that the range from which useful information can be obtained extends about 14 characters to the right of the fixation point. Again, in these experiments, since the average saccade length was just over seven character spaces, the evidence seems to be that there must be overlap of information from fixation to fixation. A similar study reported by Ikeda and Saida[40] yielded similar conclusions. Rayner[45] also found that while the information necessary to make a semantic identification of words was limited to words beginning less than six characters to the right of the fixation point, other more gross types of information were obtained beyond that region and were useful during reading.

These experiments[46,47] imply that readers are obtaining different types of information from different regions of the perceptual span during a fixation in reading. Rayner and McConkie[46] concluded that information falling on the fovea (and just to the right of it) is processed for its semantic content and information from parafoveal vision is limited to rather gross featural information such as word shape and word length. Interestingly, they also reported that there was no evidence that word shape information was obtained further from fixation than was specific letter information (the beginning and end letters of words) and there was no evidence that information beyond the parafoveal region was useful to a reader during a particular fixation. While experiments by Rayner[45,48] indicated that a combination of beginning letter information and word shape information were useful to the reader, more recent research[49,50] has indicated that the type of information that is useful and facilitative from words in parafoveal vision is confined to word length and abstract information about the beginning letters (first two or three letters of five letter words) of words. Most probably, this beginning letter information is not stored in a visual feature form, but in a more abstract code. In fact, the shape of every letter in a word can be changed on every fixation (so that one version of alternating case is replaced by another version of alternating case during eye movements) and readers are not aware of the case change, nor does it affect their eye movement behavior.[51] Thus, the type of information that is important in parafoveal vision seems to be word length and abstract information about the beginning letters of words.

In experiments which were just the inverse of the McConkie and Rayner study, Rayner and Bertera[41] and Rayner, et al.[42] found further support for the conclusion that word length information and beginning (and end) letter information is important in the parafovea. In these experiments, a visual mask moved in synchrony with the eye movement so that wherever the reader looked, the mask was centered around the fixation point. The experimenters varied the size of the mask so that sometimes it covered only the single character in the center of vision and on other occasions it was as large as 17 characters. When the mask was 7 characters, foveal vision was completely masked; when the mask was as large as 17 characters, foveal vision and a good part of parafoveal vision were masked. When foveal vision was masked, it was still possible to read, although somewhat difficult. When the mask was as large as 13 to 17 characters, coherent reading was all but impossible and the mean effective reading rate (determined by multiplying the total reading time by the number of words correctly reported) was close to zero. The errors and confabulations that occurred when subjects tried to read sentences with foveal vision masked were consistent with the partial visual information they were able to obtain from parafoveal vision. In the experiment, subjects were asked to read sentences under the masking conditions and then report whatever they could from the sentence. Errors of the following type were very common: *fliers* was misread as *fires, fuzzy* as *funny, stereo* as *store, recruits* as *relatives, customer* as *cashier, lightly painted* as *greatly pleased,* and *satisfaction* as *accommodation.* In short, the errors made when foveal vision was completely masked indicated that readers were obtaining information about the beginning letters (and sometimes ending letters) of words in parafoveal vision, as well as word length information, and trying to construct coherent sentences out of the partial information they had available to them.

In summary, the results of the experiments on the perceptual span in reading described in this section indicate that meaning is obtained from a relatively small region, namely the foveal region and just to the right. Beyond that region, readers are able to obtain beginning letter (and perhaps end letter) information and word length information. Word length information seems to be acquired further into parafoveal vision than beginning letter information. Since word length information is acquired approximately twice as far into parafoveal vision as the average saccade length, it is possible that on certain occasions more than one saccade is programmed at a time.[52] However, some data regarding regressive eye fixations to be discussed later also make it very clear that only one saccade is programmed at a time, much of the time.

B. Fixation Durations in Reading

The results of the studies dealing with the perceptual span indicate that we gain access to distinct codes during a single fixation, i.e., semantic as well as visual information seems to be available. This is in agreement with eye movement control models which allow processing to reach a semantic level during an individual fixation. In order to substantiate this position, it would be necessary to show a relationship between eye movement behavior and certain linguistic variables affecting the difficulty of the text. As indicated previously, it has been known for some time that the difficulty of the text influences fixation duration;[4] more difficult passages result in longer mean fixation durations. Syntactic structure of the text also affects fixation durations.[53,54] Likewise, when subjects are asked to read passages of statistical approximations to normal text, fixation duration decreases as the text becomes more like normal.[55,56] These demonstrations, however, reflect rather gross changes and may not reflect moment-to-moment changes.

Other research does more directly support the position that eye movements reflect cognitive activity. Infrequent and unusual words receive longer fixation times than more frequent words[14,57] and when misspellings[58] or nonwords[45] are inserted in text, there are substantially increased fixation times. Rayner[45] also reported differences in fixation duration on words that were changed during the eye movement that depended on the type of change made and Pynte[59] reported that the number of syllables in the stimulus influenced fixation duration; if more syllables were required to pronounce the stimulus, fixations were longer than when fewer syllables made up the stimulus.

In addition, a number of studies have related longer fixations to certain grammatical elements in text.[54,57,60-62] For instance, these studies have reported that the main verb in simple active sentences received longer fixations than the key nouns in the sentence. Just and Carpenter[63] found that fixation durations were longer on an agent in a sentence in which there was an indirect inference linking two concepts than one in a sentence in which there is direct inference. In some other research, Carpenter and Just[64] found that readers tend to make regressive eye movements to the referent of a pronoun. In the study, the referent of the pronoun was ambiguous, such that either of two nouns in a preceding sentence would qualify. On over 50% of the trials, readers looked back to at least one of the two nouns in the preceding sentence. The occurrence of the regressive fixation probably indicates the point in time at which the assignment of the referent was made. The assignment could occur as soon as the pronoun was encountered, or it could occur after the entire clause or sentence was read. The results of the study showed both trends, producing a clearly bimodal distribution. The fact that a regression occurred as soon as the pronoun was encountered on many trials provides strong support for the position that there is not a lag between eye fixation and cognitive processing. Further support for the position comes from studies relating fixation duration to inferential processes in reading.[65,66]

Finally, in some recent studies[42] in which the onset of a visual mask was delayed for various amounts of time after the eye movement ends, it has been found that most of the visual information necessary for reading is acquired during the first 50 msec of the fixation. Presenting the mask rather late in the fixation does provide some disruption over a control condition in which there is no mask (see Wolverton[67] for an argument that information is acquired throughout the fixation period), but it appears that most of the visual information is acquired early, leaving later parts of the fixation for integrating the semantic information.

As we indicated previously, two major positions can be taken with regard to the control of fixation duration in reading. One position, most closely aligned with minimal control and low-level models, assumes that there is no control over fixation duration. Hence, the length of a fixation is determined by oculomotor processes or determined by masking constraints. The other position, represented by high-level control and process-monitoring models, assumes that fixation duration reflects cognitive processes or difficulty level of text. Experimental evidence from both perceptual span studies and research controlling semantic or syntactic text characteristics seem to favor this latter position.

C. Eye Guidance in Reading

While there is much speculation on how eye movements may be guided during reading, the data are not as plentiful. Rayner and McConkie[12] computed the probability of a fixation landing on words of different lengths and the probability of fixating on a letter within a word of a given length. They found that as word length increased, the probability of fixating the word increased. However, when the probability of fixating on a letter within a word of a given length was computed, it was found that a letter in a word four to seven letters long was more likely to be fixated than a letter in a shorter or longer word. Rayner[68] found that fixation location within words was not random, but rather fixation frequency peaked in the middle and slightly toward the beginning of the word. Thus, for example, the median fixation point was on the third letter in five letter words and the fourth letter in ten-letter words. Thus, both of these studies indicate that where the eye was sent was related to the word length pattern of the text.

In the perceptual span experiments described previously, McConkie and Rayner found that filling the spaces between words outside of the window area resulted in longer reading times and shorter saccades than when the spacing was left intact. Spragins, Lefton, and Fisher[69] also found that filling in spaces between words resulted in longer reading times and shorter saccades. However, in this study, passages of text were prepared so that every space was filled between words and compared to the reading of passages with normal spacing. Hence, the study did not indicate where the locus of the problem is when spaces between words in the fovea are filled; that is, whether this is disruptive to the eye movement mechanisms or whether added processing is required to identify the location of words. Of course, the answer may be that both types of interference are occurring. Ahlen,[70] Ikeda and Saida,[40] Rayner and Bertera[41] and Rayner et al.[42] found that removing the text pattern outside of the window area significantly decreased saccade size.

In other studies dealing with the effect of spacing on eye movements in reading, Abrams and Zuber[71] and Ahlen[70] found that readers tended not to fixate on blank areas inserted in text. Along a similar vein, Rayner[72] reported that there were fewer fixations than usual in the region between sentences; that is, on the last letters in one sentence, the period and space between, and the function word beginning the next sentence. He also found that fixations occurring in that region tended to be of shorter durations than fixations in other regions of the text.

Finally, O'Regan[73,74] and Rayner[68] both found that the length of the word to the right of the fixated word influenced the length of the next saccade; if that word was longer, the eye tended to jump farther. Thus, if the reader was fixated on the second letter of a six-letter word and either a five-letter word or a ten-letter word occurred next, the saccade would be longer in the case of the ten-letter word. On the other hand, if the six-letter word was followed by a short word (one to three characters), the probability is rather high that the short word would not be fixated[68] resulting in a longer saccade than when a five-letter word occurred next. These results are consistent with Rayner's finding[68] that there are preferred viewing locations in words and that readers try and center their fixation on these preferred viewing locations. O'Regan[73,74] also reported that the word *the* tends to be skipped more frequently than other more substantive three-letter words. Since *the* is a function word containing little useful information, presumably the reader could detect it in nonfoveal vision and direct the saccade beyond it. The closer the eye is to the word *the* on the prior fixation, the higher is the probability that it will be skipped.

The results presented here provide strong evidence that the eye is being directed in some nonrandom fashion. Thus, as we have implied previously, these data serve to eliminate minimal control models. Of course, it is still likely that there is a random component in our eye movement control; i.e., the eye movement control is not entirely accurate no matter what its basis is. This latter point is entirely possible as Kaufmann and Richards[75] have shown that when subjects are asked to move their fixation point back and forth between two targets, they often do not fixate directly on the target even though they think they are. On the other hand, McConkie[36] has argued that in reading, fixation locations are specifically determined. The amount of variability which must be left to the explanation that there is some inaccuracy in eye movement control can only be ascertained following extensive attempts to explain it on other bases.

The data reviewed here strongly indicate that where the eye is sent is related to word length patterns. However, this data pattern could arise from any of the three types of models that assume specific control. For example, a low-level control process could adjust saccade lengths to increase the probability that longer words, as identified in parafoveal vision, would be located at the center of vision on preferred viewing locations. This could be seen as a strategy shaped during learning to read, as one learns that they can be identified at locations further from the center of vision. This tendency could be coupled with a tendency to fixate a well-known word only once, which is usually sufficient to identify it. Thus, if a longer word is in central vision, the eye mechanism would tend to cast the eye further to get beyond it on the next fixation. These tendencies would produce eye movement patterns that are consistent with the data we have reviewed here.

High-level control models could probably also account for the same type of eye movement pattern. For example, Rayner and McConkie[12] in informal studies noted that word length patterns are related to syntactic structure. They asked readers to mark phrase boundaries in mutilated text in which every letter was replaced by an *x* and found that subjects could do so with an accuracy far above chance. Thus, a model which supposes that readers make hypotheses about the syntactic structure of the text, aided partially by parafoveal and peripheral visual information, and then guide the eye in some manner on the basis of these hypotheses to bring the most information-rich segments of text into the center of foveal vision, might in some manner lead to a data pattern like that described. Such models have not yet been worked out in enough detail to make clear predictions, but it is likely that they could lead to predicted relations between fixation locations and word length. However, we also hasten to add that McConkie and Rayner[34] have strongly argued that for hypothesis testing notions to be distinct from other models of reading, readers must be making hypotheses about specific words. The results of recent studies indicate that readers are not able to obtain accurate information for making semantic identifications on the basis of partial information obtained from parafoveal vision.[45,49,50] Rayner[45] presented passages of text in which either of two visually similar words (*palace-police, chest-chart)* could occur in the same location and fit into the context of the passage. One of the two words was initially displayed in the text on the CRT, but when the reader's eye movement crossed a prespecified location, the word originally displayed was replaced by the other member of the pair. Hence, certain information the reader obtained about the word prior to the eye movement would be inconsistent with information available after the saccade; certainly, the meaning of the two words differs although visually they are quite similar. If readers are able to make semantic identifications (or partial identifications) of words in parafoveal vision, then changing from one word to the other during the saccade should lead to a certain amount of disruption, since the hypothesis would be disconfirmed and some reprocessing or reanalysis would have to occur. Rayner found that this type of disruption occurred only for words beginning less than six character spaces to the right of the fixation point. McConkie[76] has also reported data which indicate that the information necessary for semantic identification is limited to the foveal region. Furthermore, the errors subjects made in the foveal masking studies[41,42] were predictable from the visual appearance of the words in the parafovea and not from any type of semantic relationship. These findings seem to mitigate against the high-level view that semantic or partial semantic information is involved in eye guidance in reading.

Finally, process-monitoring models could lead to predictions of the same general type concerning word length and fixation location. For instance, if it were supposed that the reader identifies words as far to the right of the fixation point as possible, and then simply casts the eye some distance which reflects the termination of word recognition on the prior fixation, it is likely that a pattern of eye movements yielding a relationship between word length and fixation location would emerge. For example, Rayner and McConkie[12] in accounting for the curvilinear relationship found between word length and fixation location, suggested that two opposing tendencies operate to account for the results. First, if two words begin an equal distance to the right of the fixation point, the shorter is more likely to be identified. Thus, the longer word is more likely to be fixated on the next fixation. Second, the reader actually needs to see a smaller proportion of a longer word in order to identify it. Thus, a greater proportion of a longer word could lie outside the perceptual span region for making semantic identifications, and it could still be identified, than with a shorter word, on the average. This means that fewer fixations per letter would be required for long words. These two tendencies, which work in opposite directions, could give rise to a data pattern in which there was a curvilinear relationship between word length and the average number of fixations per letter in the word. O'Regan[73] argued for a model of this type and attempted to describe the contextual constraints and parafoveal visual information limitations which determine how far into the parafovea word identification is likely to succeed at different points in the text.

In summary then, we have reviewed the existing data on the control of eye guidance and suggested that word length patterns are strongly associated with fixation location. It would also appear that while the data provide support for the existence of some sort of specific and momentary control over eye guidance, we are not able to unambiguously select among competing models which assume control of quite different sorts. The data do seem to be more consistent with either low-level models, which assume that visual characteristics of the text are more important in eye guidance, or process-monitoring models. While high-level control models which assume that there is semantic control of eye movements are not ruled out, the position is weakened somewhat by the available data.

V. CONCLUSION

In this chapter, we have reviewed various models of eye movement control during reading and the extent to which they can assimilate currently available experimental data. We have argued that there are three basic eye movement components of reading (fixation duration, saccade length, and regressions) and that each of these characteristics have a fair amount of variability associated with them. The goal of the different models is to account for the variability. For the most part, we have focused on fixation duration and saccade length in our discussions of the various models, although most of the models can easily accomodate ideas regarding regressive eye movements. We have reached a number of conclusions regarding acceptable models of eye movement control, but we cannot unambiguously choose between certain models that account for the data in different ways.

First, we have argued that minimal control models cannot adequately account for the data that are available. In addition, we have suggested that gain control models and buffer monitoring models (which represent extensions of the minimal control and process-monitoring models, respectively) have no explanatory value, since each fixation and each saccade seem to represent a processing cycle of their own. In order to account for the data which we have reviewed, the gain control and buffer monitoring would have to operate on a moment-to-moment basis and, hence, these models become indistinguishable from models which explicitly posit that the control of eye movements in reading is made on a moment-to-moment basis. Also, the high-level model falls short in explaining data associated with saccade length while the low-level model cannot absorb experimental evidence favoring a relation between cognitive processes and fixation duration. Finally, we have argued that the process-monitoring model faces a potential difficulty if it is assumed that the programing of the next eye movement is contingent upon semantic evaluation of the foveally fixated information.

Models which remain acceptable are as follows: The high-level model, as well as a processing-monitoring model adapted to the fixation duration data, while a low-level model and a process-monitoring model can be adjusted to deal with eye guidance characteristics. However, although high-level and process-monitoring models arrive at the same predictions for fixation duration (since they share the common assumption of semantic processing of the fixated text), the models differ in the mechanisms assumed to be in operation. A high-level model seems to rely on whole word identification processes, while the process-monitoring view additionally holds that the reader projects his attention as far to the right as possible for semantic identification to occur. Thus, this model is at ease with multiple fixations within single, long words. Considering saccade length, we associate the relationship between word length and saccade length as evidence for low-level processes operating in the parafoveal region, while the importance of beginning letter information suggests a level above the visual processing (yet short of semantic processing), especially since the beginning letter information is stored independently from its visual representation.

We would argue that no unmodified eye movement control model that has been outlined is in accordance with the available experimental data. What we shall argue in the remainder of this chapter is that mixed models provide the most reasonable explanation for eye movement control. A high-level and low-level mixed model which assumes high-level processes operating in a right-biased foveal area and low-level processes controlling parafoveal information extraction from the right of fixation can account for the data. Here, word length information may serve to program the extent of the saccadic eye movement and initial letter identification may facilitate later lexical access. According to this model, the reader gains semantic, word length, and initial letter information during each individual fixation, which seems to be composed of two discrete stages. Recent data[42] suggest that visual representation processes are accomplished within an initial 50 msec interval. Following this initial period, a division of labor may follow with a foveal system specialized in semantic evaluation, while parafoveal information serves to calculate the length of the saccade. The result of this calculation is held in storage and the saccade is executed as soon as semantic identification is accomplished, i.e., saccade initiation is contingent upon termination of cognitive evaluation. As we indicated earlier, regressions may involve a different eye guidance mechanism, since the reader regresses to information he has already stored. Thus, in order to regress, the reader may call forth a storage-based parameter instead of its visually guided equivalent used to direct forward saccades. This seems to implicate that the saccade initiation is dependent upon a successful integration of information in an ongoing fixation with stored information.

The only model that initially appeared able to handle both the fixation duration and saccade length data is the process-monitoring model. However, this model does have some problems of its own in dealing with the data. First, as we indicated above, if it is assumed that programing of the next eye movement is contingent upon semantic evaluation of the currently fixated text, there are problems concerning timing constraints. That is, semantic evaluation and integration of the text at a semantic level presumably takes up a certain amount of time. In addition, the average latency period of the eye is in the range of 150 to 175 msec and, so, the combination of the time for semantic evaluation and the latency period of the eye would result in most fixations far exceeding the average duration of 200 to 250 msec. Second, if it is assumed that process-monitoring involves word identification as far to the right of fixation as possible, it is unclear how such a model can account for the findings suggesting the importance of beginning letters of parafoveal words. A way of dealing with this problem is to assume that the system identifies words as far to the right as possible and also processes the beginning letters of unidentified words prior to the initiation of the next saccade bringing a new region into foveal vision.[77] It may also well be that word length is a major cue (along with the semantic span) utilized in determining where to look next and regressions would be determined when some type of semantic evaluation failed. Thus, a mixed model combining process-monitoring and low-level models also could account for the data patterns we have described.

In essence, then, either of the two mixed models we have described here can account for the data. In fact, at some level the two models become indistinguishable in predicting the data. Both would suggest that evaluation of the foveal information influences the type of information that can be obtained from the parafovea[78] and both models would predict that fixations should be located toward the beginning of words that were previously in parafoveal vision.[68] Hence, there would be a relationship between word length and fixation location and, since fixation duration is influenced by the characteristics of the text in foveal vision, there would be lengthened fixations at certain critical places in text.

While on the one hand, both of these mixed models can be adjusted to account for the data, as we have mentioned before, the two versions are based on different assumptions. Inherent in the high-level model is a distinction between foveal and parafoveal processing or between semantic processing and semantic preprocessing. In the mixed high-level and low-level models, the dual process assumption, as well as the notion of foveal semantic processing remains basically unmodified. However, in dealing with the parafoveal system, we suggested that a different mechanism controls the timing characteristics of saccade programing than controls the duration of the fixation. Hence, the saccade is determined by visual characteristics. This mixed model also seems to leave open the possibility of global semantic processing operating during a single fixation so that a number of fixations on the same word or phrase would be lumped together representing a "gaze" on the word or phrase.[79]

The process-monitoring and low-level combination presumably would rely on individual fixation durations as major indices of cognitive processing, rather than aggregating a number of fixations together. The mixed process-monitoring and low-level model remains basically a single component (semantic span) model. Conserving the process-monitoring character for fixation duration and adding low-level processes for eye guidance makes the rather simple process-monitoring model much more intricate in the combined form. For example, it seems that saccade length, though biased by visual cues, also has to consider the output of the foveal semantic span processes. Thus, saccade length seems to be the result of two separate processes: semantic span length and visual cues about word length. In this model then, foveal and parafoveal processing seem not to follow the division of labor principle described above, but rather seem to be controlled by an interactive principle.

It also seems to us that there are two final distinctions between these two mixed models. One potential difference revolves around the accuracy of the saccadic eye movement. It would appear that the combined high-level and low-level model could allow for a certain amount of noise in terms of where the eye lands, as long as it is fairly close to the next region to be semantically evaluated (and which has received some preprocessing in terms of the beginning letters of the upcoming word). On the other hand, it would seem that even in its modified form, the process-monitoring component[36] requires that eye movements are rather strictly programmed to the specific point at which new information necessary for semantic identification can be acquired. The other potential difference relates to the concept of attention; the notion of attention is very important to the process-monitoring model and not relevant to the high-level and low-level mixed models. It is well known that attention and eye location are not always correlated.[80] However, this demonstration is based mainly on rather simple tasks and the process-monitoring model proposed by McConkie[36] assumes that in a complex task like reading, there is a fairly high correlation between eye location and attention. Attention does move around in the eye fixation according to the process-monitoring notion and generally shifts to the right in a fixation; when word boundaries are reached, an eye movement is initiated. This concept can be retained in the mixed model and serves as the basis for the interaction between process-monitoring and the use of low-level cues. The attention shift principle can also be used in explaining the finding that on return sweeps and certain regressions attention is directed to the left of the fixation.[68]

In summary then, we would argue that in the last few years a number of advances have been made toward our understanding of the control of eye movements in reading. However, many unanswered questions remain and are obvious from our discussions throughout this chapter. It does appear, as we have reviewed above, that fixation duration is determined either by high-level or process-monitoring activities and that saccade length is determined by low-level or process-monitoring activities. We have suggested that some type of mixed model of eye movement control can most adequately explain the data and future research and theorizing will have to spell out more specifically the characteristics and limitations of how our eyes are controlled as we read text.

REFERENCES

1. Javal, L. E., Essai sur la Physiologie de la Lecture, *Ann. Ocul.*, 82, 242, 1878.
2. Huey, E. B., *The Psychology and Pedagogy of Reading,* Macmillian, New York, 1908.
3. Woodworth, R. S., *Exp. Psychology,* Holt, Rinehart & Winston, New York, 1938.
4. Tinker, M. A., Recent studies of eye movements in reading, *Psychol. Bull.,* 55, 215, 1958.
5. Rayner, K., Eye movements in reading and information processing, *Psychol. Bull.,* 85, 618, 1978.
6. Blumenthal, A. L., *Language Psychol.,* John Wiley & Sons, New York, 1970.
7. Gray, C. T., The anticipation of meaning as a factor in reading ability, *Elementary School J.,* 1923.
8. Schmidt, W. A., *An Experimental Study with the Psychology of Reading,* University of Chicago Press, Chicago, 1917.
9. Hochberg, J., Components of literacy: speculations and exploratory research, in *Basic Studies on Reading,* Levin, H. and Williams, J. P., Eds., Basic Books, New York, 1970.
10. Tinker, M. A., Eye movements in reading, *J. Educ. Res.,* 30, 241, 1936.
11. Tinker, M. A., The study of eye movements during reading, *Psychol. Bull.,* 43, 93, 1946.
12. Rayner, K. and McConkie, G. W., What guides a reader's eye movements?, *Vision Res.,* 16, 829, 1976.
13. Andriessen, J. J. and deVoogd, A. H., Analysis of eye movement patterns in silent reading, *IPO Ann. Prog. Rep.,* 8, 29, 1973.
14. Bouma, H., Visual search and reading: eye movements and functional visual field, in *Attention and Performance VII,* Requin, J., Ed., Erlbaum, Hillsdale, N.J., 1978.
15. Kolers, P. A., Buswell's discoveries., in *Eye Movements and Psychological Processes,* Monty, R. A. and Senders, J. W., Eds., Erlbaum, Hillsdale, N.J., 1976.
16. Shebilske, W., Reading eye movements from an information-processing point of view, in *Understanding language,* Massaro, D., Ed., Academic Press, New York, 1975.
17. Bouma, H. and deVoogd, A. H., On the control of eye saccades in reading, *Vision Res.,* 14, 273, 1974.
18. Hochberg, J., On the control of eye saccades in reading, *Vision Res.,* 15, 620, 1975.
19. Antes, J. R., The time course of picture viewing, *J. Exp. Psychol.,* 103, 62, 1974.
20. Mackworth, N. H. and Morandi, A. J., The gaze selects informative details within pictures, *Percept. Psychophys.,* 2, 547, 1967.
21. Saida, S. and Ikeda, M., Useful visual field size for pattern perception, *Percept. Psychophys.,* 25, 119, 1979.
22. Gould, J. D., Pattern recognition and eye-movement parameters, *Percept. Psychophys.,* 2, 399, 1967.
23. Engel, F. L., Visual conspicuity, visual search and fixation tendencies of the eye, *Vision Res.,* 17, 95, 1977.
24. Fitzgerald, R. E. and Kirkham, R., Backward visual masking as a function of average uncertainty of the masking pattern, *Psychonomic Sci.,* 6, 469, 1966.
25. Cox, S. I. and Dember, W. N., Backward masking of visual targets with internal contours, *Psychonomic Sci.,* 19, 255, 1970.
26. Jacobson, J. Z., Interaction of similarity to words of visual masks and targets, *J. Exp. Psychol.,* 102, 431, 1974.
27. Jacobson, J. Z. and Rhinelander, G., Geometric and semantic similarity in visual masking, *J. Exp. Psychol.: Hum. Percept. Performance,* 4, 224, 1978.
28. Levin, H. and Kaplan, E. L., Grammatical structure and reading, in *Basic Studies on Reading,* Levin, H. and Williams, J. P., Eds., Basic Books, New York, 1970.

29. Smith, F., *Understanding Reading,* Holt, Rinehart & Winston, New York, 1971.

30. Kolers, P. A., Three stages of reading, in *Basic Studies on Reading,* Levin, H. and Williams, J. P., Eds., Basic Books, New York, 1970.

31. Lewis, J. L., Semantic processing of unattended messages using dichotic listening, *J. Exp. Psychol.,* 85, 225, 1970.

32. Lackner, J. R. and Garrett, M. F., Resolving ambiguity: effects of biasing context in the unattended ear, *Cognition,* 1, 359, 1972.

33. Kolers, P. A. and Lewis, C. L., Bounding of letter sequences and the integration of visually presented words, *Acta Psychologica,* 36, 112, 1972.

34. McConkie, G. W. and Rayner, K., Identifying the span of the effective stimulus in reading: literature review and theories of reading, in *Theoretical Models and Processes of Reading,* Singer, H. and Ruddell, R. B., Eds., International Reading Association, Newark, Del., 1976.

35. Gibson, E. J. and Levin, H., *The Psychology of Reading,* MIT Press, Cambridge, 1975.

36. McConkie, G. W., On the role and control of eye movements in reading, in *Processing of Visible Language 1,* Kolers, P. A., Wrolstad, M., and Bouma, H., Eds., Plenum Press, New York, 1979.

37. Rayner, K., Eye movement latencies for parafoveally presented words, *Bull. Psychonomic Soc.,* 11, 13, 1978.

38. Rayner, K., Eye movements and the perceptual span in reading, in *Neuropsychological and Cognitive Processes in Reading,* Pirozzolo, F. J. and Wittrock, M., Eds., Academic Press, New York, 1981.

39. McConkie, G. W. and Rayner, K., The span of the effective stimulus during a fixation in reading, *Percept. Psychophys.,* 17, 578, 1975.

40. Ikeda, M. and Saida, S., Span of recognition in reading, *Vision Res.,* 18, 83, 1978.

41. Rayner, K. and Bertera, J. H., *Reading without a fovea, Science,* 206, 468, 1979.

42. Rayner, K., Inhoff, A. W., Morrison, R., Slowiaczek, M. L., and Bertera, J. H., Masking of foveal and parafoveal vision during eye fixations in reading, *J. Exp. Psychol., (Human Perception and Performance),* 6, 167, 1981.

43. McConkie, G. W. and Rayner, K., Asymmetry of the perceptual span in reading, *Bull. Psychonomic Soc.,* 8, 365, 1976.

44. Rayner, K., Well, A., and Pollatsek, A., Asymmetry of the effective visual field in reading, *Perception Psychophys.,* 27, 537, 1980.

45. Rayner, K., The perceptual span and peripheral cues in reading, *Cognit. Psychol.,* 7, 65, 1975.

46. Rayner, K. and McConkie, G. W., Perceptual processes in reading: the perceptual spans, in *Toward a Psychology of Reading,* Reber, A. and Scarborough, D., Eds., Erlbaum, Hillsdale, N.J., 1977.

47. McConkie, G. W., The use of eye-movement data in determining the perceptual span in reading, in *Eye Movements and Psychological Processes,* Monty, R. A. and Senders, J. W., Eds., Erlbaum, Hillsdale, N.J., 1976.

48. Rayner, K., Foveal and parafoveal cues in reading, in *Attention and Performance VII,* Requin, J., Ed., Erlbaum, Hillsdale, N.J., 1978.

49. Rayner, K., McConkie, G. W., and Ehrlich, S., Eye movements and integrating information across fixations, *J. Exp. Psychol.: Hum. Percept. Performance,* 4, 529, 1978.

50. Rayner, K., McConkie, G. W., and Zola, D., Integrating information across eye movements, *Cognitive Psychol.,* 12, 206, 1980.

51. McConkie, G. W. and Zola, D., Is visual information integrated across successive fixations in reading?, *Percept. Psychophys.,* 25, 221, 1979.

52. Levy-Schoen, A. and Blanc-Garin, J., On oculomotor programming and perception, *Brain Res.,* 71, 443, 1974.

53. Klein, G. A. and Kurkowski, F., Effect of task demands on relationships between eye movements and sentence complexity, *Percept. Motor Skills,* 39, 463, 1974.

54. Communale, A. S., Visual selectivity in reading: The relationship between eye movements and linguistic structure, Ph.D. thesis, University of Massachusetts, 1973.

55. Vanacek, E., Fixations dauer und Fixations frequenz bein stillen lesen von Sprachapproximationen. *Z. Exp. und Angew. Psychol.,* 19, 671, 1972.

56. Jacobson, J. Z. and Dodwell, P. C., Saccadic eye movements during reading, *Brain Language,* 8, 303, 1979.

57. Rayner, K., Visual attention in reading: eye movements reflect cognitive processes, *Mem. Cognit.,* 4, 443, 1977.

58. Zola, D., The effects of context on the visual perception of words in reading, paper presented at the meetings of the Am. Educ. Res. Assoc., San Francisco, 1979.

59. Pynte, J., Readiness for pronunciation during the reading process, *Percept. Psychophys.,* 16, 110, 1974.

60. Mehler, J., Bever, T. G., and Carey, P., What we look at when we read, *Percept. Psychophys.,* 2, 213, 1967.

61. **Wanat, S. F.,** Language behind the eye: some findings, speculations, and research strategies, in *Eye Movements and Psychological Processes,* Monty, R. A. and Senders, J. W., Eds., Erlbaum, Hillsdale, N.J., 1976.

62. **Zargar-Yazdi, A.,** An investigation of reading: eye movements and word recall, Ph.D. thesis, Stanford University, 1973.

63. **Just, M. A. and Carpenter, P. A.,** Inference processes during reading: reflections from eye fixation, in *Eye Movements and the Higher Psychological Processes,* Senders, J. W., Fisher, D. F., and Monty, R. A., Eds., Erlbaum, Hillsdale, N.J., 1978.

64. **Carpenter, P. A. and Just, M. A.,** Reading comprehension as eyes see it, in *Cognitive Processes in Comprehension,* Just, M. A. and Carpenter, P. A., Eds., Erlbaum, Hillsdale, N.J., 1977.

65. **Scinto, L. F.,** Relation of eye fixations to old-new information of texts, in *Eye Movements and the Higher Psychological Processes,* Senders, J. W., Fisher, D. F., and Monty, R. A., Eds., Erlbaum, Hillsdale, N.J., 1978.

66. **Kennedy, A.,** Eye movements and the integration of semantic information during reading, in *Practical Aspects of Memory,* Gruneberg, M. M., Morris, P. E., and Sykes, R. N., Eds., Academic Press, London, 1979.

67. **Wolverton, G. S.,** The acquisition of visual information during fixations and saccades in reading, paper presented at the meetings of the Am. Educ. Res. Assoc., San Francisco, 1979.

68. **Rayner, K.,** Eye guidance in reading: fixation locations within words, *Perception,* 8, 21, 1979.

69. **Spragins, A. B., Lefton, L. A., and Fisher, D. F.,** Eye movements while reading spatially transformed text: a developmental study, *Mem. Cognit.,* 4, 36, 1976.

70. **Ahlen, J.,** Spatial and temporal aspects of visual information processing during reading, Ph.D. thesis, University of Illinois Medical Center, 1974.

71. **Abrams, S. G. and Zuber, B. L.,** Some temporal characteristics of visual information processing during reading, *Reading Res. Q.,* 12, 41, 1972.

72. **Rayner, K.,** Parafoveal identification during a fixation in reading, *Acta Psychologica,* 39, 271, 1975.

73. **O'Regan, K.,** Structural and contextual constraints on eye movements in reading, Ph.D. thesis, University of Cambridge, 1975.

74. **O'Regan, K.,** Saccade size control in reading: evidence for the linguistic control hypothesis, *Percept. Psychophys.,* 25, 501, 1979.

75. **Kaufman, L. and Richards, W.,** Spontaneous fixation tendencies for visual forms, *Percept. Psychophys.,* 5, 85, 1969.

76. **McConkie, G. W.,** Where do we read?, paper presented at the meetings of the Psychonomic Soc., San Antonio, 1978.

77. **Rayner, K.,** Eye movements in reading: eye guidance and integration, in *Processing of Visible Language 1,* Kolers, P. A., Wrolstad, M., and Bouma, H., Eds., Plenum Press, New York, 1979.

78. **Lee, Y. A.,** Parafoveal processing during reading, Ph.D. thesis, University of Rochester, 1979.

79. **Just, M. A. and Carpenter, P. A.,** Eye fixations and cognitive processes, *Cognit. Psychol.,* 8, 441, 1976.

80. **Klein, R.,** Does oculomotor readiness mediate cognitive control of visual attention?, in *Attention and Performance VIII,* Nickerson, R., Ed., Erlbaum, Hillsdale, N.J., 1979.

Chapter 12

CLINICAL DISORDERS OF OCULAR MOVEMENT

Louis F. Dell'Osso and Robert B. Daroff

TABLE OF CONTENTS

I. INTRODUCTION

A. Definition of Approach

The study of "experiments of nature" (i.e., ocular motor pathology) can provide valuable insights into *normal* ocular motor physiology which may be impossible to learn from the study of normals. After nature has stressed the ocular motor system in various specific ways, its responses demonstrate inherent abilities, adaptabilities, and limitations not obvious from the study of normal subjects. The extension of clinical studies in patients by a modeling approach has further added to our knowledge of the abnormal and normal ocular motor system.

The model, to the bioengineer, is like the experimental animal to the physiologist; both are substrates upon which hypotheses can be tested quantitatively. The distinct difference between the physiologist's animal and the bioengineer's model is the fine control one has over the exact type, placement, and extent of the lesions administered to the latter. All of the constraints required for a good model of normal ocular motor function (close conformity to known anatomy and neurophysiology), apply to models of ocular motor pathology. In addition, models of disturbed eye movements must respond to appropriate "lesions" in a manner which duplicates the clinical manifestations in patients. If the model (hypothesis) is a good one, it will respond normally before it is "lesioned" and exhibit the appropriate specific abnormalities after the "lesion" is placed.

B. Value of Approach

With the modelling approach to ocular motor pathology, one is forced to think logically about function and interactions of subsystems in a framework defined by specific quantitative assumptions. As much can be learned from a negative test of the hypothesis (model) as from a positive test; the redefinition of its parts caused by the model's failure to respond properly to a stimulus may yield more insight into ocular motor function than a proper response.

In this chapter, we will discuss models of eye movement disturbances starting at the plant (the extraocular muscles) and working rostrally through the cranial nerves to the central nervous system.

II. PLANT DISORDERS

A. Ocular Myasthenia

Myasthenia gravis (MG) is a motor disorder believed to be secondary to blockade of the acetylcholine receptor at the neuromuscular junction.[1] The extraocular muscles seem preferentially involved, as almost all cases ultimately manifest, in eye muscle weakness. The study of ocular myasthenia is complicated by the fact that the neuromuscular deficit in the ocular motor plant is nonstationary resulting in saccade-to-saccade variability. Plastic changes in the central saccadic gain can only correct for some average deficit, however. The resultant eye movements, although predominantly hypometric, are at times orthometric or even hypermetric. An adequate model of such stochastic variation requires nonstationary coefficients in the plant parameters. An attempt to match the temporal randomness of the neuromuscular junction efficiency would result in an extremely complex model. We therefore chose to model the system by simulating the different states of plant efficiency with specific parameter adjustments and then study the system response to each state separately. This simpler model common in myasthenic patients. Figure 1a is a block diagram of the model, which was simulated on a Systron Donner SD-80 analog computer.[2] Both retinal feedback and simulated on a Systron Donner SD-80 analog computer.[2] Both retinal feedback and internal monitoring (efference copy) were included in the model; proprioception (dashed line) was not. Provisions for selectively causing plant deficits were included as was the ability to simulate the increased central gain (i.e., saccadic plasticity) which occurs in MG and serves to partially compensate for the peripheral deficits. With this model, we could study saccadic metrics in MG, but not the variations in saccadic trajectories.[3]

The primary changes in MG occur in the eye plant. We simulated the plant by two cascaded "leaky" integrators (first-order lag elements) as shown in Figure 1b. Without deficit, the transfer function of the normal plant was:

$$\frac{\theta_E}{\theta_M} = \frac{K}{(T_1 s+1)\,(T_2 s+1)} \quad , T_1 = .150, T_2 = .007 \text{ and } K = 7 \qquad (1)$$

Thus, for our particular simulation, the steady-state transfer function was:

$$\left.\frac{\theta_E}{\theta_M}\right|_{t \to \infty} \to K = 7 \qquad (2)$$

Note: The value of $K = 7$ has no physiological significance and was chosen because of voltage constraints of the analog computer.

Two specific types of plant disorders were simulated (also indicated in Figure 1b). One is a deficit in the tonic fibers of the extraocular muscles, with relative sparing of the phasic fibers. This was simulated by placing a resistor (R_L) around the first integrator (A1) which greatly increased its "leakiness". Although this reduced its transient response somewhat, the main effect was an inability to maintain a tonic level. When simulating a tonic deficit ($R_L = 10^6$, $R_s = \infty$) the transfer function was:

$$\frac{\theta_E}{\theta_M} = \frac{.4K}{(T_L s+1)\,(T_2 s+1)} \quad , T_L = .06 = .4T_1 , T_2 = .007 \text{ and } K = 7 \quad (3)$$

which yielded the steady-state solution:

$$\left.\frac{\theta_E}{\theta_M}\right|_{t \to \infty} \to .4K = 2.8 \qquad (4)$$

Thus, the eye would not hold the proper tonic level and would decay to 40% of the level required by the saccadic motor command (pulse step). The net result of this plant deficit in the model is a series of hypometric saccades, with overshooting trajectories spaced in time by the reaction time of the visual feedback loop (200 ms in our model), which eventually bring the eye to the target. This was a commonly observed response of MG patients.

A second plant disorder in MG is a paresis of the extraocular muscle. This was simulated by placing a saturation circuit (R_s, θ_s, and a diode) around the output integrator (A2). Small saccades (less than θ_s) would be accurate but those larger than θ_s would not. Both the point of onset (θ_s) and degree of hardness of the saturation (R_s) are adjustable. When simulating a paresis ($R_L = \infty$ and $10^6 \leqslant R_s \leqslant 10^3$), the transfer

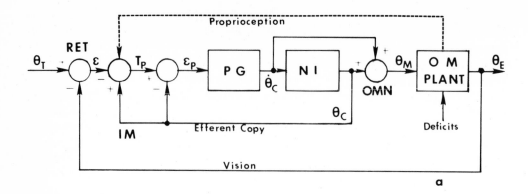

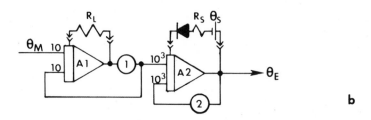

FIGURE 1.   (a) Block diagram of model used to simulate eye movements of patients with myasthenia gravis; (b) analog simulation of ocular motor plant with deficits. θ_T is target angle; ε is retinal (RET) error; T_p is perceived target angle generated by the internal monitor (IM); ε_p is perceived error; PG is pulse generator; NI is neural integrator; $\dot{\theta}_C$ is velocity command; θ_C is position command; θ_M is motor command from the ocular motor nuclei (OMN) and θ_E is eye angle in this and subsequent figures.

function was:

$$\left. \frac{\theta_E}{\theta_M} \right|_{\theta_M > \theta_S} = \frac{(.571-.00143)K}{(T_1 s+1)\,(T_S s+1)} , \quad T_1 = .150, \quad .004 \le T_S \le 10^{-5} \text{ or}$$

$$.571T_2 \le T_S \le .00143T_2, \quad K = 7 \tag{5}$$

which yielded the steady-state solution:

$$\left. \frac{\theta_E}{\theta_M} \right|_{t \to \infty} \to (.571-.00143)\, K = .4-.01 \tag{6}$$

For $\theta_M < \theta_S$, the transfer function

$$\left. \frac{\theta_E}{\theta_M} \right|_{\theta_M < \theta_S} = \left. \frac{\theta_E}{\theta_M} \right|_{normal} , \text{ which is given in Equation 1.} \tag{7}$$

The net results of a hard saturation ($R_s = 10^3$) was a large series of very hypometric (gain = .00143K) saccades spaced at 200 ms which never reached the target. The softer saturation ($R_s = 10^6$) yielded a smaller series of less hypometric (gain = .571K) saccades which also never reached the target.

In addition to simulating the primary plant disorders caused by MG, we also used the model to simulate the secondary, central compensatory mechanisms responsible for an increased innervation level. In the MG patient, this is observed by the administration of the drug edrophonium chloride which transiently improves the deficit at the neuromuscular junction. What results are hypermetric saccades (ocular dysmetria) and, if the central gain increase is sufficient, macro saccadic oscillations. These eye movements resemble those seen with cerebellar dysfunction.[4,5] A gain between one and two produced static hypermetria and a gain which transiently rose above two caused a burst of macro saccadic oscillations.

Thus, this model stimulated both the primary neuromuscular deficit and the dysfunction secondary to central plastic changes and their dual effects on saccadic metrics in myasthenia gravis.

Our studies of myasthenia revealed frequent multiple, closely spaced saccades and dynamic overshoots. These trajectories could not be the result of efference copy by an internal monitor of eye position commands, since such commands would be larger than normal; nor could visual feedback be responsible, since this loop requires a minimum of 85 ms. Only the rapid proprioceptive loop (shown dashed in Figure 1) seemed a feasible alternative. Proprioceptive feedback was also the most reasonable explanation for our observation of saccadic intrusions during maintained gaze fatigue and increased saccadic gain after maintained gaze.[6] This presumption of the role of the proprioceptive loop is supported by the fact that in normal subjects, both closely spaced saccades and dynamic overshoots increased in occurrence with fatigue.[7] Although proprioception is known to be present, this is the first time that a function for this loop has been convincingly presented; the hypothesis resulted from the study of the ocular motor system's responses to plant pathology.

B. Strabismus

Although the primary defect resulting in malalignment of the optical axes (strabismus) is innervational, this disorder is conventionally regarded as due to muscle imbalance primarily because its treatment often involves surgery of the extraocular muscles. Models which simulate the normal plant, such as those described in an earlier chapter by Robinson, can also be used to simulate strabismus if the innervation is adjusted appropriately. Robinson addressed this topic specifically by mathematically modeling the six extraocular muscles and orbital tissues for all eye positions.[8] His modeling utilized data obtained from, and in collaboration with, the Smith-Kettlewell group who have been at the forefront of plant modeling.[9,10] Although the complexity of the mathematics requires the use of a digital computer, the program can be used to estimate the correction which would result from any particular muscle surgery. The need for a more accurate approach to strabismus surgery is evident from the number of repeat operations necessary (in the U.S., 40%). What is needed now are interdisciplinary studies using the model and, when necessary, modifying it to conform to actual surgical results. If the model proves capable of predicting the efficacy of a specific surgical procedure, it may become extremely useful to strabismus surgeons.

III. NERVE PALSIES

A. Saccadic Plasticity

A discrete cranial nerve lesion which, unlike myasthenia gravis, is time invariable, allows one to study the extent and dynamics of central adaptation (plasticity). As with MG, the ocular motor system adjusts its gain to overcome deficits which impair performance. Figure 2a outlines, in block diagram, how an automatic gain control system (AGC) might alter saccadic gain utilizing retinal error (ε), efference copy, and proprioceptive information as performance measures. We studied the dynamics of saccadic gain changes in a patient with an abducens nerve lesion.[11] By alternately patching, for several days, the good and paretic eyes, we were able to force the gain of the saccadic system to change in both directions. When the changes were plotted over time, we were able to approximate the transfer function as a first-order exponential with a time constant of approximately one day (Figure 2b). Any model of the adaptive gain circuitry of the *normal* saccadic system should follow the same exponential time course obtained from this study of a patient with a unilateral and uniocular paresis.

IV. CENTRAL DISORDERS

A. Pulse Generator
1. Slow Saccades

Some patients with spinocerebellar degenerations make abnormally slow saccades. There was some question as to whether the slow refixational movements were saccades or a form of substituted slow eye movement, but Zee et al.[12] found that they were, indeed, slow saccades. The long time course of these slow saccades reveal details about the mechanism involved in creating the pulse of innervation which could not be obtained from studying normally fast saccades. The two major conclusions were (1) Saccades were not preprogramed (i.e., ballistic), but could be modified in flight; and (2) Saccades were driven to an orbital position, rather than a given distance from the point of origin.

Zee et al.'s study of patients with slow saccades prompted the model of the normal pulse generator shown in Figure 3. The model used a bootstrap circuit in which the eye position command was fed back and determined pulse width. Pulse height (i.e., saccadic velocity, $\dot{\theta}_c$) was determined by a saturation nonlinearity to the forward path. By proper scaling of the velocity-amplitude nonlinearity, they were able to duplicate the responses of different patients to short and long pulses, as well as double steps of target position. Although their model used the same neural integrator as part of the pulse generator and also to generate the efferent position command and (θ_c), we have indicated in Figure 3 that perhaps these functions are separately performed (θ_c'). The reasons for this change will be discussed in the following section on gaze-paretic nystagmus.

Although patients with spinocerebellar generations may have brainstem lesions, those with slow saccades who have been studied pathologically have not been found to have lesions of the paramedian pontine reticular formation (PPRF) where the pulse generator is located. Furthermore, the other clinical conditions associated with slow saccades (congenital ocular motor apraxia, Huntington's chorea, Wilson's disease, Gaucher's disease, and progressive supernuclear palsy) do not typically have pontine lesions. In most of these cases, therefore, the slow saccades seemed to result from disturbed inputs to the pulse generator rather than a defective generator per se. It is possible that the gains of the bootstrap loop or of the $\dot{\varnothing}$ vs. θ element in the forward path are under extra-pontine control (i.e., cerebellar, basal ganglia, etc.) and that deficits in these structures or in their interconnections with the pulse generator are responsible for the saccadic slowing.

B. Integrator
1. Gaze-Paretic Nystagmus

Gaze-evoked nystagmus is characterized by slow centripetal drifts from eccentric eye positions interrupted by centrifugal saccades back to the target. The slow phases of the nystagmus may be linear (as in vestibular and pursuit-defect nystagmus) or have a decreasing-velocity exponential shape. The latter is referred to as "gaze-paretic" nystagmus which has been modeled by creating a defect in the neural integrator (Figure 4).[13]

In gaze-paretic nystagmus, the fast phases are *normal* saccades indicating that the pulse generator functions normally despite the deficiency of the position-holding integrator. The magnitude of the centripetal drift (and hence, the nystagmus) varies directly with gaze angle from primary position. As alluded to in the previous Section, and as shown in Figure 4, the bootstrap circuit in the pulse generator utilizes a neural integrator that is distinct from the integrator responsible for generating eye position commands. In this way, deterioration of the latter produces gaze-paretic nystagmus without affecting refixation saccades and fast phases. The internal monitor (utilizing efferent copy of the position command) is responsible for making corrective eye movements in the absence of vision and is the driving stimulus for the fast phases of the gaze-paretic nystagmus. Neuronal pools (simulated by two integrators in parallel) were made deficient by either a "leak" or saturation circuit. Thus, variable deficits could be simulated by proportionally using both an unaffected integrator and one with either deficit. This simulated the percentage of affected neurons in the pool of neurons performing neural integration. The model duplicated normal saccades when no deficit was present and gaze-paretic nystagmus when either a leak or saturation occurred in a percentage of the integrator pool. Comparison of the transition areas between the nystagmus-free range of gaze angles and those with nystagmus produced by each method (leak or saturation) revealed subtle differences. The model, therefore, not only duplicated known clinical phenomena, but also suggested further studies on patients to elucidate the actual deficit present in such cases. In addition, since some portion of the total neural integrator pool was functioning normally, the internal monitor not only stimulated the pulse generator, but also directed the fast-phase pulses only to those integrator neurons whose output was deficient. Neural integration must be accomplished by many neurons whose outputs supply the large numbers of motoneurons with eye position commands. When a subset of these neurons is made to function inadequately by disease or trauma, only the neurons in that subset should receive additional neural pulses from the pulse generator. The healthy neurons in the integrator pool must not, lest they produce a position command greater than the correct output which they generated as a result of the initial saccadic velocity pulse. This model, therefore, also provided some insight into the complex control of redundant neuronal circuitry which would not have been apparent from modeling normal saccadic function.

C. Pause Cell

Zee and Robinson[14] attributed several saccadic abnormalities to pause cell dysfunction. Before considering these disorders, we will review the role of the pause, burst, and tonic neurons in the generation of saccadic control signals. Figure 5 (which is equivalent to the model shown in Figure 3), is a modification of a hypothetical neural network put forth by Zee and Robinson.[14] Using the perceived target position (T_p) as the desired eye position, a perceived error (ε_p) is generated by subtracting an estimate of eye position from T_p. This estimate is given by the position command (θ'_c) which is the integral of the velocity command ($\dot{\theta}_c$). The burst neurons are driven by ε_p when the pause cell (P) is inhibited by the trigger signal shown. Once the pulse is initiated, the pause cell is latched off via interneuron B_i until ε_p is driven to zero by θ'_c. The bias shown then excites P to fire at a constant rate between saccades which inhibits B. Finally, when the contralateral burst neurons fire, B_c inhibits B_i allowing P to inhibit the ipsilateral burst neurons (B). The Zee and Robinson model is compatible with the known properties of saccade-related neurons identified in monkey brainstems. Since

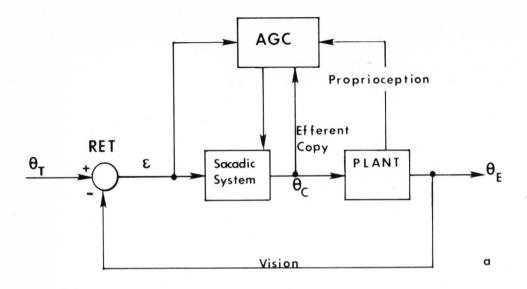

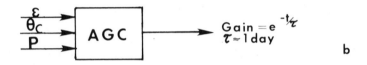

FIGURE 2.   (a) Block diagram of saccadic system with automatic gain control (AGC); (b) Transfer function of AGC with a time-constant of 1 day.

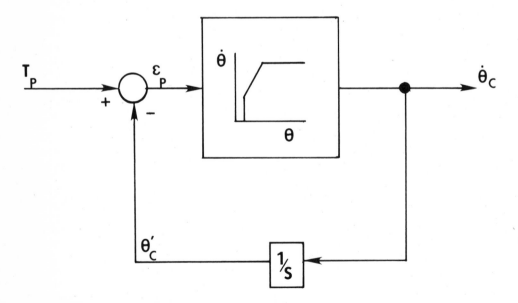

FIGURE 3.   Model of pulse generator. (Adapted from Zee, D. S., Optican, L. M., Cook, J. K., Robinson, D. L., and King-Engel, W., *Arch. Neurol.*, 33, 243, 1976.).

it allows for continuous control of the pulse, a change in T_P (or a proprioceptive input as described in the myasthenia gravis section) could result in a saccade interrupted or

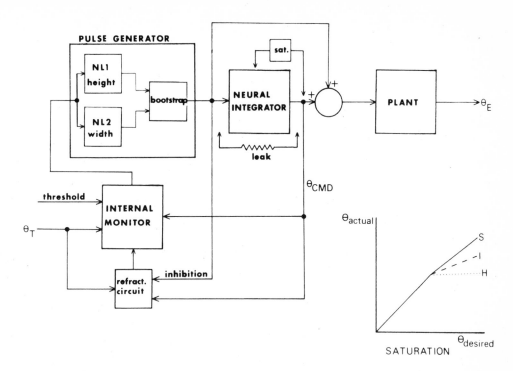

FIGURE 4. Block diagram of the model used to simulate gaze-evoked nystagmus. The input target (θ_T) is compared by the internal monitor to the eye position command (θ_{CMD}) and the necessary saccade initiated in the pulse generator. The monitor contains an error threshold below which no correction is called for. It also is prevented by a refractory circuit from calling for a correction during a saccade. The pulse generator contains nonlinearities that reproduce the physiological variations in pulse height and duration. The output of the pulse generator is integrated in the neural integrator. The pulse and step are summed, with the resulting innervation used to drive the plant to produce the desired eye position (θ_E). Both a leaky integrator and saturating integrator (SAT) are indicated as ways to produce gaze-evoked nystagmus. The inset shows typical saturation characteristics used (soft, S; intermediate, I; Hard, H). (From Abel, L. A., Dell'Osso, L. F., and Daroff, R. B., *IEEE Trans. Biomed. Eng.*, 25, 71, 1978. With permission.)

otherwise modified in flight. One additional change included in the model of Figure 5 is the positive intercept of the $\dot\theta$ vs. θ curve which determines B. This was proposed in the Zee and Robinson model based on the neurophysiological evidence of Keller[15] and Van Gisbergen and Robinson.[16] They found that burst neurons fire minimally (e.g., 100 spikes/sec) for ipsilateral and contralateral microsaccades, for vertical saccades, and toward the end of large contralateral saccades. The modeling implications were the positive intercept of the B curves on each side of the brainstem and that the ipsilateral and contralateral burst neurons must be connected to the ocular motoneurons in a push-pull fashion. Such a model corresponds to the correlation between saccadic velocity and difference between B_i and B_c burst rate.[15] Analysis of this model led Zee and Robinson to postulate mechanisms for flutter, "flutter dysmetria," opsoclonus, and voluntary "nystagmus."

1. Flutter

Ocular flutter is a disorder in which fixation is interrupted by bursts of high-frequency saccadic oscillations. These alternate in direction without intersaccadic intervals which creates a pendular-looking appearance. Zee and Robinson demonstrated how their model could simulate ocular flutter when a short delay is introduced into the θ'_c feedback loop. The high gain of B makes the pulse generator inherently unstable

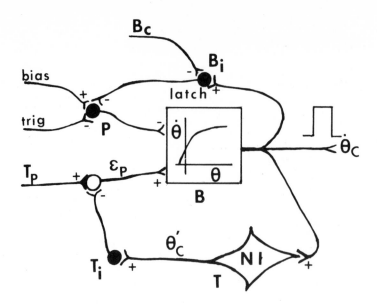

FIGURE 5.   Neural model of pulse generator. (Modified from Zee, D. S. and Robinson, D. A., *Ann. Neurol.,* 5, 405, 1979.)

so that it will oscillate with such a delay. Intermittent bursts of oscillation were produced by reducing the level of tonic inhibition of the burst cells which is normally provided by the pause cells. This could be due to (a) a prolonged trigger signal; (b) an inadequate bias; or (c) unresponsive pause cells.

2. Flutter Dysmetria

Flutter dysmetria is a term which we are introducing to describe ocular flutter occurring after a refixation saccade prior to the eyes coming to rest at a new target position. The Zee and Robinson model simulates this condition by adjustment of the gain of the B curve and varying the pause cell bias to produce a variation in the number of dysmetric flutter oscillations.

3. Opsoclonus

Opsoclonus describes seemingly random, chaotic, multidirectional, conjugate saccadic oscillations. This can be regarded as secondary to simultaneous instabilities in both horizontal and vertical pulse generators and were so simulated by Zee and Robinson in their model.

4. Voluntary "Nystagmus"

Voluntary "nystagmus" is the name given to the voluntary ocular oscillation in the horizontal plane that some normal subjects are able to accomplish. As with flutter, this oscillation looks pendular, but Shultz et al.[17] demonstrated that the eye movements were back-to-back saccades and, therefore, not truly a nystagmus oscillation. The Zee and Robinson model easily simulated this oscillation when the pause cells were turned off allowing the burst cells to oscillate. This corresponds to the report of subjects who, when asked to explain how they make their eyes oscillate, generally reply that they "let it happen," suggesting that the oscillation was a natural phenomenon that only needed to be released.

Thus, the Zee and Robinson model for saccadic pulse generation led to insightful hypotheses concerning the mechanisms of three pathological and one artificially created saccadic oscillations.

D. Medial Longitudinal Fasciculus

1. Internuclear Ophthalmoplegia

Lesions of the medial longitudinal fasciculus (MLF) result in impairment of adduction in the eye ipsilateral to the lesion and abduction nystagmus in the contralateral eye. This is called internuclear ophthalmoplegia (INO). The adduction deficit can range from complete inability to move the eye past the midline (loss of both pulse and step of innervation) to a slight decrease in saccadic velocities (loss of some of the pulse). Commonly, adducting saccades appear to have a truncated fast portion followed by a slow exponential drift to the target; this corresponds to a partial loss of the pulse. This initial loss of pulse, resulting in slowed adduction saccades, is due to the inability of demyelinated fibers to transmit the high-frequencies of the pulse as well as they transmit the low-frequencies of the step. Since excitation of the agonist is responsible for most of the pulse of muscle force and only part of the step, the pulse will always be affected to a greater extent.[18] Simple superposition of the slow adduction saccadic motion and the linear slow phases induced by an optokinetic stimulus was used by Dell'Osso et al.[19] to explain the asymmetry of OKN response in INO. In the same paper, the illustration of simultaneous saccades of the abducting and adducting eyes shows both the truncated adduction saccades with following glissade and the nystagmus of the abducting eye. Careful inspection of that figure reveals small hypometric saccades superimposed on the glissade of the adducting eye; these correspond to the fast phases of the abduction nystagmus. Note that both disappear when the adducting eye reaches the target. Thus, abduction "nystagmus" may merely be pulse responses (i.e., stepless saccades) of the abducting eye corresponding to the hypometric saccades of the adducting eye which are attempting to bring it to the target. If the target is within the patient's range of adduction, the nystagmus will diminish and cease as the target is reached by the adducting eye; if not, abduction nystagmus will continue. Recordings in our laboratory with high bandwidth (DC-100 Hz) position and velocity channels have always shown the corresponding hypometric adducting saccades. Further studies of this nystagmus are required to determine if our hypothesis is valid in explaining the abduction nystagmus in patients with INO. Other hypotheses have been proposed. Pola and Robinson[18] constructed a model which included both excitatory and inhibitory fibers in the MLF. The excitatory fibers went to the ipsilateral medial rectus subnucleus and the inhibitory fibers were destined for the contralateral medial rectus, crossing at the nuclear level. Thus, an MLF lesion not only causes impaired excitation of the ipsilateral medial rectus, but disinhibition of the opposite medial rectus. This disinhibited medial rectus has a tonic innervational level incompatible with the eccentric gaze deviation and, therefore, causes a centripetal drift which is the basis for their explanation of the abduction nystagmus.

E. Vestibular

1. Alexander's Law

Inner ear disease of a variety of causes induces an imbalance between the two sides which is responsible for pathological vestibular nystagmus. The diseased end organ almost always has a decreased rate of tonic firing. The slow phase of the nystagmus, which has a linear slope, drifts toward the abnormal side and the fast phase beats in the opposite direction (i.e., toward the normal ear). Warm or cold caloric stimulation induces convection flows of the endolymph of the semicircular canal on the side of irrigation. The direction of flow depends upon the temperature of the water. Warm water results in an increase in tonic firing frequency, whereas cold water induces a decreased frequency and, therein, mimics the effect of a diseased semicircular canal. In either instance, however, an imbalance between the two sides is created, the eyes drift to one side, and nystagmus is induced. The amplitude of vestibular nystagmus grows as gaze is increased in the direction of the fast phase and diminishes with gaze in the opposite direction. This phenomenon was described by Alexander in 1912 and is known as "Alexander's Law."

In an attempt to better understand the interaction between gaze and the vestibulo-ocular system, we modeled Alexander's Law utilizing relevant brainstem anatomy and physiology.[20] The model shown in Figure 6 represents the brainstem mechanisms that determine the gaze-dependent slope variation of the slow phase of vestibular nystagmus. Therefore, it was not necessary to explicitly model the generation of the fast phases; they were assumed to occur with a constant frequency. A model has been proposed for fast phase generation during head rotation[21] and will be presented subsequently in this chapter.

Figure 6 is a block diagram of our model. Neural signals from the semicircular canals (SCC) pass to the vestibular nuclei (VN) before being integrated by the neural integrators (NI). The NI outputs then lead to stimulation of the extraocular eye muscles (EOM) via the ocular motor nuclei (OMN). The position of the eyes is represented by θ_E. The net effect is an idealized vestibulo-ocular reflex (VOR).

In order to include a gaze-dependent variation, however, we added a slow phase modulator (SϕM) which modulates vestibular nuclei activity with desired gaze (θ_D) and a constant tone signal (T). In this manner, we were able to simulate the variation of slow phase velocity with canal imbalance and desired gaze. The fast phase stimulator (FϕS) and pulse generator (PG) are connected by dashed lines to illustrate that they were not *explicitly* modelled, although their role in the fast phase of the vestibular nystagmus was represented. The waveforms shown indicate neural firing frequencies and the resulting nystagmus of the eyes.

A signal flow diagram of the model is shown in Figure 7. The terminology *Neural Summer* is utilized to emphasize the true correspondence with actual neurons which fire with positive frequency only when the net input stimulation is excitatory.

Several characteristics were required of this brainstem model: (a) equal and opposite neural tone from each side should exist when the eyes are in primary position; (b) when a vestibular imbalance is present, a gaze angle signal should modulate the value of the drift velocity produced by the imbalance; (c) the gaze angle signal must not induce a drift velocity when no vestibular imbalance exists; and (d) the modulated imbalance must result in a constant-velocity, linear drift of the eyes.

These considerations resulted in specific model characteristics. The constant tone output requirements from each of the eye position integrators and the necessity for the integrator outputs to track each other in a push-pull fashion about that steady-state tonic level, gave rise to the push-pull connection of first-order lag elements shown in Figure 7. This solution was taken from an earlier, more complete, model of brainstem circuitry developed by Dell'Osso in 1974 (unpublished). It has the unique characteristics that yield a constant output for equal innervation to each of the integrators and an integrated output for a differential input. Satisfaction of requirements b and c resulted in a gated modulation which was present only when a vestibular imbalance exceeded a threshold. To maintain linear slow phases, desired gaze signals, rather than feedback of the output of the integrators (actual gaze commands), had to be used, as the latter would have resulted in nonlinear slow phases. As an initial simplifying assumption, the frequency of the nystagmus was held constant (at 3.33 Hz). The computer was adjusted to automatically zero, its output approximately every 0.30 sec, thereby simulating the action of the fast phases of nystagmus. During this time, the slow drift increased at a rate determined by the model output.

The model suggested a possible neural configuration (Figure 8) which would produce nystagmus from vestibular imbalance which varied with gaze. The vestibular nu-

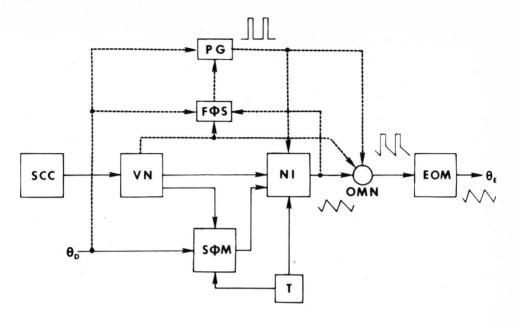

FIGURE 6. Functional block diagram of model to simulate vestibular nystagmus. Solid lines represent slow phase generation; dashed lines represent fast phase aspects. (From Doslak M. J., Dell'Osso, L. F., and Daroff, R. B., *Biol. Cybern.,* 34, 181, 1979. With permission.)

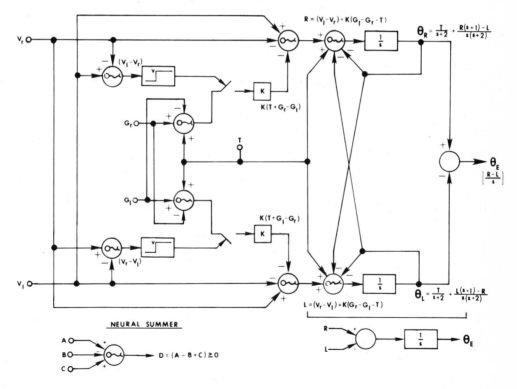

FIGURE 7. Signal flow diagram of the model shown in Figure 6 containing the necessary quantitative interaction among signals. Mathematical relationships utilize Laplace notation where applicable. (From Doslak, M. J., Dell'Osso, L. F., and Daroff, R. B., *Biol. Cybern.,* 34, 181, 1979. With permission.)

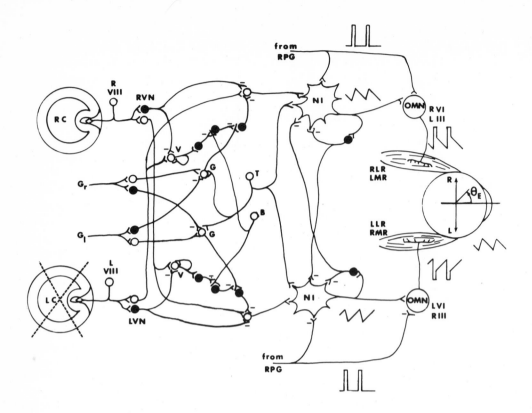

FIGURE 8.   A possible neural "wiring diagram" suggested by the model
in previous two figures. The upper half of the diagram corresponds to the
right side of the brainstem and the lower half to the left side. Open circles
represent excitatory neurons; filled circles represent inhibitory neurons. Dysfunction of the left semicircular canal is signified by a large X through LC.
(From Doslak, M. J., Dell'Osso, L. F., and Daroff, R. B., *Biol. Cybern.*,
34, 181, 1979. With permission.)

clei (RVN, LVN) transfer excitatory signals contralaterally and inhibitory signals ipsilaterally to the neural integrators (NI). Prior to synapsing with the integrators, these
signals are modulated by desired gaze (G_r, G_l) and tone (T) signals. When no imbalance
between vestibular nerve activity from each side is present, the summed gaze and tone
signals (G) are prevented from passing by means of the presynaptic inhibition supplied
by a postulated bias (B). When an imbalance of vestibular activity occurs, this inhibitory bias is turned off by additional presynaptic inhibition. Such inhibition of inhibitory signals is not unusual in other areas of neurophysiology.[22] Also shown are the
ocular motor nuclei (OMN) and the eye muscles. With dysfunction of the left canal
(LC), the right canal (RC) leads to increased stimulation of the left lateral rectus (LLR)
and right medial rectus (RMR) causing the eyes (represented here as one eye) to drift
to the left. Intervening saccadic pulses from the right pulse generator (RPG) move the
eyes back to their predrift position. The waveforms shown represent changes in the
neural firing frequencies and eye position (θ_E).

2. Fast Phase Generation

The model for fast phase generation during head rotation proposed by Chun and
Robinson[21] utilized their pulse generator (Figure 5) which was driven by two internal
signals that specified the eye positions at the beginning and end of each fast phase.
Both signals were generated internally and varied with the head velocity signal from

the vestibular system. One specifying signal created a "center of interest" to which fast phases drove the eyes, and a second signal was an error signal which sensed the deviation of the eyes from the "center of interest." When this difference exceeded a threshold (also determined by head velocity), a fast phase was initiated by triggering the pulse generator. The nonlinearities and dynamics incorporated into these circuits, as well as their interconnections to the pulse generator are sufficiently complex to prevent further discussion of this excellent model in this chapter.

The generation of fast phases of pathological vestibular nystagmus and the variation of their timing and amplitude with gaze angle has not been studied and, therefore, cannot be modeled adequately at this time. Studies of patients with vestibular nystagmus and normals with caloric-induced nystagmus are necessary to answer the following questions prompted by our model of Alexander's Law: (1) Is the relationship between the amplitude of the nystagmus actually linear?; (2) For a given gaze angle, is the change in nystagmus amplitude a linear function of canal deficit?; and (3) How does nystagmus frequency vary with gaze? Until answers to these questions are found, further modelling of the phenomena associated with slow and fast phase variations in vestibular nystagmus must, of necessity, be highly speculative.

F. Cerebellar

Ocular flutter, flutter dysmetria, and opsoclonus are oscillations, discussed earlier, which occur in patients with cerebellar disease. Other cerebellar eye signs are (1) macro square wave jerks (MSWJ); (2) overshoot dysmetria; and (3) macro saccadic oscillations (MSO).

1. Macro Square Wave Jerks (MSWJ)

MSWJ are spontaneous saccades which cause the eyes to move from the object of fixation to some point in space lateral to that object. After a short latency (50 to 150 msec), a corrective saccade returns the eyes to the target. Such saccades may occur singly or in bursts during fixation or following a voluntary refixation. Our study of a patient with cerebellar signs due to multiple sclerosis led us to postulate the model shown in Figure 9.[23] An ipsilateral disturbance (presumably from the cerebellum) to the pulse generator initiated the MSWJ and the corrective return saccade was mediated by an internal monitor which compared the efferent position signals from the neural integrator with the desired eye position. MSWJ are not simply square wave jerks of larger amplitude, as the name suggests, but represent a mechanistically different instability.[24]

2. Ocular Dysmetria

Ocular dysmetria is a conjugate overshooting of a refixation saccade followed by a corrective saccade after a normal intersaccadic latency of 125 to 200 msec. The correction may also be hypermetric leading to an oscillation of saccades of diminishing amplitude before the eyes come to rest on the new target. Overshoot dysmetria differs from flutter dysmetria which has no intersaccadic latency.

Selhorst et al.[4] studied overshoot dysmetria and identified the responsible control system abnormality as a gain increase in the feed-forward path to a value greater than 1.0, but less than 2.0. They simulated the disorder using the Young-Stark[25] sample-data model of the saccadic system and postulated that a lesion of the cerebellar vermis was responsible for the disturbed gain modulation in the saccadic system.

3. Macro Saccadic Oscillations (MSO)

MSO consist of a burst of to-and-fro saccades, with normal intersaccadic latencies,

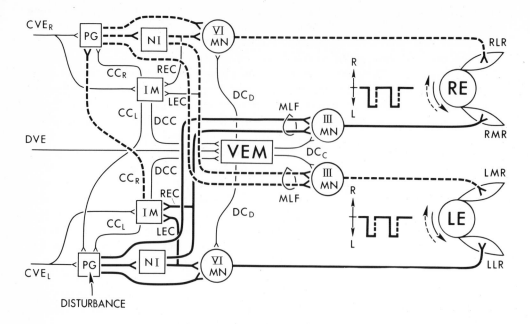

FIGURE 9.   Binocular model of brainstem output portions of the horizontal fast eye movement and vergence eye movement (VEM) subsystems illustrating the functional operation of an internal monitor (IM) in
the generation of corrective eye movements. Conjugate visual errors to the right and left (CVE_R and CVE_L,
respectively) drive the pulse generators (PG) on their respective side to produce saccades.

The output of the pulse generator is integrated in the neural integrator (NI) and the resulting step of
innervation is summed with the original pulse from the pulse generator at the motoneuron (MN). (Motoneuronal summing is provided for simplicity only; summing may actually occur at a prenuclear level.) Signals
then go to the respective extraocular muscles (RLR, RMR, LMR, LLR) to drive the right (RE) and the left
(LE) eyes. Disconjugate visual errors (DVE) drive the vergence eye movement subsystem to produce disconjugate commands of convergence (DC_C) and divergence (DC_D).

The IM monitors the commands to both eyes (REC and LEC), compares them with the desired output
(CVE), and directs the required conjugate correction to the right (CC_R) or left (CC_L) pulse generator, as
well as any required disconjugate corrective command (DCC) to the vergence eye movement subsystem. The
disturbance input for this patient and the pathways for the consequent abnormal leftward saccade are in
heavy solid lines, with the pathways for the corrective rightward saccade in dashed lines. The resulting
macrosquare wave jerks are shown next to each eye. (From Dell'Osso, L. F., Troost, B. T., and Daroff, R.
B., *Neurology*, 25, 978, 1975. With permission.)

which gradually increase and then decrease in amplitude.[5] Unlike MSWJ, MSO strad-
dles fixation.[24] Again, using the Young-Stark[25] sample-data model, Selhorst et al.[5]
produced constant amplitude saccadic oscillations when the gain was 2.0 and increasing amplitude oscillations at greater gains. By varying the gain between 2.25 and 1.75,
they created oscillations which increased and then decreased in amplitude. This closely
simulated the MSO recorded in their patients.

Thus, Selhorst et al.[4,5] demonstrated that both overshoot dysmetria and macro saccadic oscillations result from high loop gains in the saccadic system with the difference
being the magnitude of the gain increase.

G. Basal Ganglia
1. Progressive Supranuclear Palsy (PSP)

PSP is a basal ganglionic and midbrain disorder resembling Parkinsonism. The most
prominent eye signs are paralysis of downward, followed by upward gaze (pursuit and
saccades) with preservation of vestibulo-ocular movements. The progression of the
vertical gaze disturbance leading to paralysis has never been studied quantitatively.

Volitional horizontal eye movements may also become paralyzed and these have been studied carefully prior to the stage of total paralysis. The horizontal eye signs include: square wave jerks (SWJ); slow, hypometric, long-duration saccades; low pursuit gain (cogwheel pursuit); and inability to enhance or suppress the vestibulo-ocular (VOR) gain.[26] The pons is pathologically spared in this disease; the horizontal eye signs must be explained by lesions elsewhere. From Figure 1, it is evident that a supranuclear disorder could interfere with the generation of the signals T_p or ε_p and result in diminished saccadic gain, or stimulate the pulse generator causing SWJ. In a similar manner, such a disorder could lower the pursuit gain and, therein, prevent variation of VOR gain. However, the mechanism by which a supranuclear disorder could modify saccadic peak velocity or duration, if the pulse generator is hard-wired in the pons, as shown in Figure 5, is not as apparent. Given the model of Figure 5, we must postulate supranuclear influences impinging directly on the network responsible for the $\dot{\theta}$ vs. θ transfer function of B. This is supported by the observation that slow saccades are present in other basal ganglionic disorders such as Huntington's chorea and Wilson's disease, as well as spinocerebellar degenerations (discussed earlier). The two mechanisms postulated for the slow saccades,[26] defective pulse (pulseless) and unsustained pulse, both require malfunction of the pulse generator (Figure 5) circuitry. At present, there are not sufficient data about supranuclear connections from basal ganglia and cerebellum to the PPRF pulse generator neurons for construction of a meaningful model.

2. Parkinson's Disease

Parkinson's disease is also associated with saccadic pursuit reflecting defective pursuit gain. Saccades are hypometric, but there is disagreement as to saccadic velocities. Shibasaki et al.[27] found them to be slow, which is at variance with the normal speeds previously reported by Melville Jones and DeJong.[28] If the former authors are correct, a model for Parkinsonian saccades would have to be similar to that of PSP and require supranuclear control of the pulse generator transfer characteristics. If the saccades are not slowed, a simpler model would be applicable with only saccadic gain under supranuclear control.

V. NYSTAGMUS

Nystagmus is a biphasic ocular oscillation which begins with a slow (nonsaccadic) movement and in which both phases are approximately equal amplitude. Thus, SWJ, MSWJ, MSO, opsoclonus, flutter, flutter dysmetria, and voluntary "nystagmus" (all of which are saccadic) are not forms of nystagmus. Traditionally, nystagmus is divided into pendular and jerk types. The former is sinusoidal and in the latter, the initial slow phase is away from the object of fixation (or intended gaze angle); it is followed by a saccadic fast phase in the direction of the target. By convention, the fast phase direction defines the nystagmus direction. The waveforms of jerk nystagmus may be further subdivided on the basis of slow phase shape (Figure 10) which may be linear, increasing-velocity exponential or decreasing-velocity exponential.[29] These differences imply different control system abnormalities.

A. Congenital

Twelve distinctive forms of congenital nystagmus (CN) have been identified[30] and fall into three categories: pendular (three waveforms), jerk (eight waveforms), and dual jerk (one waveform). These waveforms, some of which are complex, are the result of basic instabilities in the slow subsystem of ocular motor control and the secondary

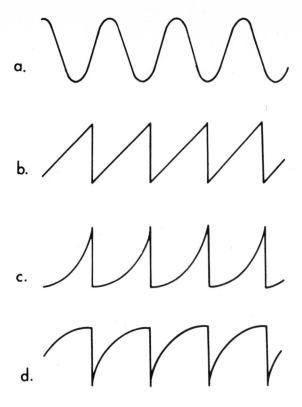

FIGURE 10.   Oculographic representation of (a) pendular nystagmus and the three major types of jerk nystagmus (b, c, d). Jerk nystagmus classification is based upon the shape of slow phase: (b) linear, (c) increasing-velocity exponential, and (d) decreasing-velocity exponential. (From Daroff, R. B., *Weekly Update: Neurol. Neurosurg.*, 1, 1, 1978. With permission.)

plastic adaptations designed to maximize foveation time, thereby decreasing the visual impairment resulting from the nystagmus. Basically, all of the waveforms are variations of one of two distinct instabilities or, in the case of dual jerk, a combination of both types of instability. The waveforms of Figure 10a and 10c are the basic instabilities of CN. The pendular waveform is a high-gain instability of the slow subsystem whose roots must lie on the jω-axis as shown in Figure 11.[31] Pendular nystagmus disappears with visual inattention (low-gain) and increases proportional to greater visual attention or effort to see (high-gain). Increasing the gain appears to drive the poles up the jω-axis, since the frequency of the oscillation may increase along with the amplitude. Jerk CN behaves in a similar manner with increasing effort (gain) driving a pole further into the right half plane on the σ-axis (Figure 11). Dual jerk nystagmus supports the contention that the pendular and jerk waveforms are independent oscillations caused by different instabilities. This is a high-frequency, low-amplitude pendular oscillation superimposed on a low-frequency, high-amplitude jerk nystagmus. At times, one or the other component can be reduced or eliminated without affecting the other; one component may spontaneously diminish or increase.

Pendular CN may merely require increasing the loop gain of a normal slow subsystem with its inherent transport lags. Robinson[32] found sinusoidal oscillations of 2.9 Hz when the gain of a normal system was increased. When this was done experimen-

s-PLANE

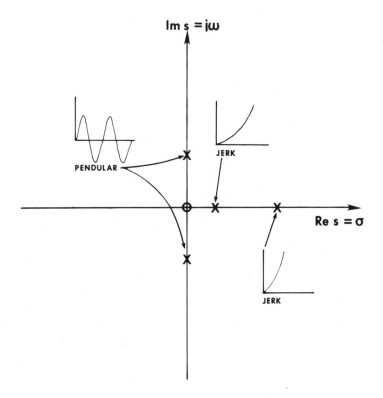

FIGURE 11.   Plot of various system pole positions (X) on the complex frequency plane (s-plane) and the types of oscillations which result. See text for
explanations. (From Daroff, R. B. and Dell'Osso, L. F., *Topics in Neuro-
Ophthalmology,* Thompson, H. S., Daroff, R. B., Glaser, J. S., Frisen, L.,
and Sanders, M. D., Eds., Williams & Wilkins, Baltimore, 1979, 286. With
permission.)

tally on a patient with CN, the amplitude of his existing pendular oscillations increased.[33] For the patient with pendular CN, a pair of j-axis poles with the transfer
function $\frac{\omega_0}{s^2+\omega_0^2}$ (Figure 12a) might become manifest when input variables associated
with effort, psychological set, and other factors surpass a threshold. It is not clear
whether these inputs, which do not cause instability in the normal system, are ineffec-
tively opposed by the system with CN or whether distinct pathology introduces the
poles (not present in the normal system) that cause oscillations as gain is increased.

A possible model of jerk CN (Figure 12b) includes the addition of a positive-feedback loop around the position command (i.e., the neural integrator).

The transfer function of this model is:

$$\frac{\theta_c}{T} = \frac{\left(\dfrac{\tau}{1-\tau c}\right)}{\left(\dfrac{\tau}{1-\tau c}\right)s+1} \tag{8}$$

When $c = 1/\tau$, the transfer function is $1/s$, an ideal integrator. If, however, c becomes
greater than $1/\tau$, the pole moves into the right half plane and an increasing-velocity

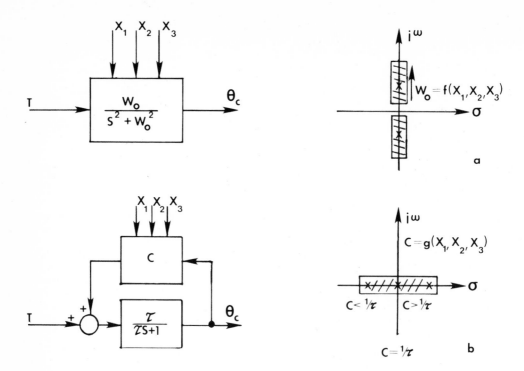

FIGURE 12. (a) Partial model for pendular congenital nystagmus and locus of pole positions; (b) Partial model for jerk congenital nystagmus and locus of pole positions. $X_1 - X_3$ are inputs from other physiological systems which affect the oscillations (see text).

exponential runaway results. If c were a function of the same factors discussed above for pendular CN, this could be the underlying mechanism for jerk forms of CN. Recently, Zee et al.[34] have proposed such a model for cerebellar-induced gain changes which caused increasing-velocity runaway slow phases in nystagmus acquired by a patient with cerebellar dysfunction. Their model was based on the known interaction of the cerebellum and the neural integrator. Since no lesions have ever been associated with CN, the exact anatomical localization of the poles discussed above is unknown.

The root locus plots of Figure 12a and b cannot be combined easily, since they represent subloops (or part of subloops) in a multiloop control system, the exact form of which is still not known. The gains of each (ω_o and c) are presumably different functions of the input variables x_1, x_2, and x_3 and, therefore, a family of root locus plots would be generated by the variations in ω_o and c; such an analysis is beyond the scope of this section.

B. Latent and Manifest Latent

Latent nystagmus (LN) and manifest latent nystagmus (MLN) have recently been studied and distinguished from CN by the slow phase waveform.[35] LN and MLN slow phases are decreasing-velocity exponentials (Figure 10d) in contrast to the increasing-velocity slow phases (Figure 10c) of the jerk form of CN. The fast phases are always directed toward the viewing eye and true binocular vision abolishes the nystagmus.

An explanation for this nystagmus was hypothesized[36] based upon the perceived angle of a target in space which, under conditions of true binocular vision, is shown in Figure 13a to be

$$\theta_{T_B} = \frac{\theta_T\big|_R + \theta_T\big|_L}{2} \qquad (9)$$

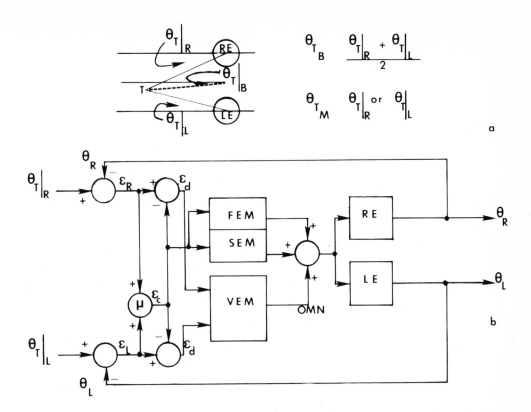

FIGURE 13. Explanation of latent and manifest latent nystagmus. (a) Definitions of target angles referenced to each eye and computation of binocular (θ_{T_B}) and monocular (θ_{T_M}) direction; (b) Model illustrating how conjugate retinal error (ε_c) and disconjugate retinal error (ε_d) might be generated from target angles referenced to the right ($\theta_T|_R$) and left ($\theta_T|_L$) eyes and their respective retinal errors (ε_R and ε_L). Their use by the version (fast eye movement [FEM] and slow eye movement [SEM]) and vergence (VEM) subsystems is indicated. The factor μ is 0.5 for binocular vision and 1.0 for monocular vision (see text for further explanation).

where, $\theta_T|_R$ and $\theta_T|_L$ are the angles of the target with respect to the right and left eyes, respectively. When only one eye is viewing, the perceived target angle is equal to its angle with respect to that eye. Thus, the brain must mathematically accomplish a switch from a summation of error signals divided by two to a unity gain acceptance of one error signal. Figure 13b is a model of how this might be done to generate conjugate error (ε_c) and disconjugate error (ε_d) signals for use by the version (comprised of fast and slow modes) and the vergence subsystems, respectively. If the mathematical switching is performed improperly when monocular vision is imposed (both LN and MLN occurred during monocular viewing conditions), a discrepancy between perceived target angle and actual target angle would be created and the eyes would move conjugately towards the improperly calculated target position (always towards the non-viewing eye). This would generate a true retinal error in the viewing eye (which was on target during binocular vision) and stimulate a conjugate saccade to refoveate the target. Repetition of this sequence could produce LN (or MLN). The decreasing-velocity slow phase may merely reflect the plant dynamics subjected to a step difference in position commands (i.e., the proper and improper target directions).

C. Pursuit-Defect
1. Downbeat, Upbeat, and Horizontal
Zee and coworkers[37] found that patients with primary position downbeating nystag-

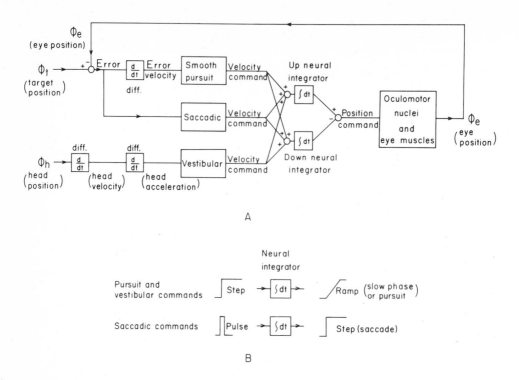

A

B

FIGURE 14.   Relationship between the vestibular, pursuit, and saccadic control systems. Each system generates a velocity command that is transmitted to the neural integrators. From the integrators, a position command is then transmitted to the final common pathway. (From Zee, D. S., Friendlich, A. R., and Robinson, D. A., *Arch. Neurol.*, 30, 227, 1974. Copyright 1974, American Medical Association. With permission.)

mus had a unidirectional absence of pursuit in the downward direction. Vestibulo-ocular movements were intact, seemingly establishing the specificity of the pursuit abnormality. The nystagmus was of the jerk type with a linear slow phase (Figure 10b). They created a computer model of downbeat nystagmus by abolishing all downward pursuit commands (Figure 14). This model duplicated the linear slow phase nystagmus found in their patients. Subsequently, primary position upbeating,[31,38,39] as well as a horizontal primary position jerk nystagmus with a linear slow phase,[40,41] have been attributed to a pursuit-defect in the direction of the quick phases of the nystagmus. Modelling upbeat nystagmus would represent a mirror image of that for downbeat and the model for horizontal pursuit defect would merely require relabelling the up and down pursuit integrators of Figure 14 as right and left.

There is reason to question the basic concept of "pursuit-defect" nystagmus. We recorded a patient with spinocerebellar degeneration and periodic alternating nystagmus in whom we found alternating pursuit defects. The unlikelihood of such an alternating defect raised the question of how pursuit should be manifest in the direction of the fast phase of an on-going jerk nystagmus. The nystagmus persists and pursuit can only be expected to decrease the slow phase velocity (decrease slope) in the opposite direction. We confirmed this in a normal subject during caloric-induced nystagmus. For pursuit to be regarded as absent, no change in slope should result. This occurred in the computer model of Zee et al.,[37] but not in their patients or, convincingly, in any of the others reported. Determination of true pursuit gain would require careful study with varying velocity ramps. This must be done before causality can be established in these cases of "pursuit-defect" nystagmus.

REFERENCES

1. Drachman, D. B., Myasthenia gravis, Part I, *New Engl. J. Med.,* 298, 136, 1978.
2. Abel, L. A., Dell'Osso, L. F., Schmidt, D., and Daroff, R. B., Myasthenia gravis: Analog computer model, *Exp. Neurol.,* 68, 378, 1980.
3. Schmidt, D., Dell'Osso, L. F., Abel, L. A., and Daroff, R. B., Myasthenia gravis: Saccadic eye movement waveforms, *Exp. Neurol.,* 68, 346, 1980.
4. Selhorst, J. B., Stark, L., Ochs, A. L., and Hoyt, W. F., Disorders in cerebellar ocular motor control. I. Saccadic overshoot dysmetria: an oculographic, control system, and clinico-anatomic analysis, *Brain.* 99. 497. 1976.
5. Selhorst, J. B., Stark, L., Ochs, A. L., and Hoyt, W. F., Disorders in cerebellar ocular motor control. II. Macrosaccadic oscillation: an oculographic, control system and clinico-anatomical analysis, *Brain,* 99, 509, 1976.
6. Schmidt, D., Dell'Osso, L. F., Abel, L. A., and Daroff, R. B., Myasthenia gravis: Dynamic changes in saccadic waveform, gain and velocity, *Exp. Neurol.,* 68, 365, 1980.
7. Bahill, A. T. and Stark, L., Overlapping saccades and glissades are produced by fatigue in the saccadic eye movement system,., *Exp. Neurol.,* 48, 95, 1975.
8. Robinson, D. A., A quantitative analysis of extraocular muscle cooperation and squint, *Invest. Ophthalmol.,* 14, 801, 1975.
9. Collins, C. C., The human oculomotor control system, in *Basic Mechanisms of Ocular Motility and Their Clinical Implications,* Lennerstrand, G. and Bach-y-Rita, P., Eds., Pergamon Press, Oxford, 1975, 145.
10. Scott, A. B., Strabismus — muscle forces and innervations, in *Basic Mechanisms of Ocular Motility and Their Clinical Implications,* Lennerstrand, G. and Bach-y-Rita, P., Eds., Pergamon Press, Oxford, 1975, 181.
11. Abel, L. A., Schmidt, D., Dell'Osso, L. F., and Daroff, R. B., Saccadic system plasticity in humans, *Ann. Neurol.,* 4, 313, 1978.
12. Zee, D. S., Optican, L. M., Cook, J. K., Robinson, D. A., and King Engel, W., Slow saccades in spinocerebellar degeneration, *Arch. Neurol.,* 33, 243, 1976.
13. Abel, L. A., Dell'Osso, L. F., and Daroff, R. B., Analog model for gaze-evoked nystagmus, *IEEE Trans. Biomed. Eng.,* 25, 71, 1978.
14. Zee, D. S. and Robinson, D. A., A hypothetical explanation of saccadic oscillations, *Ann. Neurol.,* 5, 405, 1979.
15. Keller, E., Control of saccadic eye movements by midline brain stem neurons, in *Control of Gaze by Brain Stem Neurons,* Baker, R. and Berthoz, A., Eds., Elsevier/North-Holland, New York, 1977, 327.
16. Van Gisbergen, J. A. M., and Robinson, D. A., Generation of micro and macrosaccades by burst neurons in the monkey, in *Control of Gaze by Brain Stem Neurons,* Baker, R., and Berthoz, A., Eds., Elsevier/North-Holland, 1977, 301.
17. Shults, W. T., Stark, L., Hoyt, W. F., and Ochs, A. L., Normal saccadic structure of voluntary nystagmus, *Arch. Ophthalmol.,* 95, 1399, 1977.
18. Pola, J. and Robinson, D. A., An explanation of eye movements seen in internuclear ophthalmoplegia, *Arch. Neurol.,* 33, 447, 1976.
19. Dell'Osso, L. F., Robinson, D. A., and Daroff, R. B., Optokinetic asymmetry in internuclear ophthalmoplegia, *Arch. Neurol.,* 31, 138, 1974.
20. Doslak, M. J., Dell'Osso, L. F., and Daroff, R. B., A model of Alexander's Law of vestibular nystagmus, *Biol. Cybern.,* 34, 181, 1979.
21. Chun, K. -S. and Robinson, D. A., A model of quick phase generation in the vestibuloocular reflex, *Biol. Cybern.,* 28, 209, 1978.
22. Eccles, J. C., *The Physiology of Synapses,* Springer-Verlag, Berlin, 1964.
23. Dell'Osso, L. F., Troost, B. T., and Daroff, R. B., Macro square wave jerks, *Neurology,* 25, 975, 1975.
24. Dell'Osso, L. F., Abel, L. A., and Daroff, R. B., "Inverse latent" macro square wave jerks and macro saccadic oscillations, *Ann. Neurol.,* 2, 57, 1977.
25. Young, L. R. and Stark, L., Variable feedback experiments testing a sampled data model for eye tracking movements, *IEEE Trans. Hum. Factors Electron.,* 4, 38, 1963.
26. Troost, B. T. and Daroff, R. B., The ocular motor deficits in progressive supranuclear palsy, *Ann. Neurol.,* 2, 397, 1977.
27. Shibasaki, H., Sadatoshi, T., and Yoshigoro, K., Oculomotor abnormalities in Parkinson's disease, *Arch. Neurol.,* 36, 360, 1979.
28. Melville Jones, G. and DeJong, J. D., Dynamic characterics of saccadic eye movements in Parkinson's disease, *Exp. Neurol.,* 31, 17, 1971.

29. Daroff, R. B., Nystagmus, *Weekly Update: Neurol. Neurosurg.,* 1, 1, 1978.
30. Dell'Osso, L. F. and Daroff, R. B., Congenital nystagmus waveforms and foveation strategy, *Doc. Ophthalmol.,* 39, 155, 1975.
31. Daroff, R. B. and Dell'Osso, L. F., Nystagmus — a contemporary approach, in *Topics in Neuro-Ophthalmology,* Thompson, H. S., Daroff, R. B., Glaser, J. S., Frisen, L., and Sanders, M. D., Eds., Williams & Wilkins, Baltimore, 1979, 286.
32. Robinson, D. A., The mechanics of human smooth pursuit eye movement, *J. Physiol.,* 180, 569, 1965.
33. Dell'Osso, L. F., Gauthier, G., Liberman, G., and Stark, L., Eye movement recordings as a diagnostic tool in a case of congenital nystagmus, *Am. J. Optom. Arch. Am. Acad. Optom.,* 49, 3, 1972.
34. Zee, D. S., Leigh, R. T., and Mathieu-Millaire, F., Cerebellar control of ocular gaze stability, *Ann. Neurol.,* 7, 37, 1980.
35. Dell'Osso, L. F., Schmidt, D., and Daroff, R. B., Latent, manifest latent, and congenital nystagmus, *Arch. Ophthalmol.,* 97, 1877, 1979.
36. Daroff, R. B., Troost, B. T., and Dell'Osso, L. F., Nystagmus and related ocular oscillations, in *Neuro-Ophthalmology,* Glaser, J. S., Ed., Harper & Row, Hagerstown, 1978.
37. Zee, D. S., Friendlich, A. R., and Robinson, D. A., The mechanism of downbeat nystagmus, *Arch. Neurol.,* 30, 227, 1974.
38. Gilman, N., Baloh, R. W., and Tomiyasu, U., Primary position upbeat nystagmus, *Neurology,* 27, 294, 1977.
39. Mehdorn, E., Kommerell, G., and Meienberg, O., Primary position vertical nystagmus: "Directional preponderance" of the pursuit system?, *Albrecht v. Graefes Arch. Klin. Exp. Ophthalmol.,* 209, 209, 1979.
40. Abel, L. A., Daroff, R. B., and Dell'Osso, L. F., Horizontal pursuit defect nystagmus, *Ann. Neurol.,* 5, 449, 1979.
41. Sharpe, J. A., Lo, A. W., and Rabinovitch, H. E., Control of the saccadic and smooth pursuit systems after cerebral hemidecordication, *Brain,* 102, 387, 1979.

Chapter 13

THE VESTIBULO-OCULAR REFLEX: CLINICAL CONCEPTS

David S. Zee

TABLE OF CONTENTS

I. INTRODUCTION

The patient with dizziness and vertigo is one of the more difficult and puzzling diagnostic problems in the practice of neurology and otolaryngology. Only in the past decade have clinicians begun to feel confident when dealing with patients who have disorders of the vestibular system. The reason is that physiologists and control systems engineers have provided new information and concepts about the function of the vestibulo-ocular reflex that have direct bearing on neurological disease. This chapter will review these new ideas using, when possible, specific disease entities to illustrate how physiology can be directly applied to the analysis of clinical problems.

II. CLINICAL EVALUATION OF DISORDERS OF THE VESTIBULO-OCULAR REFLEX

New techniques of clinical examination, both at the bedside and in the laboratory, reflect the influence of the physiologist. For example, the strategy underlying vestibular testing is based upon a relatively straightforward concept of the function of the vestibulo-ocular reflex (VOR).* The VOR generates an eye movement in the orbit equal, but opposite to a head movement in space, so that the position of the eye in space (gaze) does not change. In this way, the image of the visual world upon the retina is stabilized to insure best visual acuity during head rotation. The concept of gain (output/input ratio) naturally follows and, in fact, measurement of VOR gain is now a standard part of the quantitative examination of patients with ocular motor disorders of all types.

Clinically, abnormalities of the VOR can be separated into those that affect gain (amplitude) and those that produce bias (imbalance). Gain is usually defined as the ratio of peak eye velocity to peak head velocity and is normally 1.0 so that eye movement is equal (but opposite) to head movement. Decreased gain usually occurs with severe peripheral vestibular lesions while increased gain usually reflects an abnormally increased sensitivity of central vestibular mechanisms.

Disorders that create imbalance produce static and/or dynamic bias. Static bias is manifest as spontaneous nystagmus which reflects a difference between the resting discharge rates of the vestibular nuclei on either side of the brain stem. Dynamic bias is manifest as a "directional preponderance" during vestibular stimulation (the VOR gain is greater in one direction than the other) which reflects a differential sensitivity of vestibular mechanisms to oppositely directed labyrinthine inputs.

A. Bedside Testing
1. Disorders of Gain
A remarkable amount of information about vestibular function can be gleaned at the bedside without sophisticated recording techniques if one keeps in mind several basic concepts about vestibular physiology.

For example, the gain of the VOR can be qualitatively assessed using several simple tests. First, instruct the patient to move his head back and forth while fixating a small object or a letter on a Snellen visual acuity chart. The head should be moving at a frequency of at least 1 to 2 Hz in order to eliminate the ability of the smooth pursuit system (which functions poorly at high-frequencies) to make a significant contribution to image stabilization. The patient should view a target at distance because the VOR

---

*   Unless otherwise stated, VOR refers to the semicircular canal mediated reflex used to compensate for head rotations as opposed to the otolith mediated reflex used to compensate for head translations.

gain must be increased above 1.0 for clear vision during near-viewing due to the difference between the centers of rotation of the head and the globes. (In fact, the central nervous system's ability to modify the VOR as a function of the state of accommodation and/or vergence can be tested by comparing results of VOR testing when viewing near and distant targets.)

During head rotation with distance fixation one should look carefully for corrective saccades. If the VOR is *hyperactive* (gain > 1), corrective saccades in the same direction as head movement will be required to continue fixate the target. If the VOR is *hypoactive* (gain < 1), corrective saccades in the direction *opposite* to head movement will appear. If the VOR is normal (gain about 1.0), no corrective saccades will be necessary and eye movements will be smooth.

Subjectively, one can also inquire about the direction of image motion during head movement. This can best be assessed during a brief, rapid turn of the head while the patient attempts to maintain fixation. If the fixation target appears to move oppositely to the direction of head movement, the VOR is *hypoactive*. If the fixation target appears to move in the direction of head movement, the VOR is *hyperactive*. The apparent target movement will, of course, elicit a corrective saccade and, hence, the above two tests are complementary.

Finally, one can also determine the VOR gain during ophthalmoscopy.[1] If the VOR is functioning normally, the position of the eye in space (gaze) does not change during head rotation. During ophthalmoscopy, the position of the eye in space is reflected by the position of the optic disc (or any other particular part of the retina) relative to the observer (who is stationary in space). Hence, during oscillation of the head, if the VOR is normal, the optic disc will not appear to move relative to the observer even though the head in space and the eye in the orbit are oscillating back and forth. However, if the VOR gain is abnormal, the eye will move in space and the optic disc will appear to oscillate relative to the observer. If the VOR gain is *hyperactive,* the disc will oscillate *in phase* (in the same direction) with head rotation; if the VOR is *hypoactive*, the disc will oscillate *out of phase* (oppositely directed) to head rotation. This test is best done with dilated pupils and with the nonvisualized eye covered. The patient is instructed to oscillate the head at a frequency of about 1 to 2 Hz and amplitude (peak to peak) of about 20 degrees. Quick phases or saccades are ignored as the slower drifts of the optic disc reflect the slow phase of the VOR. Head translations (as opposed to rotations) may give rise to falsely positive tests.

2. Disorders of Bias

Imbalance can also be detected at the bedside. Dynamic bias causes a directional preponderance and can be assessed using the same tests described above. For example, during head rotation with attempted fixation, if the VOR gain is greater than 1.0 in one direction and less than 1.0 in the other, corrective saccades and apparent target movement will always be directed toward the side to which head rotation elicits a hyperactive (gain > 1.0) response. Similarly, during ophthalmoscopy, the disc will always appear to be drifting in the direction of head movement which elicits the hyperactive response.

Static bias causes spontaneous drift (and nystagmus) and can be best appreciated during ophthalmoscopy. In fact, one can detect saccades as small as 0.2 deg in amplitude using the ophthalmoscope. If drift or nystagmus is of *peripheral* vestibular origin, it is usually *diminished by fixation* as the central visual following reflexes are intact. Hence, during ophthalmoscopy, one can cover the nonvisualized eye and look for an increase in or appearance of drift and nystagmus as a sign of peripheral vestibular dysfunction. One should remember that the disc lies behind the center of rotation of the globe and will, therefore, move in a direction opposite to that of the visual axis. One can also evaluate the effect of fixation upon nystagmus using Frenzel glasses (+ 20 or + 30 lenses). The slow phase velocity of nystagmus increases when the ability to fixate is impaired by the lenses.

3. Visual-Vestibular Interaction

Finally, another helpful bedside test can be used to determine the effect of fixation upon inappropriate vestibular nystagmus.[2] Usually, this is performed during caloric stimulation by recording nystagmus with eyes open and eyes closed. Normally, caloric-induced nystagmus is diminished by fixation. If not, a central disorder is implied, often of the cerebellum. At the bedside, the effect of vision upon inappropriate vestibular nystagmus can be accomplished easily by instructing the patient to fixate an object rotating with his head. For example, the patient is asked to fixate a finger of his outstretched arm as he is rotated *en block* in a wheel chair. Normally, fixation is steady as the slow phase of the VOR is cancelled ("suppressed") by an equal but opposite tracking (pursuit) command. If pursuit is impaired, the eye is taken off target by the intact slow phase of the VOR and repetitive saccades are necessary to reacquire the target. This results in an easily observable nystagmus pattern with quick phases (or saccades) in the same direction as head motion. This test actually assesses smooth pursuit but, unlike tracking with the head stationary, has the advantage that the eyes are continually near the primary position of gaze. Hence, if the patient has nystagmus on eccentric gaze, it will not interfere with the interpretation of smooth pursuit function.

Finally, another helpful bedside test can be used to determine the effect of fixation upon inappropriate vestibular nystagmus.[2] Usually, this is performed during caloric stimulation by recording nystagmus with eyes open and eyes closed. Normally, caloric-induced nystagmus is diminished by fixation. If not, a central disorder is implied, often of the cerebellum.

B. Rotational Testing

Vestibular testing using chair rotations has undergone a renaissance as both a research and, more recently, a diagnostic tool. Rotational stimuli are more natural and less discomforting than caloric irrigations and can be more precisely measured. Microprocessor computer techniques can be used to analyze the velocity, frequency, and amplitude of both slow and quick phases of nystagmus. Therefore, more quantitative information about central vestibular data-processing and visual-vestibular interaction can be gleaned using rotational testing and, in turn, mathematical control systems analysis can be used to interpret vestibular responses. Both frequency and time domain analyses have been applied to vestibular testing and terms such as gain, phase, and time constant are now in the clinician's vernacular. However, it still has not been convincingly shown that rotational testing can detect subtle degrees of peripheral labyrinthine hypofunction that are usually easily revealed by caloric testing.

1. Diagnostic Applications

Three types of rotational stimuli are used clinically. In the impulsive test (similar to what Bárány originally described), an impulse of acceleration is applied by abruptly changing the velocity of the vestibular chair to a new level. In the clinical setting, perrotatory (acceleration) rather than postrotatory (deceleration) nystagmus is usually measured, since the former usually gives more consistent responses. During a constant velocity rotation, nystagmus slow phase velocity decays approximately exponentially as the cupula returns toward the primary position. One can determine both the gain (peak eye velocity/peak head velocity) and the dominant time constant of the VOR. Because there is a late reversal phase of nystagmus during constant velocity rotation, an adaptation time constant can also be calculated.

Baloh and colleagues have evaluated the clinical efficacy of the impulsive test.[3] They found that a complete unilateral peripheral vestibular paralysis can usually be identified if high rotational velocities are used.* However, only 35% of patients with hypoactive (but not absent) caloric responses were appropriately identified by rotational testing. Impulsive tests also helped identify patients with normal vestibular function who had artifactually reduced caloric responses due to unusual geometrical configurations of their external auditory canals or temporal bones. Likewise, residual vestibular function can occasionally be detected during rotation in patients with absent caloric responses.

Wolfe and colleagues[8,9] and Barnes[10] have used frequency-domain analysis to investigate the vestibular responses during sinusoidal head rotations. Directional differences in slow phase velocity usually identify patients with a complete unilateral vestibular paralysis. The presence of an abnormal phase lead during low-frequency oscillation (0.1 Hz or less) also reliably indicates the presence, but not the side, of a complete unilateral paralysis. Interestingly, phase shifts (but not gains) were independent of both the stimulus amplitude and the patient's state of alertness.

The phase lead at low-frequencies may be related to change in the dominant time constant of the VOR caused by the peripheral labyrinthine lesion. However, this hypothesis is unproven, since different groups who have studied the effects of peripheral lesions upon the dominant VOR time constant have found different results.[11-13] The discrepancies may be related to the use of different types of rotational stimuli. Whatever the explanation for the low-frequency lead in patients with peripheral labyrinthine disorders, analysis of phase holds promise that rotational tests can be used to detect subtle degrees of labyrinthine hypofunction.

Finally, Wall and colleagues[14] have used rotational testing with a pseudorandom binary sequence of white noise acceleration stimuli. With this test, a wide range of stimulus frequencies can be presented almost simultaneously, greatly shortening testing time. However, the diagnostic reliability of this test does not appear to be better than those using sinusoidal stimuli.

2. Research Applications

Rotational testing has been especially helpful in clinical vestibular research. For example, Gresty and coworkers[15] studied the VOR in patients with central vestibular dysfunction and showed that patients with cerebellar disease often have abnormal VOR phase, whereas patients with lesions in the brain stem and especially the medial longitudinal fasciculus, have abnormal VOR gain. Zee, et al.[16] and Baloh, et al.[17] have shown, however, that VOR gain may be increased in patients with cerebellar lesions. Rotational testing has also provided data for the development of mathematical models of vestibular and ocular motor pathology (*vide infra*).

One important *caveat* should be emphasized in human vestibular testing — the influence of mental set upon the vestibular response. Naturally, maintenance of a constant state of alertness is essential for consistent, reliable testing results. However, equally important is the patients' imagined spatial frame of reference. For example, Barr, et al.[18] showed that during rotation at low-frequencies, the VOR gain in the dark can be

---

* This finding confirms Ewald's second law — for a given semicircular canal the response to an excitatory stimulus is greater than to an inhibitory stimulus. The response asymmetry is greatest at high-amplitudes and low-frequencies of acceleration.[4-6] Honrubia, et al. have presented a theoretical analysis of this problem.[7]

modulated up or down according to whether the patient attempts to visualize an imagined target which is either stationary on the wall in front of him or attached to the chair moving with his head.

III. DISORDERS OF THE VESTIBULO-OCULAR REFLEX: PHYSIOLOGICAL ANALYSIS*

A. Semicircular Canal-Ocular Muscle Connections

The existence of a precise geometric relationship between the planes in which the semicircular canals lie and the planes in which the eye or head rotates in response to vestibular stimulation has been known for over a century. The canals are arranged approximately orthogonally and work in a push-pull fashion. When a canal in one labyrinth is excited (such as the right anterior canal) a corresponding canal in the other labyrinth is inhibited (the left posterior canal). These observations imply specific semicircular canal — ocular muscle connections so that the eyes always tend to rotate in the same plane as that of the stimulated canal.[23] For example, the anterior canals primarily excite the ipsilateral superior rectus and contralateral inferior oblique while the posterior canals primarily excite the ipsilateral superior oblique and contralateral inferior rectus. In fact, the VOR is phylogenetically so basic that the anatomical organization of the brain stem ocular motor nuclei appears to have evolved on the basis of the anatomical requirements for appropriate vestibulo-ocular reflexes.[24] Thus, for the vertical VOR, the ocular motor subnuclei supplying the muscles receiving excitatory inputs lie contralateral to the vestibular nuclei, while those receiving inhibitory inputs lie ipsilaterally.

Figure 1 summarizes the known anatomical connections of the three neuron arc mediating the vertical VOR as studied in the rabbit.[25,26] Presumably, a similar organization applies to primates. Based on these specific patterns of vertical canal — ocular muscle connections one can often better interpret disorders of vertical and torsional eye movements. For example, the following clinical history is typical of patients with the benign paroxysmal positional vertigo syndrome (BPPV) first described by Barany.[27] Analysis of this problem shows how a knowledge of functional vestibular anatomy can help explain a patient's pattern of nystagmus.

A 51-year-old man was evaluated for episodic vertigo and dizziness of several years duration. The patient was in good health until an accident occurred while he was working as a foreman for a land clearing company. He was looking up at a tree when a branch hit his forehead, knocking him to the ground. He was stunned and perhaps lost consciousness for a few seconds. He then noted severe neck and arm pain and was taken to a local hospital. While having X-rays taken, he experienced dizziness when turned onto his left side. He described this sensation as, "things were moving inside my head." Since that time, he has intermit-tently experienced dizziness related to changes in head position. His symptoms are especially provoked when he looks upward or turns over onto his left side.

When initially examined, the patient's symptoms were minimal and no eye movement abnormalities were noted, even after changes in head position. However, several months later he was examined again when he reported that his dizziness recurred after a long day of shoveling snow. This time the patient developed vertigo during head positioning maneuvers. Also, several seconds after the head was positioned downward and to the left, a mixed torsional-vertical jerk nystagmus appeared with slow phases directed downward and counter clockwise. On gaze left, the nystagmus was primarily torsional, on gaze right, vertical (Figure 2). After 10 to 15 seconds, the nystagmus and vertigo abated. However, when the patient sat upright, the nystagmus reappeared, but with slow phases now directed upward and clockwise. The head positioning maneuvers were repeated several times and the nystagmus became less prominent and more difficult to elicit. The patient has been treated with a set of vestibular exercises (described below) and his symptoms have abated.

* See Precht,[19,20] Wilson and Melville-Jones,[21] and Baker and Berthoz[22] for recent reviews of vestibular physiology.

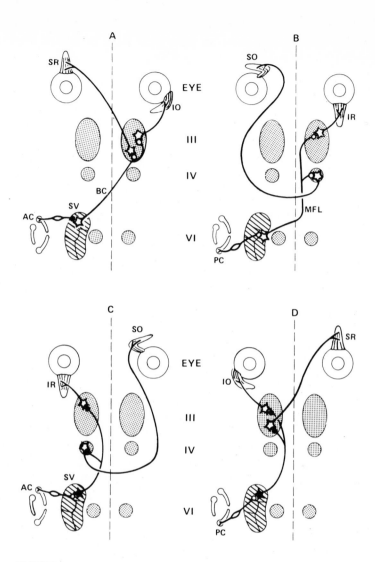

FIGURE 1. Primary pathways for the vertical VOR. A, B, excitatory, C, D, inhibitory. SR, superior rectus. IO, inferior oblique. SO, superior oblique. IR, inferior rectus. AC, anterior canal. PC, posterior canal. (From Ghelarducci, B., *Control of Gaze by Brain Stem Neurons*, Baker, R. and Berthoz, A., 1977, 167. With permission.)

To summarize, the patient showed a mixed vertical-rotatory nystagmus with slow phases directed downward and counter-clockwise, much as if one were stimulating a posterior semicircular canal. The degree of torsion or vertical rotation was related to the position of the eye in the orbit such that the muscles always tended to rotate the globe in a plane parallel to that of the posterior semicircular canal.[23] These observations, combined with the finding that patients with intractable BPPV are relieved by selective section of the portion of the vestibular nerve innervating the ampulla of the posterior semicircular canal,[26] suggest that the nystagmus of BPPV is created primarily by abnormal stimulation of the posterior semicircular canal in the offending labyrinth. Schuknecht hypothesized that BPPV occurs when the cupula of the posterior semicircular canal becomes gravity sensitive due to the lodging of fragments of displaced otoconia from the utricle — so called "cupulothiasis."[29] The cause may be trauma,

FIGURE 2.   Pattern of nystagmus in benign paroxysmal positional vertigo (BPPV). The direction of the slow phases (arrows), vertical on gaze right, torsional on gaze left, reflects excitation of the left posterior semicircular canal (black).

as in this case, or inflammatory processes due to infections or impairment of the blood supply to the labyrinth. Recently, patients with BPPV have been successfully treated by a form of mechanical therapy designed to disperse the dislodged otoconia throughout the endolymph.[30] The patients are challenged with the precipitating head positions on a repeated and serial basis until symptoms disappear. What role central compensatory mechanisms may play in the recovery of these patients is not clear.

Nystagmus from central lesions also may reflect disordered processing of the input from a specific semicircular canal. Meienberg, et al.[31] reported a patient with presumed multiple sclerosis who had nystagmus which was primarily vertical in the left eye (slow phases upward) and torsional in the right eye (slow phases counter-clockwise). One can account for this pattern by assuming a vestibular imbalance that simulates excitation of the left anterior semicircular canal or inhibition of the right posterior semicircular canal. For example, a lesion restricted to the lateral portion of the left medial longitudinal fasciculus (MLF) could interfere with excitatory projections from the right posterior canal which ascend in the MLF, but spare the excitatory projections from the left anterior canal which course through the brachium conjunctivum.

The three-neuron arc for the horizontal VOR is mediated by secondary vestibular neurons that project directly to contralateral abducens motor neurons and to the ipsilateral medial rectus subgroup of the oculomotor complex via the ascending tract of Dieters (which lies lateral to the MLF).[32,33] However, a more important pathway to the medial rectus appears to be via a direct vestibular projection to a set of internuclear neurons that lie within the abducens nucleus itself.[34] These internuclear neurons send axons that cross the midline and then ascend in the MLF to reach the medial rectus subgroup of the oculomotor nuclear complex. The internuclear neurons apparently carry information to the medial rectus for all types of conjugate eye movements — vestibular, pursuit, and saccades. The functional importance of this pathway is revealed in a common neuroophthalmologic syndrome, internuclear ophthalmoplegia (INO), usually caused by a discrete vascular or demyelinative (multiple sclerosis) lesion in the MLF. Patients with INO can not adduct the eye beyond the midline on the side of the lesion in response to any type of versional stimulus. In contrast, a vergence stimulus can still be used to drive the eye across the midline. In the vertical plane, patients with INO showed decreased VOR gain with consequent oscillopsia (illusory movement of the environment) during head movements, inadequate smooth pursuit, and impaired ability to hold eccentric positions of gaze.[35-38] In contrast, vertical saccades are normal. These findings reflect the type of vertical eye movement information carried by MLF fibers — vestibular, pursuit, and tonic activity but none related to saccades.[39,40]

The apparent inability of patients with INO to adduct the eye past the midline in response to a vestibular stimulus raises the question — What is the functional significance of the three-neuron direct horizontal VOR pathway? Do patients with complete INO also have lesions of the ascending tract of Deiters? Is recovery of function mediated by the ascending tract of Deiters? Does interruption of the MLF pathway decrease tonic input to medial rectus motor neurons so that the direct three-neuron arc via Deiters cannot effectively adduct the eye?

B. Otolith-Ocular Muscle Connections

When the head is tilted to one side, the eyes counter-roll such that the ipsilateral eye intorts and the contralateral eye extorts. During head tilt, dynamic counter-rolling is mediated primarily by the vertical semicircular canals. When the head is maintained in a tilted position, static counter-rolling is mediated by a utricular-ocular reflex. In primates, the degree of counter-rolling is relatively small, usually a maximum of 5 to 7 degrees, and is in fact, slightly asymmetrical — the downward eye torts more than the upward eye.[41,42] Presumably, otolith-ocular muscle projections parallel those of the vertical semicircular canals. Utricular reflexes must excite the ipsilateral intorters (superior oblique and superior rectus) and contralateral extorters (inferior oblique and inferior rectus).

Otolith imbalance may create both perceptual and ocular motor dysfunction. The sense of vertical upright may be distorted and disparity between the visual axes of the two eyes causes vertical diplopia, sometimes with one image tilted with respect to the other. This "skew deviation" probably reflects the phylogenetically older pattern of vertical divergence that occurs naturally during head tilt in lateral eyed animals. Skew deviation has been reported in patients with either peripheral or central vestibular disturbances.

For example, Halmagyi, et al.[43] reported a patient in whom the left vestibular labyrinth was inadvertently destroyed during a middle ear operation. The patient developed a transient vestibular disorder including horizontal nystagmus (slow phases toward the left), a head tilt to the left, vertical divergence of the eyes with the right higher than the left, and a clockwise torsion (tonic counter-rolling) of the eyes toward the left. The nystagmus reflected semicircular canal imbalance; the triad of head tilt, skew deviation, and ocular torsion reflected utricular imbalance. Rabinovitch, et al.[44] reported the same triad in a patient with multiple sclerosis and postulated paroxysmal activation of brain stem otolithic vestibular projections. Patients with lateral medullary infarction or Wallenberg's syndrome frequently have a skew deviation. In this case, the lesion usually includes the caudal aspect of the vestibular nuclear complex and probably affects otolithic-vestibular projections. See-saw nystagmus, in which the eyes rhythmically and continuously diverge and cyclovert in alternate directions, is a similar ocular motor abnormality in which the pathological lesion is thought to be in the rostral midbrain or diencephalon.

Physiological studies support the idea that skew deviation and ocular counter-rolling can occur with otolith dysfunction. Experimental stimulation of the utricle in the cat induces vertical devergence and ocular torsion.[45] Likewise, experimental stimulation of portions of the midbrain tegmentum in alert monkeys elicits the same ocular motor behavior — called the ocular tilt reaction by Westheimer and Blair.[46]

C. Disorders of Central Vestibular Mechanisms

New information about central vestibular data processing has accrued so rapidly in the past ten years that many clinical applications remain to be explored. For example, an important function of central vestibular mechanisms appears to be extension of the band width over which the vestibular nuclei reliably signal the velocity of the head. In primates, the cupula time constant is probably about four seconds (based on recording from vestibular afferents in monkeys),[5] whereas the dominant time constant of the VOR is three times as long, about 10 to 15 seconds. This transformed signal is already present on neurons within the vestibular nuclei.[47] Exactly how this transformation occurs is unknown, but several hypothesis have been suggested. Robinson[48] proposed an internal positive-feedback loop acting on the peripheral vestibular signal, while Raphan, et al.[49] suggested a neural circuit that "stores eye velocity." At any rate, measurement of the VOR time constant in patients with a variety of central lesions may provide new clinico-pathological correlations of both diagnostic and theoretical interest.

Another new concept — that of a central neural integrator — has already had significant clinical import. Neurophysiological studies have shown that primary vestibular afferents relay a head velocity signal, while ocular motor neurons discharge primarily in proportion to eye position. Hence, a neural network must exist that integrates, in the mathematical sense, vestibular velocity information into the appropriate position-coded signal for the ocular motor neurons. Skavenski and Robinson[50] have provided both a theoretical basis and experimental findings that support the idea of such a neural integration. Exactly how and where this integration is accomplished is not clear. However, it appears likely that it is mediated in part by pathways that carry information from axon collaterals of secondary vestibular neurons to the adjacent reticular formation and then back onto vestibular neurons. The latter, thus, carry both a head velocity signal from the periphery and an eye position signal created centrally.

The cerebellum also plays an important role in neural integration, since cerebellar ablation seriously impairs the ability of the brain stem neural integrator to reliably convert velocity into position-coded signals.[51] This causes the VOR to have an abnormal gain and phase.[52] Cerebellar ablation also causes an inability to hold eccentric positions of gaze resulting in the pattern of gaze paretic nystagmus.[53] After each excentering saccade, the eyes drift back toward the primary position with an exponential waveform. Thus, it appears that all conjugate eye movement systems share the same final common neural integrator.

The vestibulo-cerebellum in particular appears to play a crucial role in neural integration, since its ablation causes gaze-paretic nystagmus.[54,55] Likewise, the vestibulo-cerebellum is important for both short and long-term modulation of the VOR using vision. For example, during combined eye-head tracking, cancellation (suppression) of the VOR is necessary to fixate objects that are moving in space. In both normal subjects and patients, the ability to cancel the VOR correlates well with the ability to generate pursuit movements with the head, still making it likely that VOR cancellation is accomplished by the smooth-pursuit system.[16,56,57] In monkey, ablation of the vestibulo-cerebellum and flocculus in particular interferes with both smooth pursuit and VOR cancellation.[55] Also, a number of neurons within the flocculus discharge in relationship to eye velocity in space (gaze velocity) during tracking of targets whether the head is moving or still.[58,59] Finally, ablation of the vestibulo-cerebellum in cats interferes with their ability to make long-term adjustments in VOR gain in response to artificially induced vestibulo-ocular dysmetria (*vide infra*).[60]

1. Visual-Vestibular Interaction

Another fundamental concept of vestibular physiology has been recently reemphasized and has important clinical implications: the close relationship — perceptually, physiologically, and functionally — between vestibular and optokinetic nystagmus.* As Ter Braak suggested 40 years ago,[62] perhaps the most important function of the optokinetic system is to help the vestibular system stabilize images on the retina during head movements. The mechanical characteristics of the semicircular canals are such that they only respond transiently to angular movements of the head. Any head rotation which has a component of constant velocity will not be adequately compensated for by the VOR alone. Therefore, to insure clear vision during head movements, another image stabilizing system is needed. The optokinetic system appears to have evolved to perform this function. It supplants the fading vestibular response at low-frequencies of rotation and counteracts inappropriate postrotatory vestibular nystagmus.

When a human subject sits inside a revolving striped drum, optokinetic nystagmus is induced and is accompanied by an illusion of self-rotation (circularvection) in the direction opposite to drum rotation. When the lights are turned off, the eyes continue to beat in the same direction (OKAN) as prior drum rotation. Therefore, the direction of OKAN is *opposite* to that of perceived self-rotation. In contrast, postrotatory vestibular nystagmus occurs in the *same* direction as prior head rotation. Therefore, under natural circumstances, when one stops rotating, the optokinetic and vestibular aftereffects tend to nullify each other and, thereby, insure clear, stable vision. Figure 3 illustrates the complementary interaction between vestibular and optokinetic nystagmus.

Recently, neurophysiological studies have shown that visual-vestibular convergence takes place within the vestibular nuclei themselves, as well as in higher structures within the thalamus and parietal lobes. Henn and coworkers,[63-65] in alert behaving monkeys, showed that the discharge rates of single cells within the vestibular nuclei reflect the appropriate combination of visual and vestibular inputs so as to provide a central-best estimate of the velocity of self-rotation.

Further evidence for optokinetic-vestibular interaction comes from the observation that loss of peripheral labyrinthine function abolishes OKAN.[66,67] In fact, vestibular lesions of all types can be expected to affect optokinetic responses and especially OKAN. In foveate animals, measurement of the latter in darkness permits one to evaluate the action of the optokinetic system unobscured by smooth pursuit eye movements.

Optokinetic and vestibular signals not only combine to produce appropriate eye movements to insure image stabilization, but also provide a perceptual "best estimate" of the relationship of one's head to the physical environment. When pathology supervenes in one or the other pathway, the sensory inputs may conflict and cause vertigo, disorientation, and occasionally bizarre illusions of visual tilt. For example, a patient with an acute (unilateral) peripheral vestibular loss receives a *vestibular* signal that causes both inappropriate slow phases of nystagmus and the accompanying sensation of self-rotation in the *direction opposite* to the slow phase. However, the inappropriate nystagmus itself causes movement of the image of the world upon the retina in the direction opposite to the slow phase. This *visual* signal is often interpreted as self-rotation in the *same direction* as the slow phase. Hence, with the eyes open, the patient's central nervous system will receive opposite messages about the direction of self-rotation. Which one should the patient believe? This sensory contradiction probably accounts for the ambiguous way in which patients with acute vestibular lesions

---

*   This subject is reviewed in detail by Collewijn and Cohen and Raphan in accompanying chapters and in Dichgans and Brandt.[61]

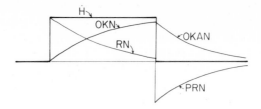

FIGURE 3. Scheme illustrating vestibulo-optokinetic interaction in response to impulsive rotational stimuli. Heavy lines represent head velocity (Ḣ). Eye velocity is the sum of the vestibular and optokinetic contribution and equals head velocity. RN = rotatory nystagmus, PRN = postrotatory nystagmus, OKN = optokinetic nystagmus, OKAN = optokinetic after nystagmus.

report the direction of self-rotation. Accordingly, when interviewing patients with vestibular dysfunction, one should inquire about the unambiguous sensory inputs — the direction of *rotation of the visual world* with the eyes open and the direction of *self-rotation* with the eyes closed. These indicators more reliably identify the nature of the vestibular imbalance.

Similar considerations apply to the sensation of tilt. The most dramatic clinical example of a distorted perception of verticality is found in patients with Wallenberg's syndrome (infarction of the dorsal lateral medulla which usually involves the caudal portions of the vestibular nuclear complex).[68,69] The following case history is illustrative:

A 57-year-old man was admitted to the hospital complaining of dizziness, nausea, imbalance, and double vision of several hours duration. On direct questioning he admitted that the visual world had transiently appeared upside down. He had several episodes of this illusion each lasting about 15 min. He also complained of vertical diplopia with the two images tilted with respect to one another so that an open angle was formed toward the left. His diplopia was relieved by lying on the left side.

General neurological examination showed the neurological signs of Wallenberg's syndrome including falling to the left, left-sided limb ataxia, paresis of the soft palate, crossed sensory loss (impaired pain sensation of the left side of the face and right side of the body) and a left Horner's syndrome (oculo-sympathetic paralysis). In addition, the patient showed a vertical divergence of the eyes, the left eye being lower, deviation of the eyes toward the left under closed lids, a mixed horizontal torsional nystagmus with quick phases to the right and hypermetric saccades toward the left. Cerebral angiography showed an occlusion of the left vertebral artery which presumably caused an infarction of the brain stem (lateral medulla) in the territory supplied by the posterior inferior cerebellar artery. Over the course of several weeks, the patient's neurological condition significantly improved.

The patient's double vision and skew deviation likely reflect utricular imbalance. The bizarre visual illusions probably reflect conflicting vestibular (otolithic), visual, and somatosensory input. In fact, some neurons within the vestibular nuclei have both visual and otolith inputs and they could provide the anatomical basis for the bizarre illusions of Wallenberg's syndrome.[70] Why the illusion is intermittent is puzzling. Perhaps the central nervous system is ambivalent about which sensory input to believe. Again, inquiry about body tilt with the eyes closed is helpful in lateralizing the abnormal vestibular input. Presumably, similar illusions may occur with lesions in the thalamic and parietal regions that also receive both vestibular and visual inputs.

IV. CENTRAL NERVOUS SYSTEM MECHANISMS FOR REPAIR OF VESTIBULAR LESIONS

The remarkable ability of the human central nervous sytem to cope with vestibular malfunction is perhaps best described in a delightful vignette written by a perceptive physician (J.C.)[71] who had permanently lost all vestibular function from streptomycin toxicity. Shortly after J.C. lost labyrinthine function, he found that he had to brace his head between two metal bars at the end of his bed in order to read clearly. Otherwise the letters on the page appeared to jump and blur at the same rate as his pulse. J.C.'s observation indicates that the VOR must be sufficiently sensitive and fast-acting to perfectly compensate for the minute, transient, head motion caused by transmission of arterial pulsations from the heart. Even so, after several years, most of J.C.'s symptoms had resolved and he summed up his experience "Is there any man-made machine designed like the human apparatus with so many alternative systems to accomplish its end"?

Recent studies by Melville-Jones and colleagues have stimulated renewed interest in the mechanisms by which the central nervous system compensates for vestibular malfunction. Gonshor and Melville-Jones[72,73] studied the effects of wearing dove-reversing prism spectables (such that during head rotation the seen world moves oppositely to what is normally observed) upon the VOR in normal human subjects. They found that subjects wearing reversing prisms first decreased the magnitude and then, after a few days to a week, actually reversed the direction of the VOR (as measured in darkness) so that slow phases moved in the same direction as head rotation. Thus, these subjects had adapted their VOR to the new requirements for image stabilization imposed by the reversing prisms. Such changes were plastic in the sense that they persisted (at least overnight) even when the subject did not have continuing visual experience. Subsequently, plasticity of the VOR has been demonstrated with other experimental paradigms. When subjects wear magnification or minification telescopic spectacles, the gain of the VOR is appropriately adjusted.[74,75] In fact, patients who wear glasses with a new prescription often have oscillopsia for a few days until their VOR gain is appropriately readjusted.

About 10 years ago, Ito[76] proposed that an important function of the vestibulo-cerebellum was to monitor and appropriately readjust the gain of the VOR in response to the effects of a pathological lesion. He hypothesized that the vestibulo-cerebellum detected movement (slip) of images upon the retina during head movements. (There should not be any if the VOR is functioning properly.) If image slip was present, the vestibulo-cerebellum would then readjust the VOR gain accordingly until image slip no longer occurred. Ito's idea required that there be both vestibular and visual inputs to the vestibulo-cerebellum. For many years, it has been known that the vestibulo-cerebellum receives an input from both primary and secondary vestibular neurons. However, after Ito presented his hypothesis, workers in his laboratory first conclusively demonstrated the visual input to the vestibulo-cerebellum.[77] Figure 4 summarizes Ito's hypothesis. Further support for Ito's hypothesis was provided by Robinson[60] who showed that vestibulo-cerebellectomy in the cat abolished the ability of the animal to modify its VOR while wearing reversing prisms. Thus, animal experiments suggest that plastic, adaptive modulation of VOR gain requires an intact vestibulo-cerebellum.

Likewise, human patients with cerebellar disorders often have enduring, inappropriate (usually increased) VOR gains; a finding which is compatible with Ito's hypothesis, since the cerebellar repair mechanism is presumably damaged in these patients. Patients with the Arnold-Chiari malformation,[78] a congenital hindbrain anomaly affecting the vestibulo-cerebellum, frequently have oscillopsia due to an abnormal VOR gain. The following case history is typical.

A 37-year old woman complained of difficulty walking and blurred vision for 6 months. She reported that when riding in an automobile, stop signs appeared to be moving up and down. When the automobile stopped at a traffic light, she could see more clearly. She also had difficulty reading the labels on canned goods while walking down an aisle in the supermarket.

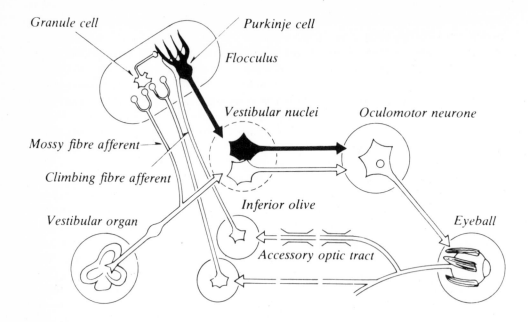

FIGURE 4. Ito's hypothesis to account for VOR plasticity. Purkinje cells receive visual information via climbing and mossy fibers and vestibular information via mossy fibers. Purkinje cells then modulate vestibular nuclei activity until image slip during head movements does not occur. Black cells are inhibitory. (From Ito, M., *Trends Neurosci.*, 2, 122, 1979. With permission.)

On clinical examination, the patient showed a very low-velocity (2.5 deg/sec) downward beating nystagmus. During rotation of the head in the vertical plane, she had to make corrective saccades in order to steadily fixate a stationary target. Saccades were always in the direction of head motion indicating a hyperactive (gain > 1) VOR in both vertical directions. In fact, the VOR gain measured in darkness was greater than 2.0 at low-frequencies and amplitudes of head rotation. The patient also had a striking pursuit deficit for downward, but not upward, moving targets.

Neurodiagnostic studies revealed an Arnold-Chiari malformation and the patient underwent a posterior fossa suboccipital boney decompression with some relief of symptoms.

A. Adaptation to Unilateral Loss of Labyrinthine Function

When faced with a unilateral peripheral vestibular lesion, the central nervous system has to do more than simply readjust the gain of the VOR. The brain must also deal with an imbalance between the vestibular nuclei creating both a static and dynamic bias. The static bias causes resting nystagmus when the head is still and the dynamic bias produces "directional preponderance" (the gain being higher in one direction than the other) when the head is rotating. To correct the static bias and null resting nystagmus, the resting discharge rates of the vestibular nuclei must be rebalanced. To correct the dynamic bias and eliminate the directional preponderance, the relative sensitivity of the vestibular nuclei to head rotation in opposite directions must be readjusted. Correction of the static bias is usually prompt and relatively complete, although a small amount of spontaneous nystagmus in darkness may persist for years after a unilateral loss of labyrinthine function.[79] On the other hand, repair of dynamic bias appears to be a slower process and a significant directional preponderance in the VOR (as measured in darkness) may persist for years.[9,10] The directional preponderance appears to be more prominent at low-frequencies of rotation. Since the visual following reflexes are capable of assisting the VOR only at relatively low-frequencies (less that 1 Hz), an organism must rely upon the VOR alone for ocular stabilization during rotation at higher-frequencies. Therefore, precise tuning of the VOR is probably necessary only for higher frequencies of rotation and one might expect adaptation at lower frequencies to be less exact.

Recent studies have shown that vestibular compensation is not just rewiring of synaptic connections, but requires active metabolic processes as well to maintain the completely compensated state. 2-deoxy-D-glucose studies in compensated hemilabyrinthectomized rats show unilaterally increased metabolic activity in portions of the cerebellar nuclei, nodulus and uvula, and inferior olive and lateral reticular neurons.[80] In addition, alcohol causes a reappearance of the signs of vestibular imbalance in the compensated hemilabyrinthectomized cat.[81] This effect is probably not solely due to the effect of alcohol upon the density gradient between the cupula and endolymph. These metabolic effects perhaps explain the fluctuating symptoms of patients who are recovering from a labyrinthine lesion.

The structures that mediate compensation for spontaneous vestibular nystagmus are still unknown. The commissural pathways between the vestibular nuclear complexes appear to be essential,[82] as are the inferior olive and its connections through the deep cerebellar nuclei.[83] Interestingly, removal of the vestibulo-cerebellum does not impair the ability of a cat to nullify spontaneous nystagmus after a vestibular lesion,[84] but does abolish the ability of the cat to change its VOR gain in response to wearing reversing prisms.[60] Thus, bias (at least the static component) and gain control have, in part, different anatomical substrates. The structures that compensate for dynamic bias are unknown.

B. Adaptation to Bilateral Loss of Labyrinthine Function

Perhaps an even more challenging problem for the central nervous system is to compensate for a complete bilateral loss of labyrinthine function. Here, no vestibulo-ocular reflex exists to modulate and, instead, alternative head movement-ocular stabilizing systems must substitute. In normal human beings, both active and passive head movements contain a number of frequency components above 1 Hz. Since the visual following reflexes (pursuit, optokinetic) normally function very poorly above 1 Hz, they only minimally help stabilize images during natural head motion. Likewise, the cervico-ocular reflex (neck-eye loop) functions poorly at high-frequencies and also makes virtually no contribution to image stabilization during natural head rotations.[85] Therefore, we rely almost exclusively on labyrinthine sensations to produce compensatory eye movements during head rotation. Consequently, a sudden, complete loss of labyrinthine function is severely disabling and accompanied by incapacitating oscillopsia. Nevertheless, most patients show a remarkable recovery by employing one or more of a number of compensatory mechanisms and behavioral strategies to assure optimal vision during head movements.

Two recent studies have quantitated the image-stabilizing mechanisms employed by labyrinthine defective human beings. Gresty, et al.[15] showed how three patients adapted to vertical oscillopsia; each developed a unique strategy to assure best vision. One patient extended the frequency range over which her visual following reflexes performed adequately, another appeared to use prediction to centrally generate compensatory eye movements, and a third potentiated his cervico-ocular reflex. Higher level, perceptual adaptations also occurred in the patient who had lost labyrinthine function at a young age. She had learned to "ignore" her oscillopsia and perceive a stationary world even though images were actually moving upon the retina.

In a complementary study, Kasai and Zee[86] investigated eye-head coordination during target acquisition in the horizontal plane. They found their patients employed a number of compensatory mechanisms, some of which had been previously described in the experimentally labyrinthectomized monkey.[87] One patient made saccades (even in darkness) in the same direction as inadequate compensatory slow phases to help stabilize gaze. In addition, during rotation of the body with the head stationary in darkness, he made slow and quick phases of nystagmus in the same direction. This patient apparently used quick phases to help stabilize gaze, rather than to redirect the center of visual attention. Another patient, to help prevent gaze overshoot, showed a decrease in the saccadic amplitude-retinal error relationship selectively during active combined eye-head movements. A third patient showed a significant amount of pre-programming of compensatory slow phases independent of actual head motion. In all patients, the passively induced cervico-ocular reflex was moderately potentiated, but still only accounted for about 25% of compensation for head motion during active target seeking.

More importantly, for all patients, "effort of spatial locatization," as shown by imagining targets in total darkness, increased the velocity of compensatory slow phases to near that of head movement during both active and passively induced head rotations. These compensatory eye movements depended upon the presence of actual head motion, since they did not occur when the head was blocked in flight or persist after the head stopped moving. In addition, since these eye movements were produced equally well during both active and passively induced head movements, their occurrence did not depend on efferent motor programs that initiate head movements. What system is actually generating these movements is not known. Finally, all subjects could better stabilize gaze during predictive tracking — either when following targets jumping periodically or during self generated tracking between two stationary targets.

Barnes[10] has pointed out an interesting feature of visual-vestibular interaction in labyrinthine defective patients which emphasizes how ingrained compensatory responses become. When his patients, who had no VOR, attempted to fixate a head fixed image during voluntary head movements at high-frequencies, they still had difficulty using pursuit to cancel slow phases generated by mechanisms substituting for the absent VOR.

The anatomic and physiological substrate for the variety of compensatory mechanisms shown by patients with bilateral labyrinthine areflexia are unknown. However, one can speculate that the vestibulo-cerebellum plays a role in the potentiation of the gain of the cervico-ocular reflex. The cervico-ocular reflex is presumably relayed through the same neurons within the vestibular nuclei that mediate semicircular canal-ocular responses.[88] Likewise, the vestibulo-cerebellum receives not only a primary vestibular afferent input, but also a short latency oligosynaptic input from cervical proprioceptors.[89] Hence, a substrate for cerebellar modulation of the cervico-ocular reflex exists in parallel to that which can change the gain of the vestibulo-ocular reflex. Experimentally, it would be of interest to study the ability of vestibulo-cerebellectomized monkeys to compensate for bilateral labyrinthectomy.

Practically, these studies suggest several possible modes of treatment for patients who have lost labyrinthine function. Firstly, since the passively induced cervico-ocular reflex is only moderately potentiated, a further increase in its gain might be achieved with exercises in which the head is passively rotated upon the body. Secondly, an attempt could be made to extend the performance range of the visual following reflexes by specifically training the pursuit system to follow targets moving at high-frequencies. Whether either or both of these rehabilitation programs would be effective is not known.

V. CLINICAL APPLICATIONS OF VESTIBULAR MODELS

A number of analytic models have been proposed to describe the generation of vestibular nystagmus, but only recently have they been successfully applied to clinical pathology. Most investigators have used the torsion pendulum analogy to describe the behavior of the cupula.[90,91] According to this formulation, the semicircular canals act as an integrating accelerometer relaying centrally an afferent signal proportional to head velocity. Further refinements of the torsion pendulum model have included an adaptation mechanism to account for the reversal phases of vestibular nystagmus,[92,93] a central mechanism to account for the extension of the lower end of the frequency range in which the vestibular nuclei reliably signal head velocity, and a central neural integrator to appropriately transform vestibular signals into ocular motor commands. More recent models have also included mechanisms for visual-vestibular interaction[56,94,95] and algorithms underlying the generation of the quick phases of nystagmus.[96-99]

A. Diagnostic Applications

Thus far, such models have had relatively little diagnostic clinical utility in the sense that they can promptly provide a correct diagnosis after a computer analysis of a patient's vestibular responses. The reason is that these models have attempted to use the results of rotational testing to differentiate peripheral from central vestibular disorders. In the context of our relative ignorance of the mechanisms by which the vestibular system compensates for peripheral lesions, that goal is perhaps more difficult to achieve than sorting out different types of central vestibular disorders. Likewise, early vestibular models did not deal with the interaction between vestibular mechanisms and the other eye movement control systems. In fact, a general principle of both bedside clinical examination and computerized vestibular testing, is that one must examine the individual performance of each of the different subtypes of eye movements systems, as well as their mode of interaction. For example, optokinetic and vestibular data-processing are so intertwined within the vestibular nuclei that vestibular lesions should and do affect optokinetic responses.

Models have another important clinical application, often not emphasized; their teaching capabilities. Models provide a conceptual framework for classification and differentiation of pathology. Once a model is understood, clinicians usually feel comfortable with it since models attempt to relate function and structure which is the strategy underlying topical neurological diagnosis. The concepts of gain, phase, and time constants have also been introduced through models and are now a part of the vocabulary and diagnostic tools of the clinician.

B. Research Applications

Two potentially fruitful areas for the clinical application of vestibular models are the investigation of patients with malfunctioning vestibular repair mechanisms and those with saccadic dysmetria. We have recently investigated several patients with periodic alternating nystagmus (PAN). PAN is a form of jerk nystagmus which changes direction every few minutes. Its usual cause is a bilateral lesion in the medulla probably involving portions of the vestibular nuclei, the commissural connections, and cerebellar-brain stem pathways. The following case history is illustrative.

A 45-year old school teacher complained of blurred vision for eight years. In 1970, the patient insidiously developed headaches, vertigo, blurred vision, and imbalance which increased in severity over the course of several months. She was hospitalized and neurodiagnostic studies showed a mass lesion within the fourth ventricle. She underwent a surgical exploration of her posterior fossa and after splitting the posterior cerebellar vermis, a granulomatous lesion in the floor of the fourth ventricle was discovered. The lesion was biopsied and histological sections and cultures subsequently demonstrated a chronic, low-grade fungal (cryptococcus) meningitis. This fungal infection had been presumably acquired the previous year while the patient and her husband were constructing their home next to a vacant building that contained pigeons (frequent carriers of cryptococcus). After diagnosis, the patient was successfully treated with antibiotics and the infec-

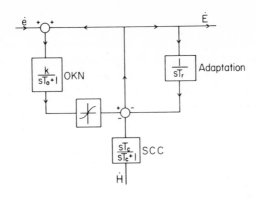

FIGURE 5. Simplified scheme of a neural circuit that will prolong the cupula time constant and generate optokinetic nystagmus, after nystagmus, and the reversal phases of vestibular and optokinetic nystagmus. If k becomes too large, the circuit will oscillate producing PAN. $\dot{e}$ = retinal slip velocity; $\dot{E}$ = eye velocity; $\dot{H}$ = head velocity; T_o = feedback loop time constant; T_c = cupula time constant; T_r = adaptation time constant.

tion was eradicated. However, she was left with permanently blurred vision. She found that objects appeared to jump and blur except for a period of a few seconds every few minutes when her vision was clear. She also noted that by turning her head first in one direction for a few minutes, then the other, she could see more clearly.

On examination, the patient had typical PAN. Before changing direction, the eyes went through a brief null period lasting a few seconds during which the eyes were quiet. During the null period, smooth pursuit was tested and found to be impaired. The patient turned her head to move her eyes into a position in the orbit in the direction of the slow phase where nystagmus intensity was least (Alexander's Law).

We have developed a preliminary model of PAN (Figure 5) using the hypothetical construct of Robinson for vestibular-optokinetic interaction.[100] By adding a saturating nonlinearity and increasing the gain of the internal vestibular-optokinetic positive feedback, as well as postulating a central adaptive mechanism that helps produce the reversal phases of vestibular and optokinetic nystagmus, we were able to produce oscillations comparable to those of our patients. Using a linear systems analysis of this model, we were able to calculate the approximate vestibular input needed to stop the oscillations. In fact, by applying an appropriately sized impulse of chair deceleration at a specific time in the PAN cycle (when eye velocity was maximum), we were able to dampen one patient's oscillations and actually stop the other's for about 8 minutes. This was the first time this patient's nystagmus had stopped in nearly eight years. Stimulated by a suggestion of Michael Gresty, we are now treating out patients with Baclofen (a drug with a presumed GABA-like action) which has effectively stopped the nystagmus of one of our patients. How Baclofen works is unknown. We are using our model in an attempt to understand its physiological mechanism of action.

Finally, several models for quick phases algorithms have been proposed which may eventually be used clinically. The quick phase algorithm should tell us what determines when a quick phase will occur and where it will take the eye. Obviously, a number of variables must be considered; the eye velocity of the slow phases, the position of the eye when the quick phase begins and ends, the frequency of quick phases, and the position of the head with respect to the body. Lau and co-workers[101] have begun examining this problem in human subjects and, using a phase plane analysis, have provided data that can be used to develop models that predict the complete eye movement trajectory during vestibular nystagmus. Once we know the complete quick phase algorithm for normal human beings, we may be able to use vestibular quick phase dysmetria much as we now use saccadic dysmetria for neuro-ophthalmologic localization. One can envision measuring and comparing the accuracy of rapid eye movements induced by visual, auditory, and vestibular stimuli. This type of analysis will likely be of both diagnostic and theoretical importance.

VI. CONCLUSION

From the viewpoint of clinicians dealing with patients who have vestibular disorders, systems analysis and computer models hold promise for major advances in accurate diagnosis and eventually development of more effective drug and rehabilitative therapies. On the other hand, the investigation of patients with vestibular disorders provides fertile ground for basic scientists attempting to understand brain mechanisms of vestibular and ocular motor control. In few other fields of neurology do basic scientists and clinicians share as much common ground than in the study of the vestibulo-ocular reflex.

ACKNOWLEDGMENTS

This work was supported in part by NIH Grants EY01849-04 and NS 11071-05. Vendetta Matthews provided editorial assistance.

REFERENCES

1. Zee, D. S., Ophthalmoscopy in the evaluation of vestibular disorders, *Ann. Neurol.*, 3, 373, 1978.
2. Zee, D. S., Suppression of vestibular nystagmus, *Ann. Neurol.*, 1, 207, 1977.
3. Baloh, R. W., Sills, A. W., and Honrubia, V., Impulsive and sinusoidal rotatory testing: a comparison with results of caloric testing, *Laryngoscope*, 89, 646, 1979.
4. Goldberg, J. M. and Fernandez, C., Physiology of peripheral neurons innervating semicircular canals of the squirrel monkey. I. Resting discharge and response to constant angular accelerations, *J. Neurophysiol.*, 34, 635, 1971.
5. Fernandez, C. and Goldberg, J. M., Physiology of peripheral neurons innervating semicircular canals of the squirrel monkey. II. Response to sinusoidal stimulation and dynamics of peripheral vestibular system, *J. Neurophysiol.*, 34, 661, 1971.
6. Baloh, R. W., Honrubia, V., and Konrad, H. R., Ewald's second law re-evaluated, *Acta Otolaryngol.*, 83, 475, 1977.
7. Honrubia, V., Kim, Y. S., Jenkins, H. A., Lau, C. G. Y., and Baloh, R. W., Ewald's second law of labyrinthine function and the vestibulo-ocular reflex, in Proc. Soc. Neurosci., Pittsburgh, 1978.
8. Wolfe, J. W., Engelken, E. J., Olson, J. W., and Kos, C. M., Vestibular responses to bithermal caloric and harmonic acceleration, *Ann. Otol. Rhinol. Laryngol.*, 87, 861, 1978.
9. Wolfe, J. W., Engelken, E. J., and Kos, C. M., Low-frequency harmonic acceleration as a test of labyrinthine function: basic methods and illustrative cases, *ORL*, 86, 130, 1978.
10. Barnes, G. R., Head-eye coordination in normals and in patients with vestibular disorders, *Adv. Otol. Rhinol. Laryngol.*, 25, 197, 1979.
11. Sills, A. W. and Honrubia, V., A new method for determining impulsive time constants and their application to clinical data, *ORL*, 86, 81, 1978.
12. McClure, J. A., Lycett, P., and Bicker, G. R., A quantitative rotational test of vestibular function, *J. Otolaryngol.*, 5, 279, 1976.
13. Stefanelli, M., Mira, E., Schmid, R., and Lombardi, R., Quantification of vestibular compensation in unilateral Meniere's disease, *Acta Otolaryngol.*, 85, 411, 1978.

14. Wall, C., Black, F. O., and O'Leary, D. P., Clinical use of pseudorandom binary sequence white noise in assessment of the human vestibulo-ocular system, *Ann. Oto. Rhinol. Laryngol.*, 87, 845, 1978.

15. Gresty, M. A., Hess, K., and Leech, J., Disorders of the vestibulo-ocular reflex producing oscillopsia and mechanisms compensating for loss of labyrinthine function, *Brain,* 100, 693, 1977.

16. Zee, D. S., Yee, R. D., Robinson, D. A., and Engel, W. K., Oculomotor abnormalities in hereditary cerebellar ataxia, *Brain,* 99, 207, 1976.

17. Baloh, R. W., Jenkins, H. A., Honrubia, V., Yee, R. D., and Lau, C. G. Y., Visual-vestibular interaction and cerebellar atrophy, *Neurology,* 29, 116, 1979.

18. Barr, C. C., Schultheis, L. W., and Robinson, D. A., Voluntary, nonvisual control of the human vestibulo-ocular reflex, *Acta Otolaryngol.,* 81, 365, 1976.

19. Precht, W., *Neuronal Operations in the Vestibular System,* Springer-Verlag, Berlin, 1978.

20. Precht, W., Vestibular mechanisms, *Annu. Rev. Neurosci.,* 2, 265, 1979.

21. Wilson, V. J. and Melville Jones, G., *Mammalian Vestibular Physiology,* Plenum Press, New York, 1979.

22. Baker, R. and Berthoz, A., *Control of Gaze by Brain Stem Neurons,* Elsevier/North-Holland, Amsterdam, 1977.

23. Cohen, B., The vestibulo-ocular reflex arc, in *Handbook of Physiology,* Vol. VI/I, Kornhuber, H. H., Ed., Springer-Verlag, New York, 1974, 477.

24. Zee, D. S., A note on the organization of the brain stem ocular motor subnuclei, *Ann. Neurol.,* 3, 384, 1978.

25. Yamamoto, M., Shimoyama, I., and Highstein, S. M., Vestibular nucleus relaying excitation from the anterior canal to the oculomotor nucleus, *Brain Res.,* 148, 31, 1978.

26. Ghelarducci, B., Highstein, S. M., and Ito, M., Origin of the premotor projections through the brachium conjunctivum and their functional roles in the vestibulo-ocular reflex, in *Control of Gaze by Brain Stem Neurons,* Baker, R. and Berthoz, A, Eds., Elsevier/North-Holland, Amsterdam, 1977, 167.

27. Barany, R., Diagnose von Krankheitserscheinungen im Bereiche des Otolithenapparates, *Acta Oto-laryngol.,* 2, 434, 1921.

28. Gacek, R., Further observations on posterior ampullary nerve transection for positional vertigo, *Ann. Otolaryngol.,* 87, 300, 1978.

29. Schuknecht, H., Cupulothiasis, *Arch. Otolaryngol.,* 90, 765, 1969.

30. Brandt, T. and Daroff, R., Physical therapy for benign paroxysmal positional vertigo, *Arch. Otolaryngol.,* 1980, in press.

31. Meienberg, O., Röver, J., and Kommerell, G., Prenuclear paresis of homolateral inferior rectus and contralateral superior oblique eye muscles, *Arch. Neurol.,* 35, 231, 1978.

32. Baker, R. and Highstein, S. M., Vestibular projections to medial rectus subdivision of oculomotor nucleus, *J. Neurophysiol.,* 41, 1629, 1978.

33. Reisine, H. and Highstein, S. M., The ascending tract of Deiters' conveys a head velocity signal to medial rectus motoneurons, *Brain Res.,* 170, 172, 1979.

34. Highstein, S. M. and Baker, R., Excitatory termination of abducens internuclear neurons on medial rectus motoneurons: relationship to syndrome of internuclear ophthalmoplegia, *J. Neurophysiol.,* 41, 1647, 1978.

35. Kirkham, T. and Katsarkas, A., An electrooculographic study of internuclear ophthalmoplegia, *Ann. Neurol.,* 2, 385, 1977.

36. Baloh, R. W., Yee, R. D., and Honrubia, V., Internuclear ophthalmoplegia. I. Saccades and dissociated nystagmus, *Arch. Neurol.,* 35, 484, 1978.

37. Baloh, R. W., Yee, R. D., and Honrubia, V., Internuclear ophthalmoplegia. II. Pursuit, optokinetic nystagmus and vestibulo-ocular reflex, *Arch. Neurol.,* 35, 490, 1978.

38. Evinger, C., Fuchs, A. F., and Baker, R., Bilateral lesions of the MLF in monkeys: effect on the horizontal and vertical components of voluntary and vestibular induced eye movements, *Exp. Brain Res.,* 20, 1, 1977.

39. King, W. M., Lisberger, S. G., and Fuchs, A. F., Responses of fibers in medial longitudinal fasciculus (MLF) of alert monkeys during horizontal and vertical conjugate eye movements evoked by vestibular or visual stimuli, *J. Neurophysiol.,* 39, 1135, 1976.

40. Pola, J. and Robinson, D. A., Oculomotor signals in medial longitudinal fasciculus of the monkey, *J. Neurophysiol.,* 41, 245, 1978.

41. Krejcova, H., Highstein, S., and Cohen, B., Labyrinthine and extra-labyrinthine effects on ocular counter-rolling, *Acta Otolaryngol.,* 72, 165, 1971.

42. Diamond, S. G., Markham, C. H., Simpson, N. W., and Curthoys, I. S., Binocular counter rolling in humans during dynamic rotation, *Acta Otolaryngol.,* 87, 490, 1979.

43. Halmagyi, G. M., Gresty, M. A., and Gibson, W. P. R., Ocular tilt reaction with peripheral vestibular lesion, *Ann. Neurol.*, 6, 80, 1979.

44. Rabinovitch, H. E., Sharpe, J. A., and Sylvester, T. O., The ocular tilt reaction: a paroxysmal dyskinesia associated with elliptical nystagmus, *Arch. Ophthalmol.*, 95, 1395, 1977.

45. Suzuki, J., Tokomasu, K., and Goto, K., Eye movements from single-utricle nerve stimulation in the cat, *Acta Otolaryngol.*, 68, 350, 1969.

46. Westheimer, G. and Blair, S. M., The ocular tilt reaction: a brain stem oculomotor routine, *Invest. Ophthalmol.*, 14, 833, 1975.

47. Buettner, U. W., Buttner, U., and Henn, V., Transfer characteristics of neurons in vestibular nuclei of the alert monkey, *J. Neurophysiol.*, 41, 1614, 1978.

48. Robinson, D. A., Linear addition of optokinetic and vestibular signals in the vestibular nucleus, *Exp. Brain Res.*, 30, 447, 1977.

49. Raphan, T., Matsuo, V., and Cohen, B., Velocity storage in the vestibulo-ocular reflex arc (VOR), *Exp. Brain Res.*, 35, 229, 1979.

50. Skavenski, A. A. and Robinson, D. A., The role of abducens neurons in the vestibulo-ocular reflex, *J. Neurophysiol.*, 36, 724, 1973.

51. Robinson, D. A., The effect of cerebellectomy on the cat's vestibulo-ocular integrator, *Brain Res.*, 71, 195, 1974.

52. Carpenter, R. H. S., Cerebellectomy and the transfer function of the vestibulo-ocular reflex in the decerebrate cat, in *Proc. R. Soc.*, (B series), 181, 353, 1972.

53. Westheimer, G. and Blair, S. M., Functional organization of primate oculomotor system revealed by cerebellectomy, *Exp. Brain Res.*, 21, 463, 1974.

54. Takemori, S. and Cohen, B., Loss of visual suppression of vestibular nystagmus after flocculus lesions, *Brain Res.*, 72, 213, 1974.

55. Zee, D. S., Yamazaki, A., and Gücer, G., Ocular motor abnormalities in trained monkeys with floccular lesions, *Soc. Neurosci. Abstr.*, 4, 168, 1978.

56. Barnes, G. R., Benson, A. J., and Prior, A. R. J., Visual-vestibular interaction in the control of eye movement, *Aviation Space Environ. Med.*, 49, 557, 1978.

57. Dichgans, J., von Reutern, G. M., and Rommelt, U., Impaired suppression of vestibular nystagmus by fixation in cerebellar and noncerebellar patients, *Arch. Psychiatr. Nerv.*, 226, 183, 1978.

58. Miles, F. A. and Fuller, J. G., Visual tracking and the primate flocculus, *Science*, 189, 1000, 1974.

59. Lisberger, S. G. and Fuchs, A. F., Role of primate flocculus during rapid behavioral modification of vestibulo-ocular reflex. I. Purkinje cell activity during visually guided horizontal smooth pursuit eye movements and passive head rotation, *J. Neurophysiol.*, 41, 733, 1978.

60. Robinson, D. A., Adaptive gain control of vestibulo-ocular reflex by the cerebellum, *J. Neurophysiol.*, 39, 954, 1976.

61. Dichgans, J. and Brandt, T., Visual-vestibular interaction: effects of self-motion perception and postural control, in *Handbook of Sensory Physiology*, Vol. 8, Held, R., Leibowitz, H. W., and Teuber, H. −L., Eds., Springer-Verlag, Berlin, 1978, 756.

62. Ter Braak, J. W. G., Untersuchungen uber optokinetischen nystagmus, *Arch. Neerl. Physiol.*, 21, 309, 1936.

63. Henn, V., Young, L. R., and Finley, C., Vestibular nucleus units in alert monkeys are also influenced by moving visual fields, *Brain Res.*, 71, 144, 1974.

64. Waespe, W. and Henn, V., Neuronal activity in the vestibular nuclei of the alert monkey during vestibular and optokinetic stimulation, *Exp. Brain Res.*, 27, 523, 1977.

65. Waespe, W. and Henn, V., Conflicting visual-vestibular stimulation and vestibular nucleus activity in alert monkeys, *Exp. Brain Res.*, 33, 203, 1978.

66. Cohen, B., Uemura, T., and Takemori, S., Effects of labyrinthectomy on optokinetic nystagmus (OKN) and optokinetic after-nystagmus (OKAN), *Equil. Res.*, 3, 80, 1973.

67. Zee, D. S., Yee, R. D., and Robinson, D. A., Optokinetic responses in labyrinthine-defective human beings, *Brain Res.*, 113, 423, 1976.

68. Hornsten, G., Wallenberg's syndrome. I. General symptomatology, with special reference to visual disturbances and imbalance, *Acta Neurol. Scand.*, 50, 434, 1974.

69. Hornsten, G., Wallenberg's syndrome. II. Oculomotor and oculostatic disturbances, *Acta Neurol. Scand.*, 59, 447, 1974.

70. Daunton, N. and Thomsen, D., Visual modulation of otolith dependent units in cat vestibular nuclei, *Exp. Brain Res.*, 37, 173, 1979.

71. J. C., Living without a balancing mechanism, *New Eng. J. Med.*, 246, 458, 1952.

72. Gonshor, A. and Melville-Jones, G., Short term adaptive changes in the human vestibulo-ocular reflex arc, *J. Physiol.*, 256, 361, 1976.

73. Gonshor, A. and Melville-Jones, G., Extreme vestibulo-ocular adaptation induced by prolonged optical reversal of vision, *J. Physiol.*, 256, 381, 1976.

74. Miles, F. A. and Fuller, J. H., Adaptive plasticity in the vestibulo-ocular responses of the rhesus monkey, *Brain Res.,* 80, 512, 1974.
75. Gauthier, G. M. and Robinson, D. A., Adaptation of the human vestibulo-ocular reflex to magnifying lenses, *Brain Res.,* 92, 331, 1975.
76. Ito, M., Neural design of the cerebellar motor control system, *Brain Res.,* 40, 81, 1972.
77. Maekawa, K. and Takeda, T., Afferent pathways from the visual system to the cerebellar flocculus of the rabbit, in *Control of Gaze by Brain Stem Neurons,* Baker, R. and Berthoz, A., Eds., Elsevier/North-Holland, Amsterdam, 1977, 187.
78. Zee, D. S., Friendlich, A. R., and Robinson, D. A., Mechanism of downbeat nystagmus, *Arch. Neurol.,* 30, 227, 1974.
79. Fisch, U., The vestibular response following unilateral vestibular neurectomy, *Acta Otolaryngol.,* 76, 229, 1973.
80. Walton, K. and Llinás, R., The role of cerebellar and brain stem nuclei in vestibular compensation in rats: a 2-deoxy-D-glucose study, *Soc. Neurosci.,* 4, (Abstr.), 70, 1978.
81. Berthoz, A., Young, L., and Oliveras, F., Action of alcohol on vestibular compensation and habituation in the cat, *Acta Otolaryngol.,* 84, 317, 1977.
82. Bienhold, H. and Flohr, H., Role of commissural connexions between vestibular nuclei in compensation following unilateral labyrinthectomy, *J. Physiol.,* 284, 178P, 1978.
83. Llinás, R., Walton, K., Hillman, D. E., and Sotelo, C., Inferior olive: its role in motor learning, *Science,* 190, 1230, 1975.
84. Haddad, G., Friendlich, A., and Robinson, D. A., Compensation of nystagmus after VIII nerve lesions in vestibulo-cerebellectomized cats, *Brain Res.,* 135, 192, 1977.
85. Barnes, G. R. and Forbat, L. N., Cervical and vestibular afferent control of oculomotor response in man, *Acta Otolaryngol.,* 88, 79, 1979.
86. Kasai, T. and Zee, D. S., Eye-head coordination in labyrinthine defective human beings, *Brain Res.,* 144, 123, 1978.
87. Dichgans, J., Bizzi, E., Morasso, P., and Tagliasco, V., The role of vestibular and neck afferents during eye-head coordination in the monkey, *Brain Res.,* 71, 225, 1974.
88. Rubin, A. M., Young, J. H., Milner, A. C., Schwarz, D. W. F., and Frederickson, J. M., Vestibular-neck integration in the vestibular nuclei, *Brain Res.,* 96, 99, 1975.
89. Wilson, V. J., Maeda, M., and Franck, J. I., Input from neck afferents to the cat flocculus, *Brain Res.,* 89, 133, 1975.
90. Steinhausen, W., Über die beobachtung der cupula in den Bogengangsampullen des labyrinths des Lebenden Hechts, *Pflügers Arch. Physiol.,* 232, 500, 1933.
91. Van Egmond, A. A. J., Groen, J. J., and Jongkees, L. B. W., The mechanics of the semicircular canal, *J. Physiol.,* 110, 1, 1949.
92. Young, L. R. and Oman, C. M., Model for vestibular adaptation to horizontal rotation, *Aerosp. Med.,* 40, 1076, 1969.
93. Malcolm, R. and Melville-Jones, G., A quantitative study of vestibular adaptation in humans, *Acta Otolaryngol.,* 70, 126, 1970.
94. Lau, G. Y. C., Honrubia, V., Jenkins, H. A., Baloh, R. W., and Yee, R. D., Linear model for visual-vestibular interaction, *Aviation Space and Environ. Med.,* 49, 880, 1978.
95. Robinson, D. A., Vestibular and optokinetic symbiosis: an example of learning by modelling, in *Control of Gaze by Brain Stem Neurons,* Baker, R. and Berthoz, A., Eds., Elsevier/North-Holland, Amsterdam, 1977, 49.
96. Chun, K-S. and Robinson, D. A., A model of quick phase generation in the vestibulo-ocular reflex., *Biol. Cybern.,* 28, 209, 1978.
97. Sugie, N. and Melville-Jones, G., A model of eye movements induced by head rotation, *IEEE Trans. Syst. Man Cybern.,* SMD-1, 251, 1971.
98. Barnes, G. R., Vestibular-ocular responses to head turning movements and their functional significance during visual target acquisition, Ph.D. thesis, University of Surrey, Guilford, 1976.
99. Schmid, R. and Lardini, F., On the predominance of anticompensatory eye movements in vestibular nystagmus, *Biol. Cybern.,* 23, 135, 1976.
100. Leigh, R. J., Robinson, D. A., and Zee, D. S., A hypothetical explanation of periodic alternating nystagmus: instability of the vestibular system, in *Recent Advances in Oculomotor and Vestibular Physiology,* Ann. N. Y. Acad. Sci., in press.
101. Lau, C. G. Y., Honrubia, V., and Baloh, R. W., The pattern of eye movement trajectories during physiological nystagmus in humans, in *Vestibular Mechanisms in Health and Disease,* Hood, J. D., Ed., Academic Press, London, 1978, 37.
102. Ito, M., Is the cerebellum really a computer?, *Trends Neurosci.,* 2, 122, 1979.

INDEX

W

Z